# International
# REVIEW OF
# Neurobiology
## Volume 80

# International
## REVIEW OF
# Neurobiology

## Volume 80

SERIES EDITORS


RONALD J. BRADLEY
*Department of Psychiatry, College of Medicine*
*The University of Tennessee Health Science Center*
*Memphis, Tennessee, USA*

R. ADRON HARRIS
*Waggoner Center for Alcohol and Drug Addiction Research*
*The University of Texas at Austin*
*Austin, Texas, USA*

PETER JENNER
*Division of Pharmacology and Therapeutics*
*GKT School of Biomedical Sciences*
*King's College, London, UK*

# Psychophysiological States: The Ultradian Dynamics of Mind-Body Interactions

BY

DAVID S. SHANNAHOFF-KHALSA
University of California
San Diego, USA

ELSEVIER

AMSTERDAM • BOSTON • HEIDELBERG • LONDON
NEW YORK • OXFORD • PARIS • SAN DIEGO
SAN FRANCISCO • SINGAPORE • SYDNEY • TOKYO
Academic Press is an imprint of Elsevier

Academic Press is an imprint of Elsevier
525 B Street, Suite 1900, San Diego, California 92101-4495, USA
84 Theobald's Road, London WC1X 8RR, UK

This book is printed on acid-free paper. ♾



For information on all Academic Press publications
visit our Web site at www.books.elsevier.com

ISBN 978-0-12-374275-9
ISSN 0074-7742

Printed and bound by CPI Group (UK) Ltd, Croydon, CR0 4YY

Transferred to Digital Print 2011

David Shannahoff-Khalsa has also authored:
Kundalini Yoga Meditation:
Techniques Specific for Psychiatric Disorders,
Couples Therapy, and Personal Growth
The Professional Book Division of W. W. Norton & Co., 2006

# DEDICATION

This book is dedicated to Guru Ram Das and Yogi Bhajan for their yogic knowledge; David and Sarah Shannahoff, my parents, for their lifelong loving support; and to Patrick, JJ, and Bubba, my three Golden Sons, for their endless loving devotion.

# CONTENTS

# FOREWORD

This remarkable and valuable book enlarges the scope of understanding psychophysiological states with a depth of scholarship and novel interpretations that are unique in the field. To explain my admiration for the achievement I offer a bit of autobiographical background. When I started my career as an independent scientist, my scientific outlook was shaped by a course in symbolic logic taught by Hans Reichenbach who was promoting the ideas of the Vienna Circle philosophers. Logical Positivism and its verifiability theory of meaning suited my temperament exactly, especially because it came to me from a professor who could casually mention conversations he had with Albert (Einstein), Kurt (Gödel), Rudy (Carnap), Otto (Neurath), and others in the analytic school of philosophy and science.

Shortly thereafter I became aware of the book by C. P. Snow based on his Rede Lecture at Cambridge University in 1959, entitled "Two Cultures and the Scientific Revolution," in which he argued that the intellectual life of all western society was increasingly being split into two polar groups: "Literary intellectuals at one pole—at the other scientists." He went on to say that "literary intellectuals" (not precisely defined) were seriously impoverished compared to their scientific coevals because they had no concept of the natural order of things as revealed by the scientific edifice of the physical world. From my Positivistic stance, this claim made good sense to me.

As we all now recognize, time has not been kind either to the manifesto of the Vienna Circle and its acolytes or to Snow's egregious dichotomization. However, the traces of their influence on me as a young, "hard-headed," medical scientist left me ill-prepared to take seriously any therapeutic claims coming from the experience and wisdom of yogis that I encountered later as examples of "alternative medicine." Some of those claims appear at the end of David Shannahoff-Khalsa's excellent book, but far from coming at the reader from the "east," tainted with mysticism, they are justified by a richness of scholarship of the "western" kind that most scientists require. Until I met David, I did not expect to see such a solid bridge between "east and west" in medical science.

In 1990, with a colleague, I published a report with a title beginning: "Ultradian adrenocortical and circulatory oscillations...." David noticed the article and called me with questions and comments that revealed a knowledge and appreciation of ultradian biological rhythms (those with periods less than 24 h) that exceeded my own. At his suggestion we became friends, colleagues, and collaborators in subsequent scientific work in the "western" style. Along the way I learned something of the content of yogic medicine and began to take it seriously because of David's scholarship. In the case of this book that scholarship appears early in the review of the history of the recognition of ultradian rhythms, and their variability's, and the speculations regarding their significance in physiology and psychology. (The book has a splendid, synoptic bibliography.)

Unusual for a review of scientific studies, in this book technical reports are displayed with clear and critical descriptions of their *protocols*: the hypotheses under test, the methods used, and the results. Such valuable detail makes demands on the reader for intense concentration, but the serious and curious reader will benefit from the honesty and maturity behind this approach.

The title of the book is perfect. The author focuses sharply on the dynamic signatures to be found in physiology, psychology, behavior, and some clinical pathology, and in various normal "states" including wakefulness at rest, and in the several different kinds of sleep. In physics, engineering, and mathematics the term "state" has formal meaning, and much of the science of dynamics (motion and change) explores rules and laws governing state transitions. When it comes to mind–body interactions, as would be expected, finding the rules and defining the states and their transitions objectively proves more difficult. Here, the text (with graphs) in this book, much of it illustrating original work by the author and his colleagues, points the way to surmounting many of those difficulties.

In biological science advances often flow from discovery of a particular organism or a special process that proves to be a promising archetype for studying aspects of complex phenomena: the fruit fly in genetics, the squid axon in neurophysiology, the small nematode *Caenorhabditis elegans* for development.... In the instance of ultradian rhythms in humans the nasal cycle, that can be monitored noninvasively, has turned out to be an enormously productive archetype in studies of states and in the design of therapeutic approaches to anxiety and depression, for example. The nasal cycle (an ultradian rhythm) is described with solid documentation throughout this book, as is the most famous ultradian rhythm—the basic rest-activity cycle (BRAC) of Kleitman. With these as guides a fresh description of asymmetries in cerebral hemispheric dominance and their alternations emerges. Throughout, the emphasis is on the lateralization of many of the structures and functions of the several branches of the autonomic nervous system, and a new explanation is given for the integrative temporal organizations within human beings, in health and disease, arising from structural and functional regionalization in the hypothalamus. This new perspective clears away prior clouds of confusion regarding the origins, character, and significance of ultradian rhythmic dynamics in mammals and invites the grand assumption that ultradian rhythms were prior to the more famous circadian rhythms (approximately 24-h periodicity) in the evolution of the nervous system. Furthermore, this work helps identify an important step in that evolution, viz., the lateralization of the rhythms of the autonomic nervous system that has otherwise been overlooked or ignored.

I close with the thoughtful language of the author at the close of his book: "Although the world of yogic medicine has a language that is different than that of modern science, it does not mean that these terms cannot be translated to help advance our understanding of the human nervous system and our ability to augment and facilitate its functions in order to improve our lives. While it is true that we need a contemporary view of ancient concepts, it is now more obvious than ever that the experimentalists of the past have more to offer than we had ever imagined."

F. Eugene Yates, MD
Emeritus Professor of Medicine and Ralph and
Marjorie Crump Professor of Medical Engineering
University of California, Los Angeles
and
Scientific Advisor
The John Douglas French Alzheimer's Foundation
Los Angeles, CA

# PREFACE

This book focuses on ultradian rhythms in the "hourly" domain—phenomena that usually exhibit with a range of 45–300 min, and characteristically with a dominant frequency at 80–140 min, and only on studies at the systems level in mammals. There is no attempt here to completely review the entire literature of ultradian rhythms for all systems. The literature for the cellular and molecular studies is not covered even though studies here are emerging that present many new insights for ultradian chronobiology. There is no doubt that many important papers are not discussed. What is attempted here is an effort to review the critical literature and synthesize a compelling and simple view for a new perspective on the autonomic regulation of psychophysiological states. Many theories and studies that I consider are peripheral to the focus here may not be included due to the complexity of the topic of psychophysiological states at large. Also, the related studies on circadian rhythms and their obvious fit toward our understanding of psychophysiological states are not included. The focus here is on the basic elements, functions, and physiology of the autonomic nervous system (ANS), and its regulation via the hypothalamus that gives rise to the phenomenon of the lateralized rhythms of the autonomic and central nervous systems during waking and sleep along with the supporting bodily systems innervated by the ANS, and how this evidence now presents us with an entirely new view on psychophysiological states. In advance, I apologize to those authors who are not cited and who have also contributed a great deal to the field of ultradian rhythms and psychophysiological states at large. There is much to add that could contribute to the complexity and scope of the field over what is presented here.

David S. Shannahoff-Khalsa

# ACKNOWLEDGMENTS

First and foremost, I thank Yogi Bhajan for sharing yogic knowledge that has made my scientific work in this book possible. Secondly, I thank Floyd E. Bloom, MD, for his efforts as my first scientific collaborator on yogic research when we were both at The Salk Institute and for helping to launch this work and making it a respectable and important scientific endeavor. His active participation inspired many others to collaborate. I am also grateful to Drs. David Schubert, Tony Hunter, and Walter Eckhart who gave me many years of institutional support at The Salk in an effort to help establish my scientific career. I express my thanks to Sheldon S. Hendler, MD, PhD, for his efforts to launch my scientific career and his sage advice over the past 37 years. I am grateful to Michael G. Ziegler, MD, for nearly 20 years of collaboration on pioneering physiological studies on waking and sleep in his laboratory and the General Clinical Research Center at the University of California, San Diego (UCSD). Michael's keen mind led to the discovery of the ultradian rhythms of alternating lateralization of catecholamine activity throughout the periphery. I am immensely grateful to F. Eugene Yates, MD, University of California, Los Angeles, for his mentoring in time series analysis and managing multivariate psychophysiological data sets and for his many years of collaboration, scholarship, and guidance that led to new insights for defining psychophysiological states. I am grateful to J. Christian Gillin, MD (deceased), Department of Psychiatry, UCSD, for his years of sleep research collaborations. I am grateful to Liana Beckett, MA, MFCC, Department of Psychiatry, UCSD, for the first invitation to collaborate using Kundalini Yoga meditation techniques for treating obsessive compulsive disorder (OCD). I am grateful to Saul Levine, MD, Department of Psychiatry, UCSD, and Children's Hospital, San Diego, for his interest and collaboration to help further the OCD clinical trial work and making the National Institute of Health (NIH)-funded randomized controlled study using Kundalini Yoga to treat OCD possible. I acknowledge with gratitude Christopher C. Gallen, MD, PhD, for his collaboration on the second OCD trial, for study design, and professional guidance throughout. I am also grateful to Christopher for initiating the research opportunities employing magnetoencephalography (MEG) for studying patients with OCD, healthy controls, and the OCD breath technique when he was director of the MEG lab at The Scripps Research Institute. His collaborative support and sage advice over the years has been priceless. I am grateful to Leslie Ellen Ray, MA, MFCC, for running the control group in the OCD clinical trial, to Barry J. Schwartz, PhD, when at The Scripps Research Institute, to John Sidorowich, PhD, UCSD, for collaboration on the OCD trial and for help on analysis of previously unpublished MEG data for Figs. 44–47. In addition, I am grateful to Henry D. I. Abarbanel, PhD, Director of the Institute for Nonlinear Science (INLS), UCSD, for providing institutional support and a home to conduct this scientific work in a most wonderful, open, rigorous, creative, and productive atmosphere. I also thank Drs. Luigi Fortuna, Maide Bucolo, Manuela La Rosa, Mattia Fresca, and Francesca Sapuppo, University of Catania, Dipartimento di Ingegneria Elettrica Elettronica e dei Sistemi, for their enduring and creative collaborative efforts on MEG signal processing for the study of yogic meditation techniques, specifically Figs. 37–43. I am grateful to Stuart W. Jamieson, MB, Head of the Division of Cardiothoracic Surgery, UCSD, and B. Bo Sramek, PhD, Czech Technical University Prague, Department of Mechanical Engineering, for collaboration on yogic techniques for altering cardiovascular function and for novel work on defining hemodynamic states. I am indeed grateful to Brian Fallon, MD, Columbia University, Department of Psychiatry, and New York State Psychiatric Institute, for inviting me to present at a 2003 symposium on OCD at the Annual American Psychiatric Association (APA) Conference that helped lead to another APA workshop and to full-day 6-h CME Courses for 2005, 2006, and 2007, where I have taught Kundalini Yoga meditation techniques specific for treating psychiatric disorders along with my basic science discoveries that are described in this book. There are many other scientific collaborators and support staff who have helped to make this work possible over the last 31 years, and I am grateful to all of them for their important key roles.

I especially acknowledge with my deepest gratitude Mr. John DeBeer and Dr. Mona Baumgartel for providing financial support to The Khalsa Foundation for Medical Science every year since its inception in 1984 to help facilitate some of this work that was all conducted at the University of California, San Diego. Their generosity has made the continuation of this work possible. In addition, I thank the Fetzer Institute, the Waletzky Charitable Lead Trust, Earl Bakken, and the National Institutes of Health for funding some of the scientific studies described in this book.

And last but not the least, I am very grateful and indebted to my editor, Hilary Rowe at Elsevier Scientific Publications, for the invitation to write this book and her patience and creative support during the process.

DAVID S. SHANNAHOFF-KHALSA

# PSYCHOPHYSIOLOGICAL STATES: THE ULTRADIAN DYNAMICS OF MIND–BODY INTERACTIONS

David Shannahoff-Khalsa

The Research Group for Mind-Body Dynamics
Institute for Nonlinear Science
University of California, San Diego, La Jolla, California 92093, USA
and
The Khalsa Foundation for Medical Science
Dei Mar, California 92014, USA



INTERNATIONAL REVIEW OF
NEUROBIOLOGY, VOL. 80
DOI: 10.1016/S0074-7742(07)80001-8




0074-7742/08 $35.00

## I. Introduction: A Historical Perspective on the Research Highlights and Basic Autonomic Essentials for Understanding Psychophysiological States

Discovering the physiological bases for mental processes, expressed as thoughts, emotions, or behavior, has always been one of the most important scientific goals. Efforts to understand the relationship of the brain, behavior, and disease go back at least to the seventeenth century BC in western civilization. Interest in this relationship is documented on an Egyptian papyrus, which is thought to be the earliest reference on this topic (Breasted, 1930). The papyrus describes the brain of two patients with head wounds and their symptoms, diagnosis, and prognosis. Therefore, we can assume man has been motivated since ancient times to learn how to control mental processes to help overcome the psychopathologies, enhance normal brain function, and to understand the basic couplings of mind and body. Research has been primarily focused in the four cardinal domains of neuroanatomy, neurophysiology, neuropharmacology, and the study of behavior, with a long-standing effort to discover the underpinnings and mechanisms of the processes of human awareness.

While the broad topic of brain and behavior is far beyond the scope of this book, the focus here is to examine new insights on how the autonomic nervous system (ANS) and hypothalamus play a central role in the modulation of the ultradian rhythms of cognition, behavior, physiological functions that support psychophysiological states during both waking and sleep, mechanisms of hypothalamic integration and regulation of the body's major systems, and the translational neuroscience that can now help exploit these new discoveries.

It has been known for almost one century that the ANS and the hypothalamus play a critical role, at the most elementary levels, in the regulation of vital physiological functions that help insure both the survival and reproduction of the species. Work at the beginning of the twentieth century, and later, established that the hypothalamus controls the sympathetic nervous system (SNS) and the parasympathetic nervous system (PNS). Electrical stimulation of specific regions in the hypothalamus evoked classical autonomic responses in pupillary diameter, salivation, heart rate, sweating, defacation, and bladder contractions (Karplus and Kreidl, 1909, 1910, 1912, 1914). Electrical stimulation in the medial parts of the tuberal region produced parasympathetic effects on heart rate, gastric motility, and bladder tone (Beattie, 1932; Beattie and Kerr, 1936; Beattie and Sheehan, 1934; Beattie *et al.*, 1932). These early findings led to the seminal studies and conclusions that the anterior region of the hypothalamus is more concerned with parasympathetic mechanisms and that the posterior region is more concerned with the sympathetic mechanisms (Hess, 1947, 1954; Ranson and Magoun, 1939; Swanson, 1987).

Both Cannon and Hess viewed the PNS as the division (Cannon, 1932; Hess, 1948) that supports "the restitution of cellular functions through anabolic processes, reduction in activity, and increase in blood supply and gastrointestinal functions, combined with the excretion of waste products" and that "the sympathetic division creates favorable conditions for the maximal performance of the somatic nervous system through cardiovascular adjustments, rises in blood sugar, delay in fatigue, etc., particularly under emergency conditions (Gellhorn, 1967)." These discoveries set the stage for formulating the early theories on psychophysiological states. While waking and sleep are the most obvious and most widely studied psychophysiological states, with all their circadian features, they are not the subject of this text, although the ANS and the hypothalamus clearly play key modulatory roles in the regulation of the sleep–wake cycle. The psychophysiological states of the ultradian domain are the focus here.

Cannon first described his theory of the "fight-or-flight" response, also known as the acute stress response, where vertebrates react to threats with a general discharge of the SNS that primes the animal for fighting or fleeing (Cannon, 1929). It soon became apparent, however, that his theory was overly simplistic and that vertebrates also employ other means to contend with life threats, and that the fight-or-flight mechanism is used only as a means of self-preservation. Nevertheless, the physiological mechanism of the fight-or-flight response was an early key to understanding psychophysiological states. That is, the extreme of the condition utilized the SNS as a means to maximize physiological "activity" and action.

Later came the notions called the ergotropic (arousal) and trophotropic (lethargy and sleep) systems and the psychophysiological states that they support via the SNS and PNS, respectively (Hess, 1949). The ergotropic system is "characterized by sympathetic discharges associated with an increased activity of the motor apparatus (skeletal and respiratory muscles)" and the trophotropic system "consisting of parasympathetic effects is associated with a lessened activity and responsiveness of the somatic nervous system" (Gellhorn, 1967). While arousal and sleep are two polar extremes, the ergotropic and trophotropic systems obviously also support, regulate, modulate, and integrate a wide variety of intermediate functions and states. Gellhorn's aim in his classic text on the underlying physiological mechanisms of the ergotropic and trophotropic systems was to "investigate their mutual relations and evaluate the significance of deviations from these patterns in special physiological and also pathological conditions, and to show the importance of these systems for the study of behavior" (Gellhorn, 1967). The discovery of the ergotropic and trophotropic systems is fundamental to an understanding of the physiology of what we call "activity" and "rest" (or sleep). The next critical discovery for understanding psychophysiological states comes from the work of Kleitman where he proposed his "Basic Rest-Activity Cycle" (BRAC) hypothesis (Kleitman, 1961, 1963, 1967b,c, 1982). The BRAC hypothesis is a dynamical view of psychophysiological states during both waking and sleep. Kleitman, Aserinsky, and Dement discovered what they called the rapid eye movement (REM) and nonrapid eye movement (NREM) sleep cycle (Aserinsky and Kleitman, 1953, 1955a,b; Dement and Kleitman, 1957a,b), where physiological changes exhibit as periods of activity and rest-like conditions that alternate during sleep with what was later termed the "ultradian" periodicity (Halberg, 1964). Kleitman proposed that the BRAC had a correlate during the waking state and continued throughout the 24-h (circadian) cycle. Kleitman, Aserinsky, and Dement, three pioneers of modern sleep research, discovered how the activities of the ANS, eye movement, dreaming, and electroencephalographic (EEG) patterns were tightly coupled during sleep. They note that "slow, rolling, or pendular eye movements" had previously been reported by others decades earlier in sleeping children and adults. But they found "a different type of eye movement-rapid, jerky, and binocularly symmetrical" (Aserinsky and Kleitman, 1953). In their seminal report in *Science*, they state:

> eye movements, EEG pattern, and autonomic nervous system activity are significantly related and do not occur randomly suggests that these physiological phenomena, and probably dreaming, are very likely all manifestations of a particular level of cortical activity which is encountered normally during sleep. An eye movement period first appears about 3 hr after going to sleep, recurs 2 hr later, and then emerges at somewhat closer intervals a third or fourth time shortly prior to awakening. This method furnished the means of determining the incidence and duration of periods of dreaming (Aserinsky and Kleitman, 1953).

This result gave birth to a flurry of studies in the following decades and was the first key finding that set the stage for a dynamical view of psychophysiological states. Hence, came the postulate of the BRAC by Kleitman for a continuous cycling of activity modes alternating with resting modes throughout both waking and sleep with a periodicity in the hourly ultradian domain.

Kleitman's BRAC hypothesis was an attempt to help organize the rhythmic patterns in sleep data, and later in waking data, that otherwise did not fit into the working model of the nervous system at that time. He provided a new framework for those patterns that fit into the evolutionary development of multilevel neurobehavioral systems and the BRAC hypothesis provided a new understanding for organization of the neuraxis. The general phenomenon of the BRAC hypothesis was believed to exhibit at all levels of the vertebrate kingdom. In the late nineteenth century, John Hughlings Jackson in his essay "Evolution and dissolution of the nervous system" wrote about the evolutionary development of neurobehavioral systems and how such systems are continued throughout evolution (Jackson, 1884). The BRAC hypothesis was one more fundamental advance in understanding the neuraxis which then includes a temporal dimension. Clearly, it was the first chronobiological model that attempted to capture the workings of all the major bodily systems during both waking and sleep, and the hypothesis also included the psychological component of dreaming, which suggested a more inclusive theory for psychophysiological states.

However, the missing link in Kleitman's BRAC hypothesis was the observation of the lateralized ultradian rhythms of the autonomic and central nervous system (CNS), and their tightly coupled relationship. One early key finding, that was apparently lost in the literature, was the early work on the nasal cycle (see Section II.A) that described "an alternation in vasomotor tone throughout the periphery on the two sides of the body" (Kayser, 1895). While Kleitman's BRAC hypothesis presented a novel view of chronobiological events, his original hypothesis also did not include the phenomenon of alternating cerebral hemispheric activity (see Section II.B), and it also lacked a component to help give it a structural framework which now helps provide a greater significance and understanding for the BRAC hypothesis, and in addition helps, in part, to explain the wobble, or nonstationary nature of ultradian phenomenon. This wobble characteristic in the ultradian data sets also led to significant confusion over time. This text is an exploration of the data from many fields of physiology and psychology, including key studies in multivariate physiology that now lead to a new view on psychophysiological states that is based on an expanded view of the BRAC and the various levels of function of the neuraxis.

## II. Toward an Integration of the Temporal and Structural Organization of Higher Vertebrates: The Lateralized Ultradian Rhythms in the Nervous System

Lateralization of function is a marker of increasing complexity in the evolution of biological systems. Bilateral symmetry is a distinguishing characteristic of invertebrates; only two groups of invertebrates, the gastropod molluscs and the decapod crustaceans, have bilateral asymmetry as a common feature (Chapple, 1977). The obvious benefit of bilateral limbs is improved movement capabilities and the benefit of bilateral sensory organs provides enhanced awareness of the environment. Any internal duplication of organs enhances survivability in the event of injury and has the potential to distribute workloads. Prior to the appearance of bilateral symmetry in evolutionary development, the primary structural organization in invertebrates was translational symmetry in which there is a segmental organization along the longitudinal axis; each successive segment is a primitive replica or serial homologue of the one before it (Chapple, 1977).

Bilateral asymmetry appeared after the evolutionary stage at which there was simultaneous activation of the contralateral limbs. Uncoupling of this rigid pattern of activation makes possible more complex functions (Chapple, 1977). The mechanisms and structures that allow for an independent activation of the two sides of the body thus lead to the possibility of a specialization of function, and thus adding to biological complexity.

The next major step in the evolution of bilateral asymmetries may be the development of the rhythmic lateralization of neural activity in paired internal structures; the two sides of the CNS and ANS may become partially independent of each other and complement each other's functions. This partial autonomy can thus lead to a specialization of each side, adding to the adaptative possibilities of the organism. Paired internal organ systems may also exhibit partial autonomy. One consequence of this autonomy could be the specialized support of different energy producing or conserving activities associated with metabolic states known as the ergotrophic and trophotropic states, or active and resting states, respectively.

While circadian rhythms subserve adaptation to the light–dark cycle, the ultradian rhythms of lateralized neural activities help to organize the functions of biological systems to meet primary bodily needs. These functions are associated with activities such as work (hunting), rest (healing), eating, and the many other behaviors that are identified by Kleitman as defining the BRAC (Kleitman, 1961, 1963, 1967a,b,c,d, 1982). Kleitman does not include lateralized neural rhythms in his definition of the BRAC, and it is the purpose here to demonstrate their relevance. Although it is not clear whether the ultradian or circadian rhythms emerged earlier in evolution, it may be that the ultradian phenomenon of the BRAC is more vital to the integrity of the organism. In the sleep–wake cycle of the newborn human, for example, the ultradian rhythm is apparently more primitive then the circadian rhythm (Hellbrugge, 1974). In fact, there are ultradian rhythms in human fetal motor activity that are the earliest signs of the BRAC (Granat *et al.*, 1979; Sterman, 1967). This may be another example of how ontogeny recapitulates phylogeny.

The relationship of the BRAC to the lateralized rhythms of the CNS and ANS is the primary focus of this book. The relationship proposed here for these phenomena provides both a new perspective and organizing principle for structural features and temporal activities in higher vertebrates and thus allows for a new perspective on understanding physiological and psychophysiological states. While metabolic activities in the body can be viewed as a sea of rhythmic changes, ultradian rhythms of lateralized neural activity may be viewed as a fundamental stage in the evolution of organizational development. These rhythms also provide clues for a better understanding of stress, adaptation, homeostasis, psychopathology, and psychophysiological states.

## A. Lateralized Rhythms of the ANS

The most obvious rhythmic shift of a lateralized autonomic function is that of the nasal cycle (Eccles, 2000; Heetderks, 1927; Kayser, 1889, 1895; Ohki *et al.*, 2005; Stoksted, 1953). Although the phenonmenon of the nasal cycle is not widely known, it has been extensively studied and is defined as an alternating congestion and decongestion of opposite nostrils where there is a vasoconstriction in one nasal turbinate paralleled by vasodilation in the other. The nasal mucosa are densely innervated with autonomic fibers and the dominance of sympathetic activity on one side produces vasoconstriction in the turbinates, while the contralateral nostril exhibits a simultaneous dominance of parasympathetic activity that causes swelling. Kayser first documented the nasal cycle in 1889 and described it as reflecting the "alternation of vasomotor tone throughout the periphery on the two sides of the body" (Kayser, 1889, 1895). This observation is only now gaining in significance. Reviews of the nasal cycle were published in 1968 (Keuning, 1968), 1986 (Haight and Cole, 1986), and 2000 (Eccles, 2000). Beickert looked at other structures in relationship to the nasal cycle and published a study on "Half-Sided Rhythms of Vegetative Innervation" (Beickert, 1951). He observed how lateralized differences in secretions of the nose and eye varied in phase with the nasal cycle and how autonomic-related pupillary changes on the two sides could vary with the lateralized changes in the nose under stellate ganglion block.

Keuning reviewed numerous studies of the nasal cycle during waking and concluded that the average cycle length is about 3–4 h and ranges anywhere from 2 to 8 h (Keuning, 1968). One study of 50 humans found a mean duration of 2.9 h, ranging from 1 to 6 h (Hasegawa and Kern, 1978). These studies were all done under laboratory conditions during the day. A more recent study with 20 healthy subjects, ages 24–77 years, measured the nasal cycle continuously under normal daily activity using a portable nonintrusive monitor for 12 h during the day and using one criterion for cyclicity found "the mean nasal cycle duration was 110 min, although variation was considerable, even in a single subject" (Ohki *et al.*, 2005). The nasal cycle has also been observed to exist throughout the 24-h period (Cole and Haight, 1986). Laboratory conditions, which impose resting states, may skew the cycle toward longer than normal periods. The frequency of sampling and what criteria define a cycle has confounded the discussion of nasal cycles. There are wide variations in the reported length. One subject exhibited a transition in dominance every 20 min for four consecutive cycles during a 90-min recording period (Werntz *et al.*, 1983). This was observed when a continuous recording was made of nasal dominance. The same subject showed a much longer cycle on a subsequent day under the same testing conditions. The question of the existence of the nasal cycle in children has also been somewhat controversial. However, in a recent study of 16 children, ages 2–11 years (mean, 6.25 years), acoustic rhinometry was used with triplicate measures every 30 min for 3 h. "All evaluated children presented nasal cycles, with five children presenting a classic pattern (31.25%), three children presenting a concert pattern (18.75%), and eight children presenting an irregular pattern (50%)" (Gallego *et al.*, 2006). They conclude "that children present nasal cycles, as well as adults. Nevertheless, the most prevalent pattern in children was the irregular pattern, whereas in adults the most frequently detected is the classic pattern." However, note that these researchers only measured 10 time points over 3 h, and the average cycle length is about 2.5 h according to most studies in adults. Therefore, it is unlikely that the observed patterns are all going to show a smooth sinusoidal cycle. The nasal cycle has also been demonstrated in rats and rabbits (Bojsen-Moller and Fahrenkrug, 1971), anesthetized pigs (Ashley and Lea, 1978), and cats (Bamford and Eccles, 1982), and no doubt occurs in all mammals with bilateral turbinates.

Another example of a normal half-sided reaction in autonomic function exists between the nose and the lung. There is a unilateral nasal-pulmonary reflex mechanism which is clearly elicited when there is a forced inhalation through one nostril producing a significant increase in inflation of the homolateral lung compared to the contralateral lung (Drettner, 1970; Samzelius-Lejdstrom, 1939; Sercer, 1930; Stoksted, 1960). Samzelius-Lejdstrom studied 182 individuals and showed that the movements of one thoracal half were much more inflated compared to the contralateral lung in 94% of subjects. She also observed that "variations in width of one-half of the nasal cavity caused variations in the amplitude of the movements of the homolateral thoracal half" (Samzelius-Lejdstrom, 1939). Whether she was aware of the nasal cycle or not, she observed how differences in nasal congestion could affect the lung. She also reported that in cases of tuberculosis where there is primarily a lateralized deficit, there is a simultaneous pathological phenomenon of the homolateral nasal and thoracal halves (Samzelius-Lejdstrom, 1939). Others have studied rabbits under experimental conditions and showed that if coal dust was inhaled through one nasal opening, it was deposited in much larger quantities in the homolateral lung (Wotzilka and Schramek, 1930). These studies all indicate that lateralized rhythms of lung inflation are likely to parallel the nasal cycle since a neural reflex exists between the nose and lung. This does not discount the central mediation of a rhythm of lateralized predominance in lung inflation. A dominant nostril on one side has greater sympathetic tone, as would the homolateral lung. However, while sympathetic activity produces vasoconstriction in the nose, it produces vasodilation in the vessels of the lung, thereby producing a unilateral relationship of predominance in activities between the nose and the lung.

Another remarkable example of lateralized autonomic tone has been reported called the "harlequin color change in the newborn" (Neligan and Strang, 1952). While this study looked primarily at premature infants, or infants born with infections, a few similar observations in normal babies were also reported. The harlequin color change occurs only on one-half of the body and lasts anywhere from 30 sec to 20 min. The baby can be in almost any position as long as it is mostly turned on one side. The upper half of the body becomes pale and there is always a clear-cut line of demarcation running exactly along the midline of the body. The attack could be abruptly curtailed by removing the baby from its side, but in some cases the pale and flushed sides could be reversed by turning the baby onto its opposite side. Neligan and Strang surmised "the precise distribution of the color changes suggests a temporary imbalance in the CNS (possibly in the hypothalamus)," and that this phenomenon might be produced by gravity in infants that had labile nervous systems. Although they were apparently unaware of the nasal cycle as a normal example of lateralized autonomic function, another researcher observed that lateral recumbency could induce a switch in autonomic tone as exhibited by a change in nasal dominance (Heetderks, 1927). He assumed that this was a gravitational effect and concluded "that the distribution of the nasal vascular contents must be largely controlled by gravitation." In 1934, one researcher described the lateralized patterns of perspiration in humans and termed this phenomenon the "hemihidrotic reflex" (Kuno, 1934), stating that "lying on one side caused a remarkable increase in sweating universally over the upper half of the body," suggesting that gravity also played a role. However, others have investigated posture and lateralized patterns of perspiration and have demonstrated that the lateral recumbent effect can be mimicked while the subject is in a vertical position by applying pressure to an axillary point near the fifth intercostal space (Ferres, 1958; Kawase, 1952; Takagi and Kobayasi, 1955; Takagi and Sakurai, 1950). Haight and Cole (1986) studied and reviewed reports on the effects of posture and pressure on the nasal cycle which showed that pressure on the axillary point, and several other areas of lesser affect, can induce the increased sympathetic tonus on the contralateral side of the body and alter the phase of the nasal cycle. This work is also discussed in Section V.B as an aspect of translational neuroscience.

Others have also studied how sympathetic tonus can differ greatly on the two sides of the body by looking for possible differences in sympathetic tone in resting subjects by assaying norepineprhine (NE), epinephrine (E), and dopamine (D) in the antecubital venous circulation in both arms using simultaneous sampling every 7.5 min (Kennedy *et al.*, 1986). Figures 1 and 2 with NE and Fig. 3 with D show how levels in plasma catecholamines can alternately rise and fall in the two arms under strict resting conditions. Figure 4 shows how NE, E, and D all covary with a similar but not identical pattern of variation on the two sides. Figures 5 and 6 show how the nasal cycle is paralleled by lateralized variations in NE levels even when there is not a complete transition in the nasal cycle. Both Figs. 5 and 6 show a left nostril-dominant mode for the nasal cycle throughout the recording period. However, there is fluctuation during that mode and the NE profile closely parallels the nasal profile. This study demonstrates that lateralized shifts in sympathetic tonus are associated with lateralized shifts in the concentrations of catecholamines in peripheral circulation.

Other researchers have studied extracellular hippocampal NE and serotonin in freely moving rats using microdialysis with a 30-min sampling rate over 24 h and found "spontaneous" or "substantial fluctuations" which correlate with the activity state of the animal (Kalen *et al.*, 1989). These fluctuations were not studied in both hippocampi, or as rhythms per se, but eight peaks are shown within the 24-h period. And others have studied ultradian rhythms in plasma NE in depressed patients and normal subjects at 30-min

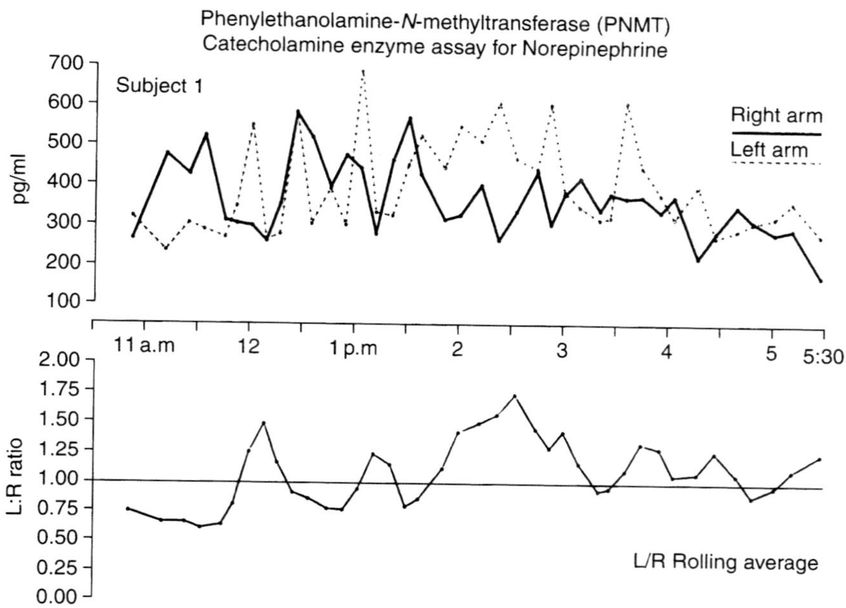


FIG. 1. Top section: Variations in plasma NE levels (pg/ml) were measured at 7.5 min intervals in both right (unbroken line) and left (hatched line) arms. Raw data for subject 1 are represented from 11 a.m. to 5:30 p.m. NE was measured by radioenzymatic assay with phenylethanolamine-*N*-methyltransferase and ([3H]SAM). Bottom section: The left:right ratio of the values of the two arms in the top section are presented as a rolling average using the formula (1:2:1). Values in the curve above 1.00 represent greater levels of NE in the left arm and values below 1.00 are greater levels in the right arm. Timescale is the same as above. Note that the values plotted in the ratio have been transformed by the smoothing function and therefore as in the first point an obvious inconsistency seems apparent. Reprinted from Kennedy, Ziegler, and Shannahoff-Khalsa; copyright (1986), with permission from Elsevier.

intervals for 24 h during complete bed rest and have found periods near 3 h (Koenigsberg *et al.*, 2004), and with 10-min sampling in healthy young men at 50–100 min (Schofl *et al.*, 1997). Ninety-nine minute rhythms of NE have also been observed in the hypothalamus in freely moving rats (Dietl *et al.*, 1993). Another study in humans with 15-min sampling over 6 h tested a range of cognitive measures and NE and found meaningful correlations in the "90 min" frequency range (Bossom *et al.*, 1983). Also, the same high-frequency ultradian rhythm was demonstrated earlier in humans (Levin *et al.*, 1979) and monkeys (Levin *et al.*, 1978).

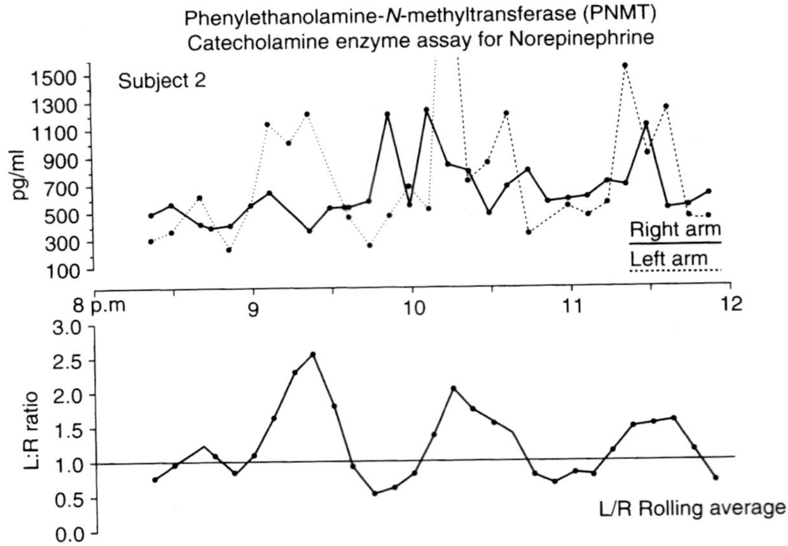


FIG. 2. Top section: Variations in plasma NE levels (pg/ml) were measured at 7.5 min intervals in both right (unbroken line) and left (hatched line) arms. Raw data are represented for subject 2 from 8:22 p.m. to 12 midnight. NE was measured by radioenzymatic assay with phenylethanolamine-*N*-methyltransferase and ([3H]SAM). The 10:08 p.m. NE value for the left arm is 2874. Bottom section: The left:right ratio of the values of the two arms from above are represented as a rolling average. Values in the curve above 1.00 represent greater levels of NE in the left arm and values below 1.00 are greater levels in the right arm. Timescale is the same as the top section. Reprinted from Kennedy, Ziegler, and Shannahoff-Khalsa; copyright (1986), with permission from Elsevier.

When Benton and Yates compared the left and right adrenal blood flows in conscious dogs at rest by simultaneously sampling from the lumboadrenal veins, they found that "there were no cases in which the mean flows were not significantly different" (Benton and Yates, 1990). They found that the right adrenal gland averaged 1.8 g in weight and the left gland averaged 1.3 g. However, they state that "paradoxically, the flows seemed unrelated to the mass of the glands" and at some points in the recording period there were transitions in which gland had higher rates of blood flow. They also observed an approximate 90-min periodicity in adrenal blood flows and cortisol secretion rates. These left/right variations in adrenal blood flow are further evidence of a lateralized rhythm in the ANS. Similar findings of lateralized differences in blood flow have also been reported for the two kidneys (Springorum and Centenera, 1938).

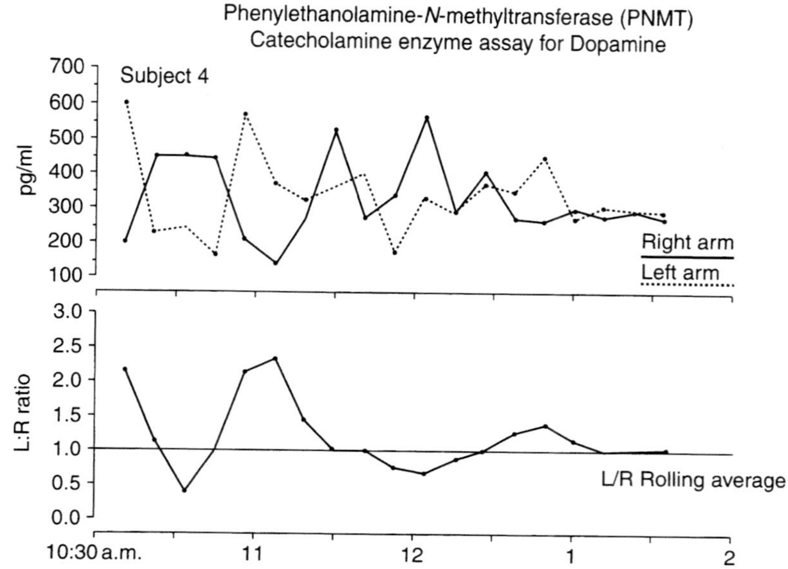


FIG. 3. Top section: Variations in plasma DA levels (pg/ml) were measured at 7.5 min intervals in both the right (unbroken line) and left (hatched line) arms. Raw data for subject 4 is represented from 10:37 a.m. to 1:37 p.m. DA was measured by radioenzymatic assay with catechol-*O*-methyltransferase and ([3H]SAM). Bottom section: The left:right ratio of the values of the two arms from above are presented as a rolling average. Values in the curve above 1.00 represent greater levels of DA in the left arm and values below 1.00 are greater levels in the right arm. Reprinted from Kennedy, Ziegler, and Shannahoff-Khalsa; copyright (1986), with permission from Elsevier.

## B. Lateralized Rhythms of the CNS

Generally, it is believed that the ANS controls only the vegetative-visceral and homeostatic systems. However, recently it has been shown that the lateralized rhythms of the ANS are also tightly coupled to and have a major regulatory influence on the activity of the CNS. Werntz *et al.* (1980, 1983) showed that the nasal cycle is tightly coupled to a newly identified ultradian rhythm of alternating cerebral hemispheric activity in humans. This ultradian rhythm of CNS activity has been reviewed (Shannahoff-Khalsa, 1993). Werntz *et al.* used the EEG to continuously record from homologous sites on the two sides of the head and the signals were then rectified, integrated, and subtracted. The right-left EEG difference in each of

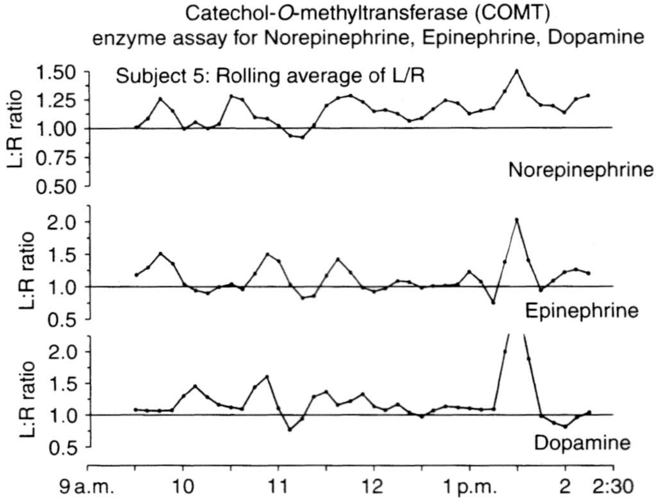


FIG. 4. Top section: The plasma variations of the left:right ratio of the two arms of subject 5 are generated by dividing the average value from the triplicate assay for norepinephrine (NE) at each time point in each arm. NE was determined by radioenzymatic assay using catechol-*O*-methyltranferase and ([3H]SAM). Timescale is 9:30 a.m. to 2:15 p.m., with plasma samples taken every 7.5 min. The rolling average of the left:right ratio is presented. Middle section: Plasma concentrations and the rolling averages of the ratios for both arms were determined as above using the same blood sample during the same assay for epinephrine (E). Bottom section: Plasma concentrations and the rolling average of the ratios for both arms were determined as in the top section using the same blood sample during the same assay for dopamine (D). Missing value at 1:30 p.m. is 2.81. Reprinted from Kennedy, Ziegler, and Shannahoff-Khalsa; copyright (1986), with permission from Elsevier.

the four major frequency bands correlates well with the nasal cycle in 19 of 19 subjects (see 3 subjects in Fig. 17). Relatively greater EEG amplitudes (power) were contralateral to the dominant nostril. Unless there was a major shift in the nasal cycle, no significant shift was observed in the EEG. Most fiber systems of the ANS travel uncrossed between the hypothalamus and periphery (Saper *et al.*, 1976) and are uncrossed from the hypothalamus to the cortex (Saper, 1985). Therefore, it seems likely that the hemisphere contralateral to the dominant nostril would have relatively greater blood flow as a result of the respective dominance in the cerebral parasympathetic influences in circulation and that the hemisphere ipsilateral to the dominant nostril would have greater sympathetic tonus. One study has been conducted that confirms this view (Klein *et al.*, 1986).

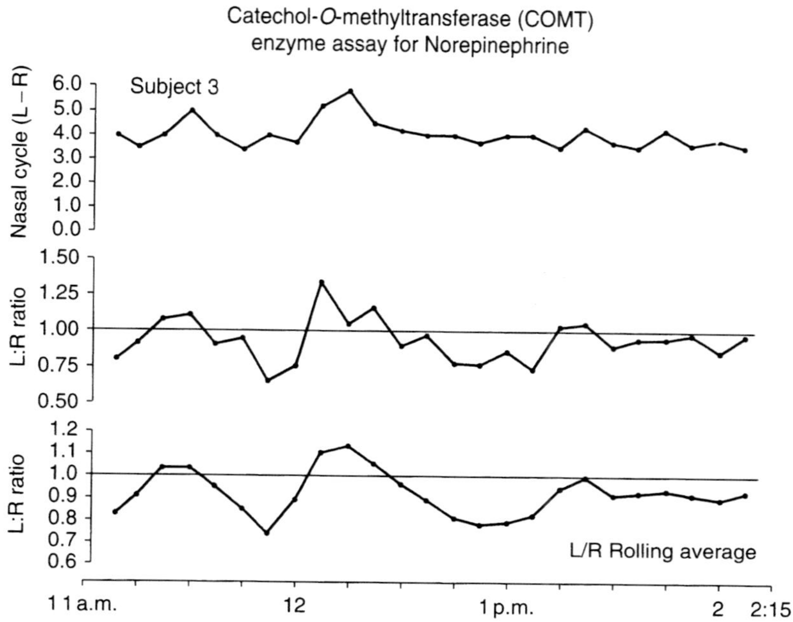


FIG. 5. Top section: The nasal cycle determination of subject 3 is plotted as the raw data of the left minus right (L − R) value versus time. The (L − R) value was assessed at each time point for blood sampling, every 7.5 min. The subject fluctuates in left nostril dominance during the recording period. The nasal cycle was shifted 7 min to the left. Middle section: The raw data of the plasma variations of the left:right ratio of the two arms of subject 3 are generated by dividing the average value from the triplicate assay for NE at each time point in each arm. Norepinephrine (NE) was determined by radioenzymatic assay using the catechol-*O*-methyltransferase and ([3H]SAM). Timescale is 11:07 a.m. to 2:07 p.m. NE values greater than 1.0 represent greater plasma levels in the left arm, values less than 1.0 represent greater plasma levels in the right arm. Bottom section: The same data as the middle section are represented here as the rolling average of the ratios, using the formula (1:2:1). Reprinted from Kennedy, Ziegler, and Shannahoff-Khalsa; copyright (1986), with permission from Elsevier.

In 1979, Klein and Armitage (1979) first reported the waking ultradian rhythms of alternating cognitive performance efficiency by studying verbal and spatial skills. They tested eight subjects with a verbal and spatial task every 15 min for 8 h. They noted ultradian variations with major peaks of activity at 37, 96, and 240 min (Klein and Armitage, 1979). The best performance on the verbal task was 180° out of phase with the best performance on the spatial task. The same cognitive tests were used to assess performance efficiency during different phases of the nasal cycle (Klein *et al.*, 1986). They observed a significant relationship between the pattern of nasal

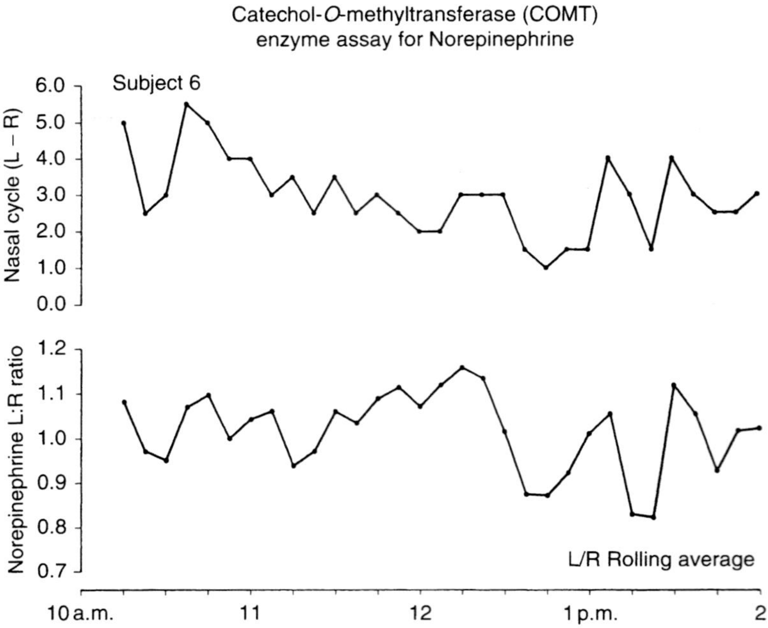


FIG. 6. Top section: The nasal cycle determination of subject 6 is plotted as the raw data of the left minus right (L − R) value versus time. The (L − R) value was assessed at each time point for blood sampling, every 7.5 min. The subject fluctuates in left nostril dominance during the entire recording period. The timescale is from 10:15 a.m. to 2:00 p.m. The nasal cycle has been shifted 15 min to the right. Bottom section: The left:right ratio of the two arms is generated by dividing the average of the triplicate value of one arm by the other. The rolling average is presented here using the formula (1:2:1). Points greater than 1.0 represent greater levels of norepinephrine (NE) in the left arm, and values below 1.0 represent greater levels of NE in the right arm. NE was determined by radioenzymatic assay with catechol-*O*-methyltransferase and ([3H]SAM). Reprinted from Kennedy, Ziegler, and Shannahoff-Khalsa; copyright (1986), with permission from Elsevier.

airflow during normal breathing and spatial versus verbal performance where right nostril dominance correlated with enhanced verbal performance, or left brain activity, and left nostril dominance correlated with enhanced spatial performance.

## 1. *Ultradian Rhythm Studies of Alternating Cerebral Hemispheric Activity Exhibited by EEG during Sleep*

The first report of lateralized hemispheric voltage asymmetries and asynchronous EEG frequencies during sleep was in a 1969 study of a pilot whale (Serafetinides *et al.*, 1972; Shurley *et al.*, 1969).

The authors report that during the waking–rest state "frequency (asynchrony) and voltage (asymmetry) discrepancies between the two sides were the rule rather than the exception" and that they exhibit with an "alternating character, that is, the electrical activity of the left and right hemispheres tended to alternate in the sense that when one showed low-voltage, alpha-like, or fast activity, the other tended to show activity of higher voltage and lower frequency" (Serafetinides *et al.*, 1972). These differences were also exhibited during sleep but to a lesser degree. No mention is made of the actual periodicity, but during two separate recordings of 6–8 h, one session showed 60% frequency asynchrony with 40% voltage asymmetry and the second session showed 45% frequency asynchrony and 55% voltage asymmetry. They concluded that "during relative relaxation the two hemispheres beat at independent electrical rates, as if each one of them functions to a certain extent independently of the other, in moments of arousal or, to a lesser extent, sleep, a certain pacemaker takes over" (Serafetinides *et al.*, 1972).

One of the early seminal EEG studies during sleep shows the ultradians of lateralized alternating cerebral hemispheric power (Goldstein *et al.*, 1970, 1972). This group found changes in amplitude relationships between hemispheres for most shifts from NREM to REM sleep in humans as well as cats and rabbits. In seven human subjects there was relatively lower EEG amplitude in the left hemisphere during NREM sleep with higher amplitude in the left during REM sleep (Goldstein *et al.*, 1972). The same directional shifts were found in three of five rabbits and three of four cats. With the rabbits and cats that were the exception, the reverse relationship was found. They concluded that "the difference in hemispheric amplitude relationships during NREM and REM sleep may eventually prove to be a neurophysiological concomitant of the change in brain function during sleep" (Goldstein *et al.*, 1972). This was the first major study providing evidence for a rhythm of alternating cerebral hemispheric activity in humans during sleep.

Webster (1977) later replicated the 1972 Goldstein *et al.* findings in six adult cats. Three cats were right-pawed and three left-pawed showing no obvious relationship between the direction of the shift and paw preference. These same shifts were seen in two 3-week-old kittens and in two adult cats with sectioned corpora callosa showing patterns that were indistinguishable from that of the intact cats. Rabbits were studied more closely and in 10 of 11 rabbits they found that the left amplitude was greater during the waking state and that during the peak periods of NREM sleep the absolute amplitude on the right was greater than on the left (Nelson *et al.*, 1977). While REM versus NREM was not the primary subject of this study, comparisons of waking versus sleep as spontaneously induced or drug induced showed "the polarity of the deviations during sedation is the opposite of that which holds during waking." They concluded "that differential lateral asymmetries of cortical activity accompany various states of consciousness, that is, normal wakefulness, REM, and NREM sleep" (Nelson *et al.*, 1977).

The Russians studied nine bottlenose dolphins for periods up to 72 h (Mukhametov *et al.*, 1977) and classified the EEG in three ways: (1) desynchronization, (2) intermediate synchronization (including sleep spindles, theta, and delta waves), and (3) maximal synchronization (2/3 of record large delta waves). In one 72-h session of sleep and wakefulness, they observed 56.8% bilateral desynchronization, 0.8% bilateral synchronization, and 42.4% unilateral synchronization with the left exhibiting 27.7% and the right showing 14.7%. They concluded that the unilaterally synchronized hemisphere was in "slow sleep" (NREM) because this wave form is so typical of slow-wave activity in all mammals. Although it is not stated, it is assumed that while one hemisphere was "unilaterally synchronized" the other was "unilaterally desynchronized," and they assume this reflects either waking or REM sleep. They stated that the "functional significance of the alternating interhemispheric asymmetry is still unclear," but "that different levels of activation in the two hemispheres result from functional independence of the two halves of some activating or deactivating system in the brain stem" (Mukhametov *et al.*, 1977).

EEG activity has also been measured during sleep in northern fur seals, both on the land and in the water (Mukhametov *et al.*, 1985). The hemispheric asynchrony was observed both in and out of the water.

When the same animal was compared in and out of the water, the relative amount of EEG asynchrony was greater during sleep in the water. The most important finding is the interhemispheric asynchrony of the EEG slow waves in the right or left hemispheres with simultaneous desynchronization in the contralateral side. Slow wave sleep accounted for 23.3% of the total record (on land) and 14.1% of this record accounted for the asynchronous hemispheric activity.

The principal difference between the dolphins and the seals was with delta-sleep. In dolphins, the delta-sleep pattern arises in either hemisphere only alternatingly in the course of delta-sleep development. In fur seals, delta-sleep patterns can develop both bilaterally and unilaterally in either hemisphere. They concluded that "the functional significance of the state characterized by unilateral slow wave EEG in the fur seal is unclear" (Mukhametov *et al.*, 1985).

In another Russian study, EEG activity and eyelid opening and closing was measured during sleep and wakefulness in a young male white whale over a 4-day period. They stated that:

> We showed that the white whale was the fifth species of Cetaceans, which exhibits unihemispheric slow wave sleep. We found that the eye contralateral to the sleeping hemisphere in this whale was usually closed (right eye, 52% of the total sleep time in the contralateral hemisphere; left eye, 40%) or in an intermediate state (31 and 46%, respectively) while the ipsilateral eye was typically open (89 and 80%). Episodes of bilateral eye closure in this whale occupied less than 2% of the observation time and were usually recorded during waking (49% of the bilateral eye closure time) or low amplitude sleep (48%) and rarely in high amplitude sleep (3%). In spite of the evident overall relationship between the sleeping hemisphere and eye state, EEG and eye position in this whale could be independent over short time periods (less than 1 min) (Lyamin *et al.*, 2002).

They concluded that "Our data support the idea that unihemispheric sleep allows Cetaceans to monitor the environment." And that unihemispheric sleep is an active state, not a result of asymmetrical sensory activation in the visual system and that it "assists in performing several functions during sleep, including sensory monitoring of the environment (first of all visual; Cetaceans, Pinnipeds, and birds), maintaining of movement (swimming in marine mammals and probably flight in some birds), and voluntary control of respiratory functions in Cetaceans" (Lyamin *et al.*, 2002). The topic of unihemispheric sleep is reviewed in depth from the perspective of behavior, neurophysiology, and evolution (Rattenborg *et al.*, 2000).

In pursuit of the findings of Goldstein *et al.* (1972), Banquet reports on alternating asymmetries in five right-handed males during sleep. He found "an alternance in the power dominance of one hemisphere on the other, mostly evident during stage 3–4 sleep for the normalized power of the delta frequency. This kind of asymmetry means usually a hemispheric alternance in the dominance of the normalized delta power and does not change the basic asymmetry but is superimposed on it" (Banquet, 1983a). Regarding REM sleep, he finds what he calls "transitional asymmetries" that occur during part or all of REM sleep. The "subjects with fundamental right-hemispheric dominance shift to left dominance during REM sleep, except for beta frequency which may remain right dominant. Subjects with left dominance keep slow frequencies left-dominant whilst beta becomes right-dominant asymmetry" (Banquet, 1983a). This type of asymmetry is the rule during REM sleep but the inverse pattern can be the exception with left hemisphere beta dominance and right hemisphere slow wave dominance.

Banquet further analyses the same five subjects from a different perspective using inter- and intrahemispheric coherence measures (Banquet, 1983b). He concludes that a steady diffuse decrease of coherence appeared during the progression from waking to NREM sleep, and that REM sleep was associated with low interhemispheric coherence and high intrahemispheric coherence. He concludes that "these findings suggest the interpretation of deep sleep in man as a state of transient partial disconnection between the hemispheres" (Banquet, 1983b).

In another approach to the study of interhemispheric relations during REM and NREM sleep, one group limited their analysis to a single parameter, the correlation coefficient between left and right activity in the various frequency bands (Barcaro *et al.*, 1986). "The major feature found in these patterns was their synchronization with the REM–NREM cycle." In 9 of 11 normal subjects they found, by both a visual comparison with the hypnogram and a statistical analysis, the existence of cyclic variations in the delta and/or sigma correlation coefficients which lasted for the whole night and were synchronized with the REM–NREM sleep cycle.

In yet another attempt to explore the REM–NREM cycle and hemispheric asymmetries, one group compared the absolute differences in interhemispheric EEG frequency bands from 23 subjects for stage 2, REM, and slow wave (stages 3 + 4 combined) sleep (Armitage *et al.*, 1989). They found that theta and delta activity during slow wave sleep was more asymmetrical than in either stage 2 or REM regardless of the hemisphere of origin. They state that "there is evidence of some asymmetry in REM sleep, but it is relatively and consistently less than slow wave sleep" (Armitage *et al.*, 1989). They interpret their results as a contrast of hemispheric symmetry versus asymmetry, where REM sleep represents the "relatively" balanced state and slow wave sleep represents the asymmetric state.

In two studies using auditory probe-evoked potentials during REM and NREM sleep, researchers computed the absolute differences in the amplitude of right- and left-evoked responses and found that asymmetries were larger in stage 4 sleep than in REM or stage 2 (Armitage *et al.*, 1990). Again how they differentiate between alternating cerebral dominance and alternations between symmetry and asymmetries is unclear.

Positron-emission tomography (PET) has been used to study the sleep of 36 normal human males to assess regional cerebral metabolic rates in nighttime sleep (Buchsbaum *et al.*, 1989). In respect to left-right asymmetries they found "a greater left than right metabolic rate in REM but a greater right than left metabolic rate in NREM and awake for the cingulum and medial frontal regions."

In an effort to test for state-specific hemispheric asymmetries, the sleep records from homologous frontocentral, centroparietal, and parietooccipital derivations were obtained from 14 young, healthy, right-handed males (Roth *et al.*, 1999). In the bipolar centroparietal montage, for the theta band (4–8 Hz), a right-hemispheric predominance prevailed in NREM sleep and a left-hemispheric predominance in REM sleep, which became more prominent over the night.

However, within the frequency range of sleep spindles (11.25–14.125 Hz), power in NREM sleep dominated in the left hemisphere in all derivations. They comment "The question is whether these results should be regarded as evidence for state related functional differences of the hemispheres during sleep." In reference to an earlier review on the ultradian rhythm of alternating cerebral hemispheric activity (Shannahoff-Khalsa, 1993), the authors comment "the data do not yield a clear picture. It may be useful in this context to recall the warning (Gazzaniga, 1995) against overpopularizing the 'left mind vs. right mind' concept. We favor an interpretation that does not attribute separate functions to the two hemispheres" (Roth *et al.*, 1999). Their study also finds power gradients along the anteroposterior axis in the high delta/theta frequency range that has a particular prominent difference between non-REM sleep and REM sleep with posterior predominance in non-REM sleep and an anterior predominance in REM sleep. This power gradient may reflect a shift from the activities of the frontal lobes in NREM sleep, which are more the lobes of our executive functions, toward the posterior regions of our brain, during NREM or deep sleep, where less conscious awareness is likely involved. In a related study, this group studied the effect of sleep deprivation on eight healthy, young, right-handed male subjects. After 40 h of sleep deprivation, which affected power spectra in all derivations, they observed hemispheric asymmetries in the delta range, where sleep deprivation enhanced the anterior predominance of delta activity in the left hemisphere but not in the right hemisphere. They conclude "This effect may reflect a functional asymmetry between the dominant and non-dominant hemisphere" (Achermann *et al.*, 2001). It may be that the left hemisphere (the hemisphere dominating during the active phase of the BRAC) after sleep deprivation requires the greatest amount of rest or deep sleep that would be correlated with delta activity.

In another study on sleep deprivation by this group, the rat was recorded in both hemispheres from frontal and parietal derivations over a 24-h baseline period followed by a 6-h sleep deprivation period and an 18-h recovery period (Vyazovskiy *et al.*, 2002):

> During the baseline 12-h light period, the main sleep period of the rat, low-frequency (<7.0 Hz) power in the NREM sleep EEG declined progressively. Left-hemispheric predominance of low-frequency power at the parietal derivations was observed at the beginning of the light period when sleep pressure is high due to preceding spontaneous waking. The left hemispheric dominance changed to a right-hemispheric dominance in the course of the 12-h rest-phase when sleep pressure dissipated. During recovery from sleep deprivation, both low-frequency power and parietal left-hemispheric predominance were enhanced. The increase in low frequency power in NREM sleep observed after sleep deprivation at the frontal site was larger than at the parietal site. However, frontally no interhemispheric differences were present. In REM sleep, power in the theta band (5.25–8.0 Hz) exhibited a right-hemispheric predominance. In contrast to NREM sleep, the hemispheric asymmetry showed no trend during baseline and was not affected by sleep deprivation. Use-dependent local changes may underlie the regional differences in the low-frequency NREM sleep EEG within and between hemispheres. The different interhemispheric asymmetries in NREM and REM sleep suggest that the two sleep states may subserve different functions in the brain (Vyazovskiy *et al.*, 2002).

They note that their study is the first to find evidence for an opposite EEG asymmetry in high-intensity NREM sleep and REM sleep in the rat. It may also be that the rat does not parallel the human and other higher species in their state-specific relationships of hemispheric dominance to sleep stages.

In an attempt to replicate the left minus right (L − R) hemisphere EEG power shifts coupled to REM and NREM sleep observed by Goldstein *et al.*, in 1972, and to also characterize the L − R EEG spectra for total EEG power, delta power, theta power, alpha power, and beta frequency band power, we took archived data with minimal movement artifact and analyzed the data from 10 young, normal, healthy adult males (Shannahoff-Khalsa *et al.*, 2001). The EEG data for left-hemisphere central 3 (C3) and right-hemisphere central 4 (C4) montage were converted to power, and the means were normalized, smoothed, and subtracted. Sleep hypnograms were also compared with L − R EEGs, and spectra were computed for C3, C4, and L − R EEG power for the total EEG power and for the respective frequency bands. Figure 7 shows the L − R

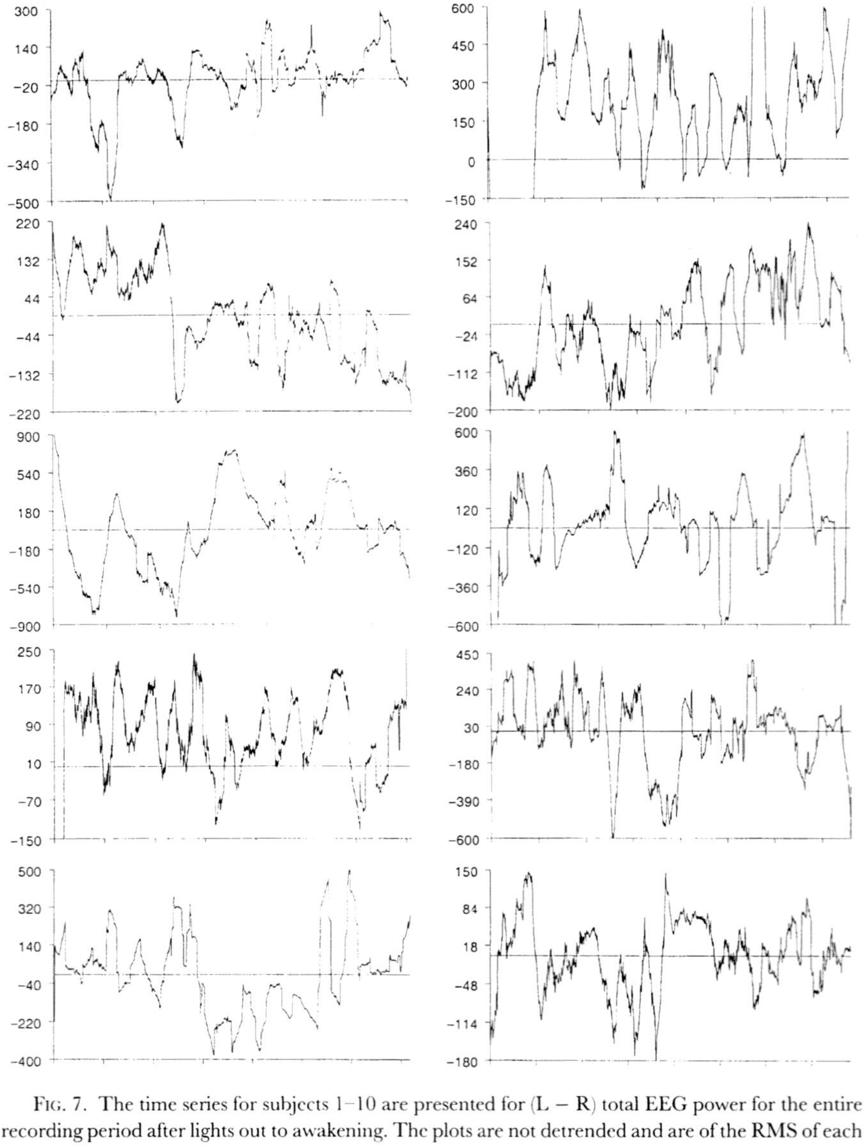


FIG. 7. The time series for subjects 1–10 are presented for (L − R) total EEG power for the entire recording period after lights out to awakening. The plots are not detrended and are of the RMS of each C3 and C4 treated for artifacts, moving average at 500, normalized means, and subtractions. The *y*-axis scaling is adjusted for each to maximize the visual appearance of the fluctuations. The *y*-axis value is the difference of power between left and right hemispheres, and 100 units is the equivalent of 0.61 mV. The average variation from the largest negative peak to the largest positive peak for the 10 subjects ranges across approximately 800 units in total or about 5 mV. Subject 1 starts at the left top and goes down through subject 5, and subject 6 starts at the right top. The *x*-axis lengths (tic marks in hours) for subjects 1 ± 10 are similar and are 7.08, 6.99, 6.75, 7.09, 7.20, 6.50, 6.86, 6.79, 7.71, and 7.96 h, respectively. Reprinted from Shannahoff-Khalsa, Gillin, Yates, Schlosser, and Zawadzki; copyright (2001), with permission from Elsevier.

hemisphere power for all 10 male subjects during the course of the entire night during sleep for total energy.

Figure 8 shows the sleep hypnogram for subject 1 in Fig. 7, and also the L − R power and C3 power for delta, theta, alpha, and beta frequency bands. It is apparent that the L − R and C3 power have sinusoidal-like activity in all frequency bands; although delta and theta power have greater power earlier in the night as expected, while alpha and beta power are more constant throughout.

The results of spectral analysis using "fast" orthogonal search (FOS) (Korenberg, 1988, 1989; Korenberg and Paarmann, 1989a,b) show that significant peaks were observed for all C3, C4, and L − R frequency bands at the 280–300, 75–125, 55–70, and 25–50 min bins with power dominating in the 75–125 min bin. Figure 9 shows the spectral plots of the time series for C3, C4, and L − R for total EEG combined as both the mean percent total mean square error (TMSE) for all 15 parameters for all 10 subjects, and also for the sum of the % MSE.

Figure 10 shows the spectral plots for all 10 subjects for total energy for C3, C4, and L − R power. While spectral plots of C3 and C4 look similar, they are not identical for total power.

Figure 11 shows the spectral plots for all 10 subjects for C3 and L − R power for the four respective frequency bands. While the general patterns are the same for the different frequency bands in the respective C3 plots or L − R plots, there are also noticeable differences.

The visually scored polysomnographic macro-architecture measures for all 10 subjects are presented in Table I showing typical sleep characteristics for a young, normal, healthy male population ranging in age from 20 to 29 years (mean = 25.3, SD = 2.58).

REM and NREM couplings to L − R EEGs for total EEG, delta, theta, alpha, and beta bands were investigated. A sleep hypnogram of REM and NREM sleep stages for the 10 subjects was first paired separately with their respective L − R EEG power time series on a single page for a visual comparison of the hypnogram with the respective L − R for delta, theta, alpha, and beta band plots. The "total EEG" value was calculated finally as the sum of all four separate bands. Calculations for comparisons of left- or

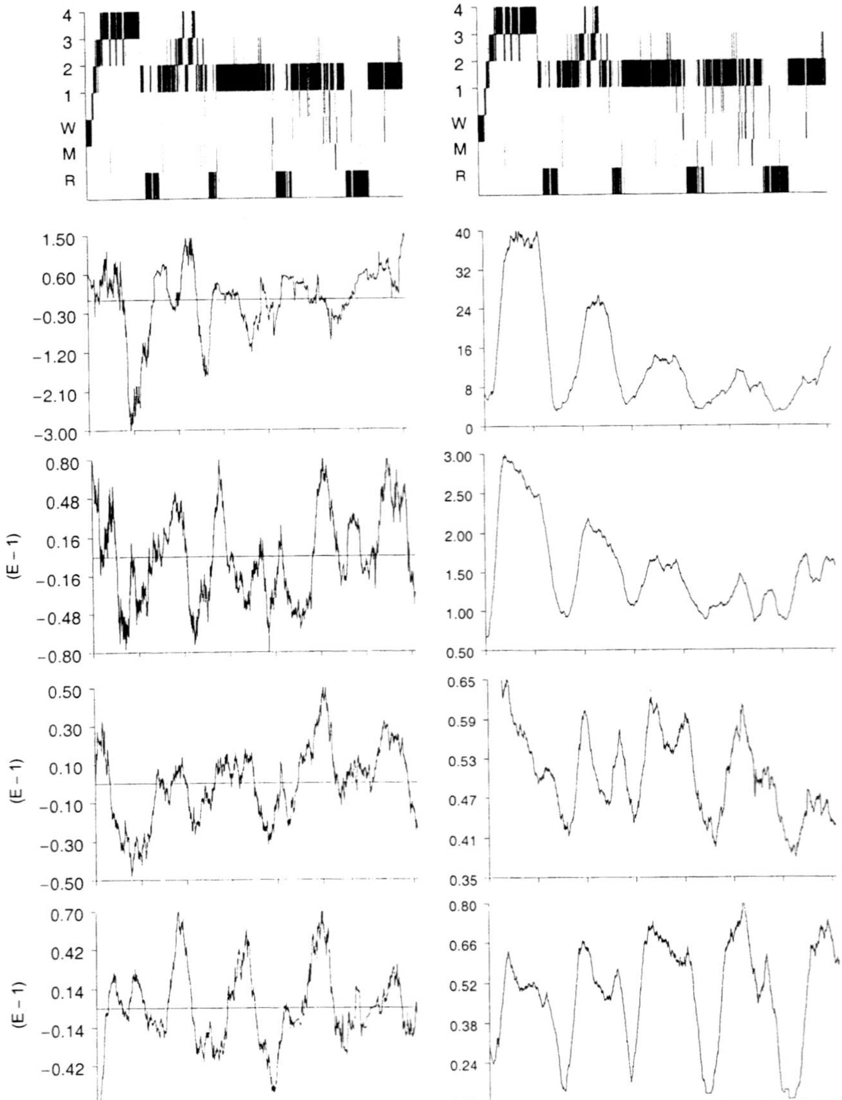


FIG. 8. Left column: The sleep hypnogram for subject 1 is at the top. The time series data for subject 1 for the (L − R) for the four different frequency bands, delta, theta, alpha, and beta, respectively, are presented below. These data are not detrended and are from the FFT power per 4 sec intervals for the entire night (7.08 h). The respective C3 and C4 were treated for artifacts, moving averages at 500, left and right means normalized and subtracted. The scaling is adjusted for each to maximize the visual appearance of the fluctuations, and the *x*-axis has markers at 1 h intervals.

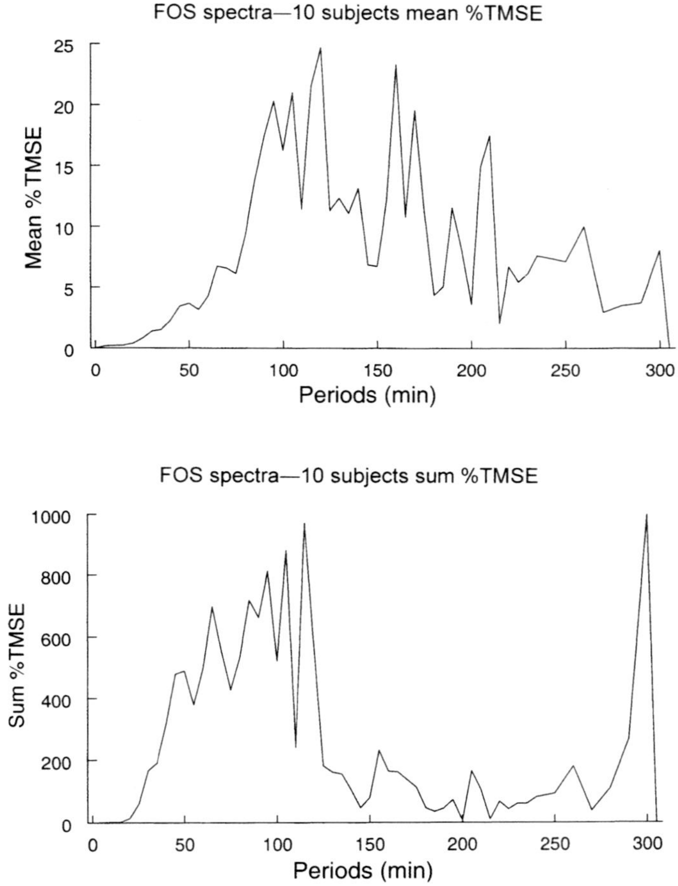


FIG. 9. Top: This spectral density plot shows the FOS time series analysis power distribution as a mean percentage of the TMSE calculation after a detrending of the data for all parameters, independent of subject and parameter. This plot combines 10 subjects and 15 parameters/subject for the 10 sleep nights. Therefore, 150 power spectrums are consolidated to produce the overall "mean" profile. Bottom: This spectral density plot shows the FOS time series analysis power distribution or sum of all individual %TMSEs calculated after a detrending of the data, independent of subject and parameter. This plot is additive for %TMSE and is the result of combining 10 subjects and 15 parameters/subject for all 10 sleep nights. Therefore, 150 power spectrums are "summed" to produce one profile. Reprinted from Shannahoff-Khalsa, Gillin, Yates, Schlosser, and Zawadzki; copyright (2001), with permission from Elsevier.

---

The $y$-axis values are in mV/Hz. Right column: The sleep hypnogram, followed by the left-hemisphere C3 counterpart to the left column L − R's presented for delta, theta, alpha, and beta bands, respectively. The $y$-axis values are in mV/Hz. Reprinted from Shannahoff-Khalsa, Gillin, Yates, Schlosser, and Zawadzki; copyright (2001), with permission from Elsevier.

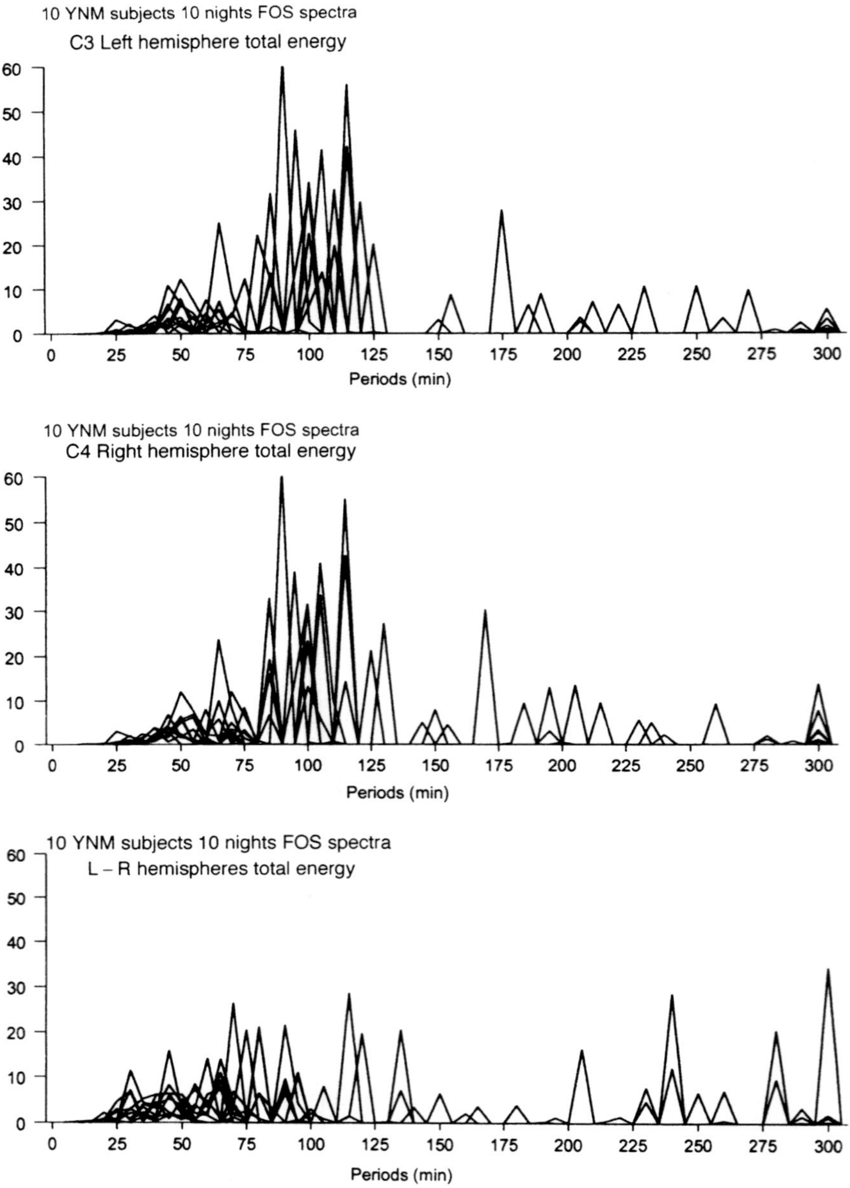


FIG. 10. Spectral density plots of 10 young normal male (YNM) subjects for all 10 nights using FOS time series analysis for the detrended data of the 3-sec RMS power intervals of the total EEG, after artifact removal and moving averages at 500 for the: (top), left-hemisphere C3-total energy;

right-hemisphere dominance were made simply by determining whether the time series was either left or right dominant during each REM period or NREM stage 4 period. Dominance was visually determined as being greater when 50% of the time series was either left- or right-hemisphere dominant during REM or stage 4 sleep. The determination had to be either a left or a right sign, since the L − R profiles were judged only as above or below the midline for L − R dominance. A trend toward a left or a right shift was not counted. Therefore, these calculations were conservative. Chi-squares (two-tailed) were used to determine significance of distributions to either left or right for the comparisons of the four separate bands and the sum of the four bands for total power.

Phase relations of the four different frequency parameters are readily apparent in Fig. 8 and help answer some important questions. The first question is how much coupling exists between the four L − R frequency bands, and second, how much exists for the four bands of C3 or C4. While this was not an immediate focus of this study, Fig. 8 shows considerable phase coupling for the four bands for either the L − R's or C3's. We also found this same "apparent" gross coupling with the other nine subjects. However, a cross-spectrum analysis for phase coupling for the various inter- and intrahemispheric relationships with the different frequency bands would be helpful to further explore other important factors of hemispheric relations as demonstrated by others that have proven helpful in differentiating normal and pathological patients (Armitage *et al.*, 1999, 2000).

Table II shows the distribution for all 10 subjects combined and the significance of the occurrence of NREM stage 4 and REM coupling to either a left or a right event for each of the four frequency bands, and the combined distribution for all four bands representing total power, for the L − R power dominance. For L − R-delta ($p < 0.001$), L − R-alpha ($p < 0.001$), and the sum of

---

(middle), right-hemisphere C4-total energy; and (bottom), L − R hemisphere total energy plots after C3 and C4 mean normalizations. The $x$-axis is (0 ± 300) min, and the $y$-axis represents (0 ± 60)% TMSE accounted for by any of the observed periods. Reprinted from Shannahoff-Khalsa, Gillin, Yates, Schlosser, and Zawadzki; copyright (2001), with permission from Elsevier.

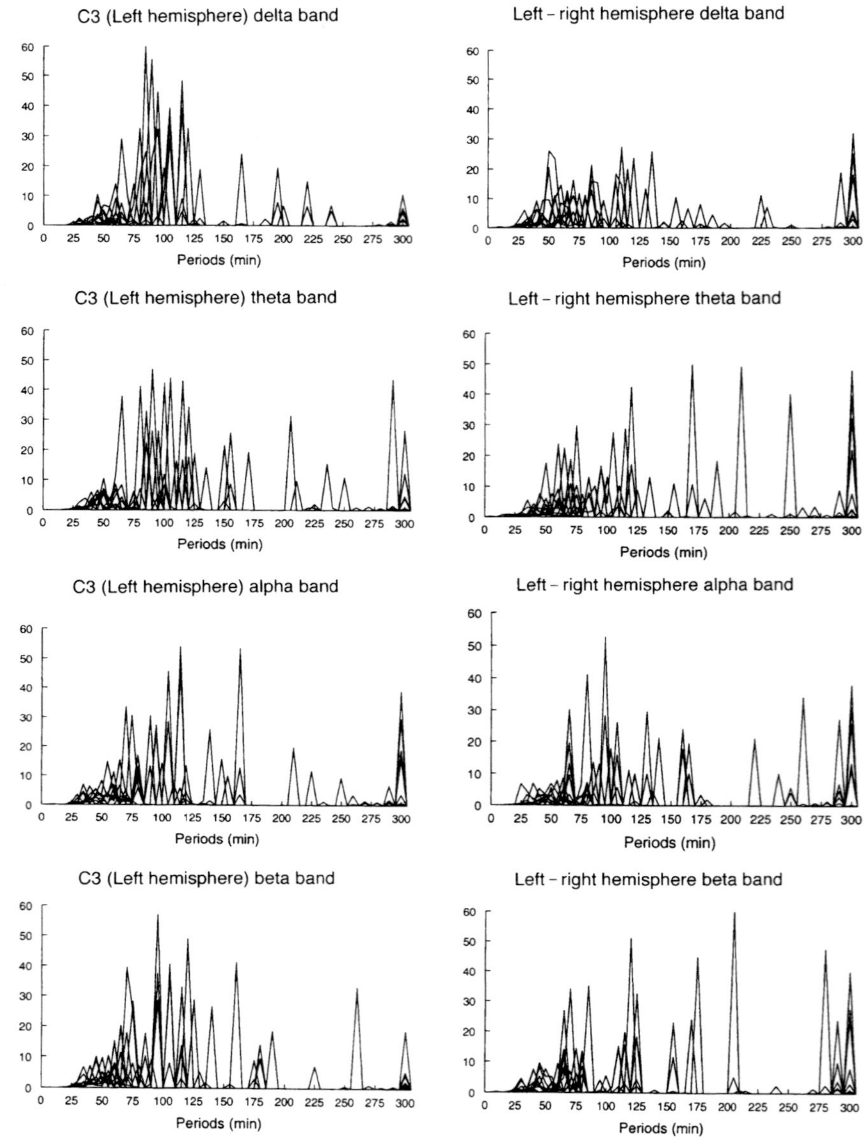


FIG. 11. The left column has four figures, each with separate frequency bands, starting down the page with the delta band FOS spectra for all 10 YNMs for the left hemisphere (C3). FFTs were first calculated to give power at 4 sec intervals, followed by artifact removal, a moving average of 500, and detrending. The second, third, and fourth figures are the theta, alpha, and beta bands, respectively. The right column presents the L – R counterparts for the four separate frequency bands, respectively. Reprinted from Shannahoff-Khalsa, Gillin, Yates, Schlosser, and Zawadzki; copyright (2001), with permission from Elsevier.

TABLE I
VISUALLY SCORED POLYSOMNOGRAPHIC MEASURES FOR 10 YOUNG NORMAL HEALTHY MALES[a]

| | Minimum | Maximum | Mean | SD |
|---|---|---|---|---|
| Sleep latency (min) | 5 | 51 | 13.2 | 14.41 |
| Time in bed (min) | 381.5 | 468 | 424.15 | 25.86 |
| Total sleep time (min) | 328.5 | 412 | 383.5 | 24.91 |
| Sleep efficiency (%) | 76.7 | 95.39 | 90.30 | 5.60 |
| Wake time after sleep onset (min) | 4 | 49.5 | 19.35 | 14.87 |
| Stage 1 (%) | 2.52 | 10.01 | 5.14 | 2.65 |
| Stage 2 (%) | 46.66 | 68.80 | 56.15 | 6.40 |
| Stage 3 (%) | 6.10 | 13.96 | 9.55 | 2.15 |
| Stage 4 (%) | 0.304 | 24.15 | 9.16 | 8.84 |
| REM latency (min) | 59 | 169 | 90.5 | 36.76 |
| REM sleep duration (%) | 9.84 | 31.07 | 20.01 | 6.513 |
| Duration of first REM period (min) | 7.5 | 40.5 | 19.05 | 9.16 |

[a]Reprinted from Shannahoff-Khalsa, Gillin, Yates, Schlosser, and Zawadzki; copyright (2001), with permission from Elsevier.

TABLE II
COMPARISONS OF REM AND NREM SLEEP STAGE 4 WITH LEFT- OR RIGHT-HEMISPHERE DOMINANCE[a]

| | REM-right | REM-left | NREM (stage 4)-right | NREM (stage 4)-left |
|---|---|---|---|---|
| L – R-Delta* | 9 | 27 | 17 | 7 |
| L – R-Theta | 13 | 23 | 13 | 11 |
| L – R-Alpha* | 5 | 31 | 17 | 7 |
| L – R-Beta | 18 | 18 | 9 | 15 |
| All four bands* | 45 | 99 | 56 | 40 |

[a]The numbers in the columns represent the number of events of REM and NREM sleep for the 10 subjects for either a left- or a right-dominant episode, that is, in row 1, the 9 + 27 = 36 gives the total number of REM events for all subjects and how L – R-delta is distributed (9 REM episodes were right dominant and 27 REM episodes were left dominant) for all 10 subjects. An asterisk (*) indicates that chi-square significance (two-tailed) was $p < 0.001$ for the distribution of greater left-hemisphere EEG power dominance during REM sleep and greater right-hemisphere EEG power dominance during NREM (stage 4) sleep. L – R-Theta showed a similar but nonsignificant trend of $p = 0.168$, and the L – R-beta band was equivocal at $p = 0.658$. Reprinted from Shannahoff-Khalsa, Gillin, Yates, Schlosser, and Zawadzki; copyright (2001), with permission from Elsevier.

all four separate bands as a measure of total L – R EEG ($p < 0.001$), there is a highly significant distribution of greater left-hemisphere EEG power dominance during REM sleep and greater right-hemisphere EEG power dominance during NREM stage 4 sleep. There was a similar but nonsignificant trend for L – R-theta ($p = 0.168$). L – R-beta showed equivocal distributions.

In an earlier multivariate waking study (see Section II.C), we observed five prominent bin ranges in the data: 40–65, 70–100, 115–145, 170–215, and 220–340 min bins (Shannahoff-Khalsa *et al.*, 1996, 1997). And in a related multivariate sleep study, we observed seven prominent ranges: 40–65, 70–100, 105–140, 145–160, 165–210, 215–275, and 280–300 min bins (Shannahoff-Khalsa and Yates, 2000). These bins were first determined by consolidating all spectral plots for all parameters for each study, respectively, as presented in Fig. 9. In the sleep study analysis presented here, using the profiles generated for Fig. 11, we determined that seven primary bin ranges were present—25–50, 55–70, 75–125, 150–180, 185–220, 235–275, and 280–300 min—and these bins were similar to our earlier waking and sleep studies and they are also those consistently reported by others for ultradian variables (Shannahoff-Khalsa *et al.*, 1996, 1997).

Table III gives the prevalence of a significant peak for the 25 min wide bin of 25–50 min, the 15 min wide bin of 55–70 min, the 50 min wide bin of 75–125 min, the 30 min wide bin of 150–180 min, the 35 min wide bin of 185–220 min, the 35 min wide bin of 235–270 min, and the 20 min wide bin of 280–300 min for the 15 parameters of C3-total, C4-total, L − R-total, L − R-delta, L − R-theta, L − R-alpha, L − R-beta, C3-delta, C3-theta, C3-alpha, C3-beta, C4-delta, C4-theta, C4-alpha, and C4-beta. Chi-square analysis was used to determine if the frequency of occurrence of different peaks was significant for each parameter for the 7 different bins for the 10 subjects. Table III lists the number of times that these periods were found for each parameter when a minimum of 5.0% of the TMSE is found for at least one nominated period in that peak range. The 5.0% level is a value that is statistically far above the background noise level and is considered here to be "physiologically significant." The TMSE of 5.0% is based, for example, on any one of the possible 3 peak values that can be identified at the three 10-min intervals between 280 and 300 min, 5 peak values of 235, 240, 250, 260, 270, between 235 and 270 min, or 8 values between 185 and 220, 7 values between 150 and 180 min, 11 values between 75 and 125 min, 4 values between 55

TABLE III

PEAK PREVALENCE FOR THE MAJOR PERIOD RANGES FOR 10 SUBJECTS[a]

| | C3-Total | C4-Total | L − R-Total | L − R-D | L − R-T | L − R-A | L − R-B | C3-D | C3-T | C3-A | C3-B | C4-D | C4-T | C4-A | C4-B |
|---|---|---|---|---|---|---|---|---|---|---|---|---|---|---|---|
| 25–50 min | 4* | 7* | 8* | 6* | 4* | 4* | 5* | 4* | 7* | 5* | 4* | 4* | 5* | $3^{\#}$ | 5* |
| 55–70 min | 4* | 6* | 8* | 7* | 8* | 6* | 7* | 4* | 3* | 7* | 9* | 5* | 3* | 6* | 9* |
| 75–125 min | 10* | 10* | 10* | 9* | 9* | 9* | 9* | 10* | 10* | 10* | 10* | 10* | 10* | 10* | 10* |
| 150–180 min | 2 | 2 | 1 | 4* | 4* | 4* | 4* | 1 | $3^{\#}$ | 4* | 4* | 1 | 5* | 2 | $3^{\#}$ |
| 185–220 min | 4* | 4* | 1 | 0 | 2 | 1 | 2 | 5* | 2 | 1 | 1 | 2 | 1 | 1 | 3 |
| 235–270 min | 2 | 2 | 3* | 0 | 1 | 3* | 0 | 1 | 1 | 1 | 1 | 2 | 4* | 3* | 2 |
| 280–300 min | 1 | 2* | 3* | 6* | 6* | 6* | 8* | 3* | 3* | 4* | 2* | 4* | 2* | 3* | 4* |

[a]Total energy for C3, C4, L − R, and C3, C4, and L − R for delta, theta, alpha, and beta bands. 5.0% is the cut off for %TMSE used to determine occurrence of a peak in a period range; the number tells how many subjects have at least one peak at >5.0% TMSE. Asterisk (*) indicates significance of peak prevalence at $p < 0.01$ (two-tailed chi-squares), or $^{\#}p < 0.05$ (two-tailed chi-squares). Reprinted from Shannahoff-Khalsa, Gillin, Yates, Schlosser, and Zawadzki; copyright (2001), with permission from Elsevier.

and 70 min, and 6 values between 25 and 50 min, all at 5-min intervals. It is not based on the %TMSE sum of neighboring peaks. The choice of a cutoff value of 5.0% is very conservative, since frequently there is significant activity at several neighboring values that are "shoulders" of the major peak in the same bin.

All 15 parameters (except C4-A in the 25–50 min range, which showed $p < 0.05$) showed significant peaks by chi-square with $p < 0.01$ in the 25–50, 55–70, 75–125 min ranges and all (except C3-total energy) showed a significant peak with $p < 0.01$ in the 280–300 min range. The 150–180 min range showed significance at $p < 0.01$ for seven parameters: L − R-delta, L − R-theta, L −R-alpha, L − R-beta, C3-alpha, C3-beta, and C4-theta; and at $p < 0.05$ only for C3-theta and C4-beta. The 185–220 min range showed significance for $p < 0.01$ for only three parameters: C3-total, C4-total, and C3-delta. The 235–270 min range showed significance ($p < 0.01$) for only four parameters: C4-alpha, C4-theta, L − R-alpha, and L − R-total. These results, in part, help differentiate the subtle spectral differences between the four frequency bands of the C3's and C4's in contrast to those of the L − R's, where the L − R's for the four separate bands all show values of $p < 0.01$ in the 150–180 min range. Note: C3-total, C4-total, and L − R-total do not have significant peaks in that range.

In sum, L − R EEG rhythms were observed for all bands. Greater right-hemisphere EEG power dominance was found during NREM stage 4 sleep and greater left during REM for total EEG, delta, and alpha bands (chi-squares, $p < 0.001$). Theta was similar but not significant ($p = 0.163$), and beta was equivocal. We concluded that earlier ultradian studies show that lateral EEG and L − R EEG power have a common pacemaker, or a mutually entrained pacemaker with the autonomic, cardiovascular, neuroendocrine, and fuel regulatory hormone systems (Shannahoff-Khalsa and Yates, 2000; Shannahoff-Khalsa *et al.*, 1996, 1997). In addition, we conclude that "these results for L − R EEG coupling to sleep stages and multi-variate relations present a new perspective for Kleitman's BRAC and for diagnosing variants of pathopsychophysiological states" (Shannahoff-Khalsa *et al.*, 2001).

In addition, one early study found fascinating changes in nasal dominance with stages of REM and NREM sleep (Alexiev and Roth, 1978). Minor changes in airflow differences may have been obscured since visual methods rather than computer-assisted analysis were used to detect changes. In healthy subjects they found that:

> During the first 3 hours of sleep slight differences in amplitude were observed in some cases: that is, respiration through the right nostril was relatively weaker than through the left, which remained at a level recorded at the beginning. This change was not permanent and changes in position of the body and movements of the head, as well as REM sleep events, led to an equalization of the amplitudes on the two sides. These periods began through NREM stage 2 and continued from several minutes up to 40 minutes. In the 4th or 5th hours of nocturnal sleep, at the end of the 3rd sleep cycle, several minutes after the onset of REM sleep, an abrupt change in the pattern of respiration took place: respiration through the left nostril was completely blocked, while that through the right nostril displayed a hyperventilatory type with an amplitude about 3 times greater than that recorded during wakefulness, which continued to the end of REM sleep, respiration through the left nostril was not restored to the original level, and respiration through the two nostrils became more equal after the subjects awakened. With two cases of hypersomnia the right nostril was blocked and hyperventilatory type of respiration took place in the left nostril during REM sleep, and in the remaining part of the night the patients breathed only through the left nostril (Alexiev and Roth, 1978).

They also analyzed two cases of narcolepsy-cataplexy and the same changes in the pattern of respiration were observed as in hypersomnia, except that during the second night in one of the subjects a sleep onset REM period was recorded during which the passage of air through the right nostril was blocked and this state remained until awakening in the morning. They apparently were not aware of the phenomenon of the nasal cycle, but concluded that "the nasal venous plexi could be a phenomenon similar to the congestion of corpus cavernosum penis leading to penile erection, which is a regular sign of REM sleep."

One study (Shannahoff-Khalsa and Yates, 2000) was conducted to compare the dynamics of multiple systems during sleep with those of earlier results during waking stationary rest that are presented in

Section II.C (Shannahoff-Khalsa *et al.*, 1996, 1997). Three consecutive nights of data were collected from three healthy adults for 10 variables: left and right central EEGs, the nasal cycle (NC), beat-to-beat measures of cardiac output (CO), stroke volume (SV), heart rate (HR), systolic blood pressure (SBP), diastolic blood pressure (DBP), mean arterial pressure (MAP), and hemoglobin-oxygen saturation (SAO2). Time series analysis detected periods at 280–300, 215–275, 165–210, 145–160, 105–140, 70–100, and 40–65 min bins with the greatest spectral power in longer periods. There was significance across subjects with all parameters at 280–300, 105–140 (except left EEG power, L − R EEG power, and HR), 70–100, and 40–65 min. Significant periods were reported earlier during waking for the NC, pituitary hormones [adrenocorticotropin hormone (ACTH) and luteinizing hormone (LH)], catecholamines (norepinephrine and epinephrine), insulin (INS), and cardiovascular function in five bins at 220–340, 170–215, 115–145, 70–100, and 40–65 min, with 115–145, 70–100, and 40–65 min common across all variables (Shannahoff-Khalsa *et al.*, 1996, 1997). These results suggest that lateral EEG power during sleep has a common pacemaker (the hypothalamus), or a mutually entrained pacemaker, with the cardiovascular and ANS, and that the waking ultradians of the neuroendocrine and fuel regulatory hormones are also coupled to lateralized rhythms of EEG activity. We concluded that "these results present a new perspective for the Basic Rest-Activity Cycle and the physiology of the ANS-central nervous system during both waking and sleep" (Shannahoff-Khalsa and Yates, 2000).

We used FOS time series analysis to characterize the spectral properties of the following parameters: the 3-sec root-mean-square (RMS) measures for left minus right (L − R) hemisphere EEG power; 3-sec RMS measures for left (L-EEG) and right (R-EEG) hemisphere EEG power; 4-Hz sampling of the NC using a moving average of 20; and beat-to-beat cardiac impedance measures of SV, HR, CO, beat-to-beat Finapres blood pressure measures for SBP, DBP, and MAP, and beat-to-beat oxygen saturation measures (SAO2) with a moving average of 20.

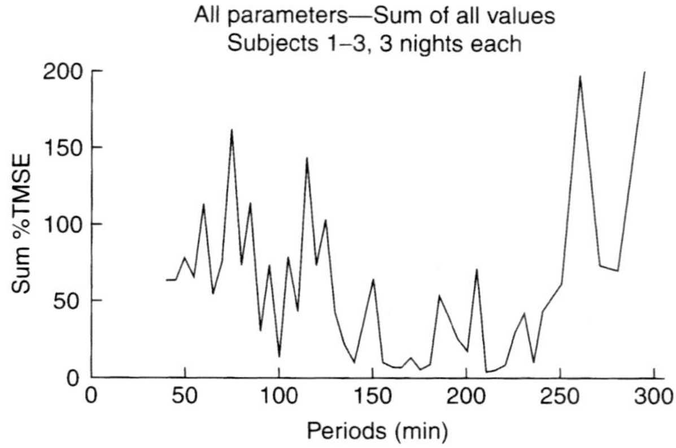


FIG. 12. This spectral density plot shows the FOS time history analysis power distribution, or sum %TMSE after detrending of the data and independent of subject, night, and parameter. This spectral plot is additive for %TMSE at each time period and combines 3 subjects and 11 parameters per subject for all 3 nights each, except subject 2, night 2 for SAO2. Therefore, 99 power spectrums are summed to produce one profile. Reprinted from Shannahoff-Khalsa and Yates; copyright (2000), with permission from Taylor & Francis.

In the earlier waking state study, we observed five prominent ranges for "bins" for consideration for FOS time series analysis: 40–65, 70–100, 115–145, 170–215, and 220–340 min (Shannahoff-Khalsa *et al.*, 1996, 1997). In this sleep study, we visually inspected a profile of the FOS data for both the sums of power for each period (Fig. 12) and the means of total power for each period (Fig. 13), when all of the parameters for each of the three subjects over the three nights (nine records) were collapsed to produce a single power spectrum as was performed earlier and presented in Fig. 9. We then arbitrarily determined that seven ranges were present. These "bands" were 40–65, 70–100, 105–140, 145–160, 165–210, 215–275, and 280–300 min. Our other sleep study also used seven primary bin ranges: 25–50, 55–70, 75–125, 150–180, 185–220, 235–275, and 280–300 min (Shannahoff-Khalsa *et al.*, 2001). These ranges are again similar to our waking study and are also consistent with that reported by others for many of these variables [reviewed in Shannahoff-Khalsa *et al.* (1996)].

The composite spectral plots of the FOS analysis for all subjects for all three nights are shown in Fig. 14 for the NC, L − R EEG,

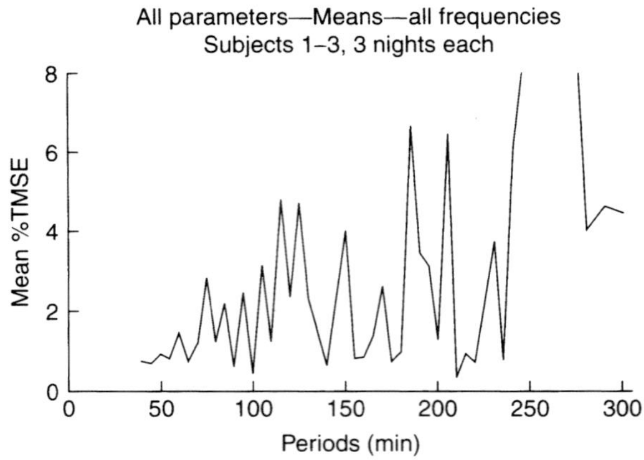


FIG. 13. This spectral density plot shows the FOS time history analysis power distribution as a mean %TMSE after detrending of the data for all parameters at any given time period, independent of subject, night, and parameter. This spectral plot combines 3 subjects and 11 parameters per subject each for 3 nights, except subject 2 for night 2 for SAO2. Therefore, 99 power spectrums are consolidated to produce the "mean" profile. Reprinted from Shannahoff-Khalsa and Yates; copyright (2000), with permission from Taylor & Francis.

L-EEG, R-EEG, HR, SV, CO, SBP, MAP, and SAO2 (DBP was omitted due to space limits). Figure 14 shows the similarity of the power spectral plots for these 10 parameters in this ultradian range.

Table IV gives the prevalence of a significant peak for the 25 min wide bin of 40–65 min, the 30 min bin of 70–100 min, the 35 min bin of 105–140 min, the 15 min bin of 145–160 min, the 45 min bin of 165–210 min, the 55 min bin of 215–270, and the 20 min bin of 280–300 min for all 11 parameters (NC, L − R EEG, L-EEG, R-EEG, HR, SV, CO, SBP, DBP, MAP, and SAO2). Chi-square analysis (two-tailed) was used to determine if the frequency of occurrence of different peaks was significant across subjects for each parameter. All 11 parameters show a significant peak with $p < 0.01$ in the 280–300 min range, and only R-EEG ($p < 0.01$) and the NC ($p < 0.05$) show marginal significance in the 215–270 min range. No parameters were significant in 165–210 min range and only HR, L-EEG, R-EEG, and SAO2 were marginally significant ($p < 0.05$) in the 145–160 min range. However, all but L-EEG, L − R EEG, and HR were significant ($p < 0.01$) in the

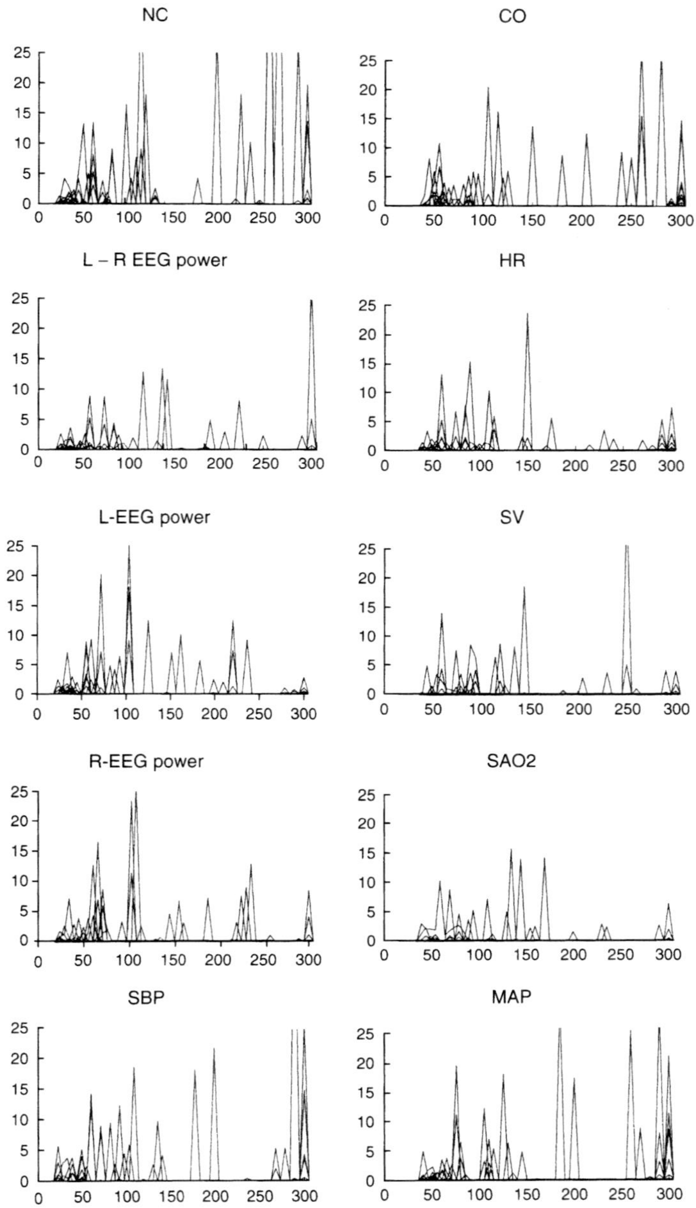


FIG. 14. Spectral density plots of three subjects for all three nights using FOS time history analysis of the nasal cycle (NC), left- minus right-hemisphere EEG power (L – R EEG power), left-hemisphere EEG power (L-EEG power), right-hemisphere EEG power (R-EEG power), systolic blood pressure

TABLE IV

PEAK PREVALENCE FOR THE MAJOR PERIOD RANGES FOR THREE SUBJECTS FOR THREE CONSECUTIVE NIGHTS SLEEP FOR THE NASAL CYCLE, EEG PARAMETERS, AND CARDIOVASCULAR PARAMETERS[a]

| | NC | L − R EEG | L-EEG | R-EEG | CO | HR | SV | SBP | DBP | MAP | SAO2 |
|---|---|---|---|---|---|---|---|---|---|---|---|
| 40–65 min | 9* | 9* | 7* | 9* | 9* | 8* | 9* | 9* | 9* | 9* | 6* |
| 70–100 min | 9* | 9* | 9* | 8* | 8* | 8* | 9* | 6* | 8* | 7* | 8* |
| 105–140 min | 7* | 4 | 3 | 6* | 5* | 4 | 5* | 6* | 8* | 8* | 5* |
| 145–160 min | 0 | 2 | 3‡ | 3‡ | 1 | 3‡ | 2 | 2 | 0 | 1 | 3‡ |
| 165–210 min | 2 | 3 | 2 | 3 | 2 | 4 | 2 | 2 | 2 | 2 | 2 |
| 215–270 min | 5‡ | 2 | 3 | 6* | 4 | 2 | 4 | 2 | 3 | 2 | 2 |
| 280–300 min | 7* | 4* | 5* | 4* | 9* | 6* | 4* | 7* | 4* | 6* | 3* |

[a] 0.40% is the cut off for %TMSE used to determine occurrence of a peak in a period range; the number tells how many subjects have at least one peak at >0.40% TMSE. Asterisk (*) indicates significance of peak prevalence at $p > 0.01$ (two-tailed chi-squares), or ‡ $p > 0.05$ (two-tailed chi-squares); [+] indicates the maximum possible number of peaks is 9 for NC, L − R EEG, L-EEG, R-EEG, CO, HR, SV, SBP, DBP, MAP and 8 for SAO2 since subject 2's data are missing for this variable for night 2. Reprinted from Shannahoff-Khalsa and Yates; copyright (2000), with permission from Taylor & Francis.

105–140 min range, and all 11 parameters were significant at $p < 0.01$ in the 70–100 and the 40–65 min ranges.

Profiles of the individual parameters were smoothed in Figs. 15 and 16 using a moving average to more clearly demonstrate the low-frequency "hourly" component relationships among these measures. The smoothed time series for seven selected parameters in three subjects are shown in Figs. 15 and 16 for the NC, L − R EEG, R-EEG, HR, SV, MAP, and SAO2. The tight inverse relationship of the NC and L − R EEG observed here was also visually apparent in at least six of the nine nights of sleep recording. Of these six nights, subject 1 exhibited two nights of tight coupling, subject 2 showed one night, and subject 3 showed visually apparent tight coupling for all three nights.

(SBP), cardiac output (CO), heart rate (HR), stroke volume (SV), hemoglobin saturated oxygen (SAO2), and mean arterial pressure (MAP). The $x$-axis is 0–300 min, the $y$-axis is in 0–25% total mean square error (TMSE) accounted for by that period. Plots of SAO2 are missing subject 2's data for night 2. Reprinted from Shannahoff-Khalsa and Yates; copyright (2000), with permission from Taylor & Francis.

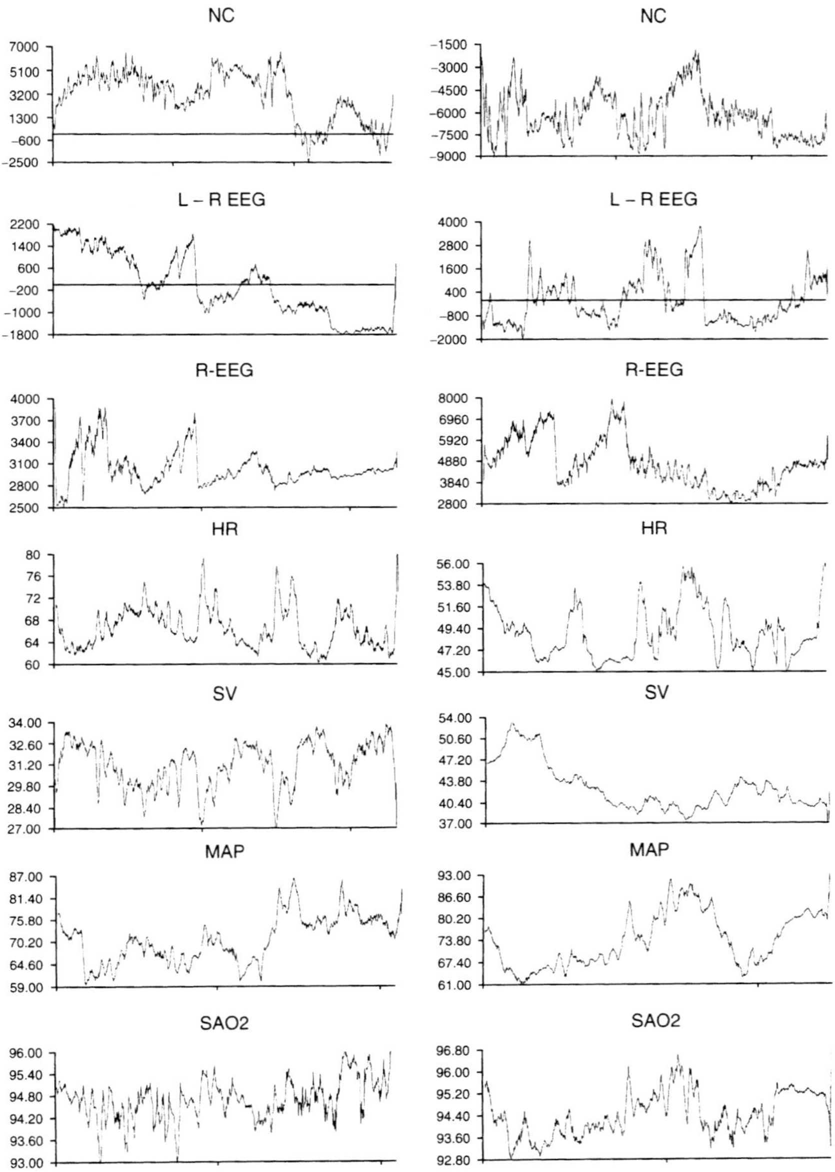


FIG. 15. The primary time series data for subject 1, night 1 (left side of figure), and subject 3, night 3, are plotted from top down for the nasal cycle (NC; left minus right nostril dominance), left-minus right-hemisphere EEG power (L − R EEG power), right-hemisphere EEG power (R-EEG power), heart rate (HR), stroke volume (SV), mean arterial pressure (MAP), and hemoglobin saturated oxygen (SAO2). The scaling is adjusted for each to maximize the visual appearance of the fluctuations.

Phase relations of the different parameters are readily exhibited here and help answer some important questions. For example, the records for subject 1, night 1 (Fig. 15) and subject 2, night 3 (Fig. 16) show within subject "mirror-images" for HR and SV as one might expect (Baust and Bohnert, 1969; Pivik *et al.*, 1996). Both subjects also show this for the other two nights (data not shown), this is less apparent for subject 3 during nights 2 and 3 (Figs. 16 and 15, respectively). But subject 3 also demonstrates this close mirror-like inverse relationship between HR and SV in night 1 (data not shown). What accounts for this cardiovascular variation in coupling in subject 3 here is unclear. MAP is also less positively coupled to HR here for nights 2 (Fig. 16) and 3 (Fig. 15) with subject 3 compared to subjects 1 (night 1) and 2 (night 3), and this is also the case for night 1 for subject 3 (data not shown) but not for subjects 1 and 2 on any night. HR is also inversely coupled to R-EEG power, a correlate of REM sleep (Goldstein *et al.*, 1972), as expected, and is fairly consistent across the night for all subjects for all nights. Subject 1 (night 1, Fig. 15) shows a tight coupling between increased R-EEG power and the left-hemisphere dominant mode of L − R EEG. This is not the case here for subjects 2 or 3 (nights 2 or 3) where the reverse is mostly true, but this does appear to be the case with night 1 for subject 3 (data not shown). The NC shows a tight inverse coupling to L − R EEG for all nights shown here and is also similarly visually very convincing in at least six of the nine nights. This coupling is further supported by the FOS results. SAO2 shows a closer coupling of higher oxygen levels with the "relative" right nostril-dominant mode and during the reduced R-EEG power modes.

---

These time series were not detrended here. The *x*-axis is for 5.83 h for subject 1 and for 5.29 h for subject 3. The *y*-axis values for the left minus right NC measures are in arbitrary electronic units related to differential thermistor activity, data above the midline indicate left nostril airflow dominance; L − R EEG is scaled as the difference of the RMS calculations after a normalization of left and right means for RMS values over the night; R-EEG is scaled as the RMS calculation from the raw primary data; the HR values are in beats/min; SV is in ml/beat; MAP is in mm Hg; and SAO2 is in % hemoglobin-oxygen saturation. Note: subject 3's NC shows only relative shifts in right nostril dominance during the entire night. Reprinted from Shannahoff-Khalsa and Yates; copyright (2000), with permission from Taylor & Francis.

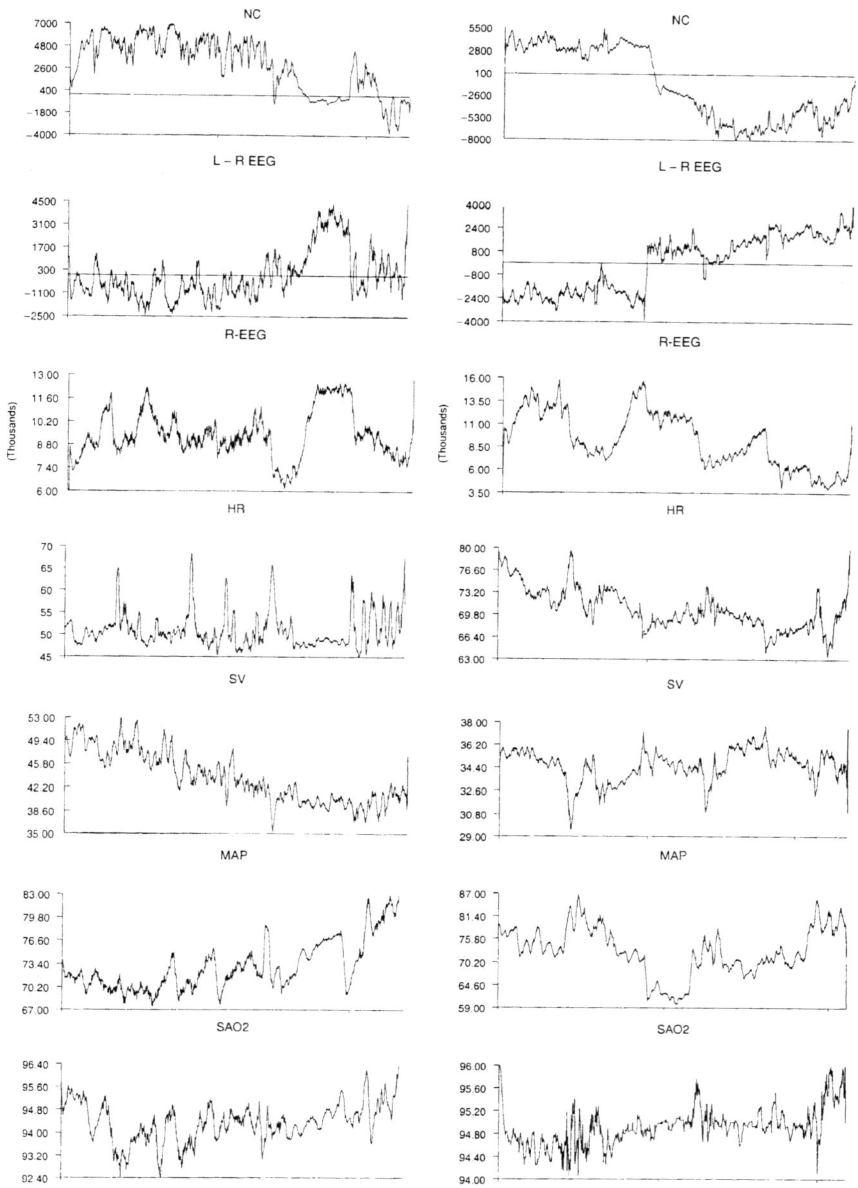


FIG. 16. The primary time series data for subject 3, night 2 (left side of figure), and subject 2, night 3, are plotted from top down for the nasal cycle (NC, left minus right nostril dominance), left- minus right-hemisphere EEG power (L − R EEG), right-hemisphere EEG power (R-EEG), heart rate (HR), stroke volume (SV), mean arterial pressure (MAP), and hemoglobin saturated oxygen (SAO2).

With 11 parameters per subject in this experiment, there are 55 possible interparameter comparisons that can be made for each subject, resulting in either an apparent positive, negative, or apparently nonsignificant relationship. However, these three possibilities do not include the possibility of phase lagging. These seven parameters were selected here to give examples of how these three systems (CNS, ANS, and cardiovascular) can compare linear time series. Other time series showing the phase relationship variance are presented in Section II.C , and many have been reported (Shannahoff-Khalsa *et al.*, 1996, 1997).

In sum, all 11 parameters had similar power spectral profiles across subjects with significance of $p < 0.01$ (chi-square, two-tailed) with peak activity in the four major bins of 280–300, 105–140 (except L − R EEG, L-EEG, and HR), 70–100, and 40–65 min. Four parameters (HR, L-EEG, R-EEG, SAO2) also show marginal significance at $p < 0.05$ in the 145–160 min range, and two parameters (NC, $p < 0.05$; R-EEG, $p < 0.01$) also show marginal significance in the wider 215–270 min range.

The study with waking subjects included all of these parameters (except EEGs and SAO2) and 14 others: luteinizing hormone (LH), adrenocorticotropin hormone (ACTH), insulin (INS), left arm norepinephrine (LNE), left arm epinephrine (LE), right arm norepinephrine (RNE), right arm epinephrine (RE), mean norepinephrine (MNE), mean epinephrine (ME), and left minus right values for norepinephrine (L − R NE), and epinephrine (L − R E), respectively; and three additional cardiac impedance measures ventricular ejection time (VET), ejection velocity index (EVI), and thoracic fluid index (TFI). The time series history analysis for the following

---

The scaling is adjusted for each to maximize the visual appearance of the fluctuations. These time series were not detrended here. The *x*-axis is for 4.78 h for subject 2 and for 6.04 h for subject 3. The *y*-axis values for the left minus right NC measures are in arbitrary electronic units related to differential thermistor activity, data above the midline indicates left nostril airflow dominance; L − R EEG is scaled as the difference of the RMS calculations after a normalization of left and right means for RMS values over the night; R-EEG is scaled as the RMS calculation from the raw primary data; the HR values are in beats/min; SV is in ml/beat; MAP is in mm Hg; and SAO2 is in % hemoglobin-oxygen saturation. Reprinted from Shannahoff-Khalsa and Yates; copyright (2000), with permission from Taylor & Francis.

22 variables in the study with waking subjects—NC, LH, ACTH, INS, SBP, DBP, MAP, TPR, LE, LNE, RE, RNE, ME, MNE, L – RE, L – RNE, CO, TFI, HR, EVI, SV, and VET—clearly showed for most variables the predominance of significant peaks in the bins of 115–145, 70–100, and 40–65 min. The exceptions are the absences of statistical significance for ACTH at 115–145 min, NC and LH at 40–65 min, the epinephrines and SBP, DBP, MAP at 115–145 min. The blood pressure parameters during the waking study were not beat-to-beat measures, but one automated cuff measure every 7.5 min (similar to the sampling for the blood plasma parameters) and perhaps would have shown rhythms in the 115–145 min bin, as were exhibited with the beat-to-beat sampled cardiac impedance variables (Shannahoff-Khalsa and Yates, 2000). While all of these 22 parameters (except TFI and HR) had some activity at 220–340 min, only the NC and LH showed significant chi-square values along with their greatest spectral power in the 220–340 min bin. While this is a wider bin than the two neighboring bins used during the sleep study (215–270 and 280–300 min), considerably less activity was observed in this longer period domain during the waking state compared to sleep even though both studies were of nearly equal length using data detrended for circadian rhythms. ACTH had its greatest power in the 170–215 min bin. See Section II.C for further discussion on these waking multivariate studies.

The broad bin of 70–140 min is the bin domain most commonly reported for the "hourly" ultradian rhythms [reviewed in Shannahoff-Khalsa *et al.* (1996, 1997)]. Here this bin was analyzed as two separate components, the 70–100 min and the 105–140 min bins (and as 70–100 and 115–145 min bins during the waking study). These two bins represent the two largest of the five during the waking study in respect to the sum total of the %TMSE. These two bins also dominate during this sleep study, but the 280–300 min bin for sum total %TMSE must be included that also existed but to a lesser extent during the waking state, as well as the 40–65 min bin for both the sleep and the waking states, but with lower %TMSE.

We suggested that "this report provides new insight to how the CNS (marked by EEG) is coupled to the autonomic, cardiovascular, neuroendocrine, and fuel-regulatory hormone systems. These results suggest that a single pacemaker or that mutually entrained pacemakers are regulating the 'hourly' ultradian rhythms under strict resting conditions during either waking or sleep" (Shannahoff-Khalsa and Yates, 2000).

This result with EEG is further evidence to suggest that all of the ultradian rhythms for the major bodily systems may be related via the proposed ANS–CNS rhythm and that the hypothalamus itself is "the pacemaker." Another result also supports this hypothalamic model of control that shows that INS secretion is positively coupled to the NREM "rest" phase of the NREM–REM sleep cycle (Kern *et al.*, 1996). They concluded that the hourly ultradian oscillations of INS are modulated by CNS mechanisms entraining this pancreatic function to the NREM–REM sleep cycle. Furthermore, others have demonstrated ultradian rhythms in humans for cytokines ranging from 80 to 240 min when sampling at 20 min intervals for 8 h during waking (Bouayad-Amine *et al.*, 1993). This result, which is temporally coincident with the above-cited studies, suggests that the immune system is also coupled to the other major systems, perhaps by coupling to the ANS–CNS rhythm through both autonomic innervation and hypothalamic-mediated humoral activity.

The above-cited work on sleep stages and EEG rhythms of alternating hemispheric activity help emphasize the important dynamic nature of left-right patterns of hemisphere dominance and how they should be more closely studied both during waking and sleep along with the other major bodily systems, that is, the autonomic, cardiovascular, fuel-regulation, neuroendocrine, and immune systems. One preliminary study demonstrated that REM sleep is coupled to the right nostril-dominant mode of the NC (Frye and Doty, 1992) and other studies have demonstrated that REM is also coupled to relatively greater EEG power in the left hemisphere, and vice versa for NREM sleep stages (Banquet, 1983a; Goldstein *et al.*, 1970, 1972; Nelson *et al.*, 1977; Shannahoff-Khalsa *et al.*, 2001; Webster, 1977). Clearly, it would be of great interest to explore large numbers of females and males, multiple age ranges, multiple EEG frequency bands and cortical sites, and various states of health and pathology to better understand the coupling of sleep stage relations to the ANS–CNS rhythm as a means to better understanding the organism as a whole and how states of health and disease may be manifested in these terms of intersystem dynamics.

### 2. *Studies of Lateralized Cognitive Performance after Awakening from REM and NREM Sleep Stages*

There is other evidence in humans which also suggests the existence of a natural rhythm of alternating dominance between the two cerebral hemispheres. Researchers have shown in some experiments that waking from either REM or NREM sleep elicits significant differences in the verbal and spatial performance skill ratios (Gordon *et al.*, 1982; Lavie and Tzischinsky, 1984; Lavie *et al.*, 1984). One study showed a significant shift in left-hemisphere cognitive performance after waking from NREM sleep relative to waking from REM sleep. The authors concluded that "these results are consistent with the observed reciprocal oscillations between left and right functions during the waking period and imply that performance of these specialized functions may be controlled by some of the same mechanisms that govern biorhythms" (Gordon *et al.*, 1982). However, while this result was significant for the group, some subjects showed the reverse finding. Another group found a significant shift in cognitive profile in the direction of right-hemisphere dominance after waking from REM sleep, and left-hemisphere dominance after waking from NREM sleep and where a "comparison of the cognitive shifts in females to that observed in males revealed a significant interaction of gender and awakening condition. Females showed a larger increase in right-hemisphere performance following awakening from REM sleep relative to NREM sleep, and a smaller increase in left-hemisphere performance following awakening from NREM sleep relative to REM sleep" and "the reverse trend was found for males" (Lavie *et al.*, 1984). These studies always used very short time (1–2 min) for cognitive testing after awakenings. These results do not hold up when awakenings are prolonged and then followed by cognitive testing. Another study with right-handed males looked at testing after 35 or 75 min (Lavie and Tzischinsky, 1984). They state that "In contrast to our previous findings in subjects tested within 1–2 min after the awakening who showed a significant sleep-stage dependent shift in cognitive asymmetry, the present results did not show significant differences in performance between the two awakening conditions for any of the groups" (Lavie and Tzischinsky, 1984). They also state that "in contrast to our previous findings in right handers, left-handers did not show any consistent shifts in cognitive asymmetry after the awakenings." So the variations here are based in part on the time of cognitive testing after awakening and handedness. We know that left-handers differ in their lateralization of cognitive skills compared to right-handers. What these researchers were not measuring was the laterality of power shifts prior to and after awakening, or the nasal cycle, a measure of lateralized ANS–CNS activity.

Interpretation of results from studies of hemisphere dominance during sleep and EEG studies in general has been difficult since many workers assumed that increasing EEG amplitudes (power) correlate with decreased mental activity. This early assumption arose from very early work on EEG using a simple arousal model in which alpha activity (8–12 Hz) was assumed to be inversely related to mental processing (Adrian and Matthews, 1934a,b). This conclusion was naive and was later shown to be a misinterpretation of results (Ray and Cole, 1985a,b), where they showed that alpha amplitudes depend on where mental attention is focused, that is, toward internal calculations or events (increased alpha) or toward external events and calculations based on external data (decreased alpha), not whether the eyes are opened or closed. It was presumably this confusion in the EEG literature that led some researchers (Goldstein *et al.*, 1972) and others to conclude that greater EEG amplitudes in the left hemisphere during REM sleep indicate that the right hemisphere is the site of REM sleep mentation. This conclusion of greater EEG amplitudes corresponding with diminished mental activity was also later based on the notion that mental activity was only possible during REM sleep and not NREM sleep, where REM sleep has much lower amplitudes compared to NREM sleep. Studies of the relationship of the EEG to the nasal cycle in awake subjects, along with the nasal cycle-cognitive studies, and studies of the nasal cycle in relation to REM and NREM sleep all suggest that the left brain is the primary site of REM sleep mentation and that the right brain is the site of NREM mentation. Part of the error in conclusion by some researchers (Gordon *et al.*, 1982; Lavie and Tzischinsky, 1984; Lavie *et al.*, 1984) results from the fact that awakenings may in fact trigger shifts in hemisphere dominance. This is in part supported by their studies where longer times did not lead to consistencies in cognitive performance links to sleep stages, and that only after immediate testing on awakening was a link found in the majority of subjects, while some, although fewer, subjects in fact showed the opposite results, which can be interpreted that they did not shift hemisphere dominance. Let us also recall a study on healthy subjects presented above where it was noted that "several minutes after the onset of REM sleep, an abrupt change in the pattern of respiration took place: respiration through the left nostril was completely blocked, while that through the right nostril displayed a hyperventilatory type with an amplitude about 3 times greater than that recorded during wakefulness, which continued to the end of REM sleep" (Alexiev and Roth, 1978). While this study did not use awakenings, it found abrupt changes in the nasal cycle could occur with abrupt changes in sleep stages. Clearly more studies are required to explore the possible shifts in the nasal cycle and cerebral rhythm during spontaneous and forced awakenings and in falling asleep. What we can definitely conclude here is that right- and left-hemisphere cognitive performance skill testing is differentially coupled to the awakenings from REM and NREM sleep.

### 3. *Ultradian Rhythm Studies of Alternating Cerebral Hemispheric Activity Exhibited by EEG During Waking*

The first study to demonstrate an ultradian rhythm of alternating cerebral hemispheric dominance using EEG during waking also showed that this CNS rhythm is tightly coupled to the ANS rhythm of the nasal cycle (Werntz *et al.*, 1980, 1983). Relative airflow through the nostrils was measured with two identically matched thermistors that were attached to a small clip that fits over the septum of the nose. Standard methods using 10–20 electrode placements were used for EEG. The raw EEG signal was rectified and integrated from 1 to 35 Hz in one hemisphere and compared to the overall integrated EEG activity of the other hemisphere. Both the airflow and EEG recordings were subjected to continuous subtraction and integration in time by an analogue integrator which produced a continuous output directly proportional to the difference in the amplitude between the left and right recordings. Naive subjects sat in a comfortable chair in a quiet private room and were instructed to remain motionless and to think of anything they wished excluding any specific mental exercises. The length of the recording period was determined by both the subject's ability to remain awake, but immobile, and by the time required to exhibit at least one transition in the nasal cycle. Figure 17 shows that there is a direct relationship of cerebral hemispheric EEG activity and the ultradian rhythm of the nasal cycle (Werntz *et al.*, 1983). Relatively greater integrated EEG activity in one hemisphere is positively correlated with predominant airflow in the contralateral nostril. Figure 17 displays the nasal dominance and EEG amplitude/power dominance relationships for three subjects. For subject GF, a right-handed male, three complete transitions in nostril airflow dominance occurred within the analysis period and it is clear that the total EEG pattern is tightly coupled to the cyclical pattern of the nasal cycle. Also, this figure shows that the alpha, theta, delta, and beta frequency bands all show the same general pattern and coupling to the nasal cycle that is consistent with the total EEG pattern. However, close examination also shows subtle differences among the various frequency bands. In addition, we also observed that the EEG from the occipital, parietal, and central regions all demonstrate a similar relationship to the nasal cycle, and this suggests that the observed correlation with the nasal cycle is unlikely due to only olfaction, since such activities would tend to be more restricted to areas around the olfactory cortex. It is also clear that changes in

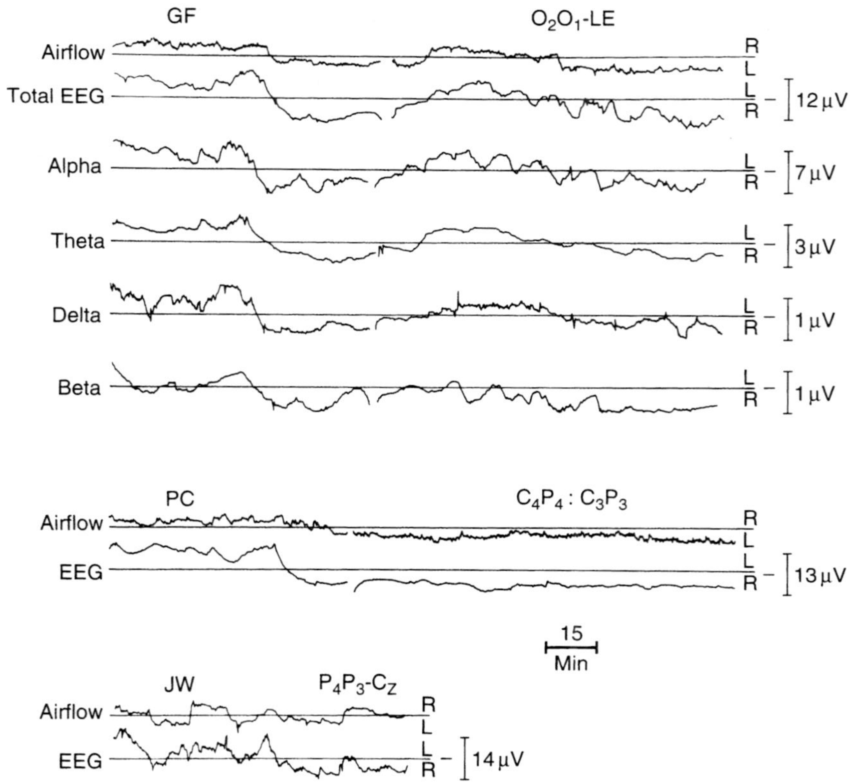


FIG. 17. Airflow tracings: Points above the baseline indicate greater right nostril airflow and points below indicate greater left nostril airflow. Total EEG is 1–35 Hz. Alpha (8–13 Hz), theta (4–8 Hz), delta (1–4 Hz), and beta (13–35 Hz) tracings were filtered through an analogue filter before integration. The baseline is drawn to visually enhance the similarity of the basic correlation of the two phenomena. The dash to the right of the EEG tracings indicates the true zero line where the right and left EEG amplitudes are equal. The bar and its numerical equivalent next to the integrated EEG tracings represent the actual calibrated amplitudes in microvolts. Reprinted from *Human Neurobiology*, 2, 1983, 39–43, Alternating cerebral hemispheric activity and the lateralization of autonomic nervous function, Werntz D. A., Bickford R. G., Bloom F. E., Shannahoff-Khalsa D. S., Figure 1. With Kind permission of Springer Science and Business Media.

cerebral dominance occasionally occur prior to changes in nostril dominance, which further argues for a centrally mediated (hypothalamus) regulator, and that the cerebral shifts are not only a result of olfactory activity. Figure 17 also shows two additional subjects, where subject PC exhibits comparatively a very long nasal cycle (>200 min) and the tightly coupled relationship to cerebral dominance remains. With subject JW, the cycle is very short, about 25 min, and the correlations of tight coupling are again obvious. Subject JW was also studied on another day and showed much longer cycling. These results showed that the correlation of EEG dominance and the nasal cycle is independent of the cycle length. This study also showed that the CNS–ANS linkage is independent of sex and handedness.

In total, 43 subjects were recorded for periods ranging from 40 to 215 min (mean 90 min), and once excessive muscle artifact was observed due to movement, the recordings were terminated. Of the 43 subjects, 22 exhibited nasal cycles during this relatively short interval, and 19 were analyzed in detail. Three of these 22 subjects had too much muscle artifact to obtain enough data for analysis. The remaining 21 subjects did not show shifts in their nasal cycle. All of the 19 subjects demonstrated the same relationship between the nasal cycle and EEG dominance, that is, when right nostril dominance occurs, there is relatively greater EEG amplitudes in the contralateral hemisphere, and when left nostril dominance occurs, there is relatively greater EEG amplitudes in the right hemisphere. No significant changes in EEG dominance occurred unless accompanied by a transition in nasal dominance and vice versa. Of the 19 subjects, 12 were right-handed males, 2 left-handed males, 2 left-handed females, and 3 right-handed females. Statistical analysis of coupling between the nasal cycle and pattern of cerebral dominance showed a median measure of correlation for all subjects of 85%, the mean was 83%, and the range was 67–100%, and the correlations of all individuals were significant at $p < 0.05$.

Of the 21 subjects with abbreviated recording sessions due to excessive muscle artifact or no transitions in nasal dominance, only 15 of these had artifact-free data to analyze. Of the 15, 10 individuals demonstrated a correlation of the dominant nostril with greater EEG amplitudes in the contralateral hemisphere. The remaining five exhibited an ipsilateral relationship in dominance. However, in these 15 subjects, essentially two straight lines were observed as tracings for both activities, including no transition in either the nostril or hemispheres. In general, the recordings are based on the relative changes in EEG amplitude measurement values and not on absolute values of hemispheric dominance. Therefore, subjects exhibiting an ipsilateral relationship in dominance do not present contradictions to the observed relationship. For example, subject JW (see Fig. 17) demonstrates a tight coupling of the phasic shift in patterns of activity for the nasal cycle and cerebral dominance, while maintaining the absolute values of EEG activity in the left hemisphere during the entire recording period. Note the small horizontal slash next to the microvolt measure on the right side of the figure for each EEG profile. This marker shows the actual or real midline for dominance, as opposed to the constructed or artificial midline in Fig. 17 for subject JW, indicating that dominance throughout the recording is showing greater activity in the left hemisphere. Again, the relative shifts of dominance and tightly coupled relationship here are the key to understanding this phenomenon.

This study was the first in a series of multivariate CNS–ANS physiology. In our paper (Werntz *et al.*, 1983), we interpreted these findings and postulated a range of relationships during waking and sleep. We stated the following:

> These experiments demonstrate a previously undescribed relationship between cerebral hemispheric activity and the nasal cycle. Since alternating stages of the ultradian sleep patterns have been closely correlated with the activities mediated by the ANS such as stomach contractions (Baust and Rohrwasser, 1969), neuroendocrine secretions, dreaming, locomotor activity and genital engorgement (Kripke, 1974), it is possible that cerebral hemispheric activity is also functionally coupled with autonomic nervous activity other than the nasal cycle. These rhythmic changes in physiology and dreaming have been the major components for the formulation of the BRAC (Kleitman, 1963, 1967d). Our work makes the point that an understanding of peripheral autonomic nervous function might reflect activity in the separate hemispheres. Since it is known that the majority of autonomic nerve fibers travel ipsilaterally (Eccles and Lee, 1981; Netter, 1972; Saper *et al.*, 1976) a sympathetic dominance in activity of the nasal mucosa on one side would correlate with a sympathetic dominance of activity in the vasculature of the hemisphere on the same side. Since cerebral circulation is known to be diminished during increased sympathetic activity (Gomez *et al.*, 1976), it is possible that breathing through one nostril would correlate with increased metabolic or mental activity in the

contralateral hemisphere. However, increased amplitudes have generally, but not exclusively (Dolce and Waldeier, 1974; Grabow *et al.*, 1979) been considered a reflection of mental inactivity (Rebert and Low, 1978). Therefore, future correlative studies of the nasal cycle in relation to spatial and verbal performance are required to resolve this question.

The predominant sympathetic activity on the right side of the body reflects a relative and concurrent predominance of EEG activity in the left hemisphere. Therefore, the nasal cycle becomes a clear indicator for the relative sympathetic-parasympathetic influences associated with the lateralization of activity. It follows that a unilateral dominance of sympathetic activity as exhibited by decongestion of one nostril and its concurrent enhancement of the contralateral cerebral hemispheric EEG amplitude could be viewed as a left-brain:right-body lateralization alternation. This relationship between the peripheral autonomic and lateralized cerebral activites would correlate with the BRAC hypothesis (Broughton, 1975; Jouvet, 1973; Kleitman, 1963, 1967d). Greater relative EEG amplitudes in the left hemisphere correlated with REM sleep which is considered to be the "active" phase during the cycle (Goldstein *et al.*, 1972). Right-brain: left body dominance would therefore be expected to correlate with NREM sleep, or the "rest" phase of the BRAC since it is known that NREM sleep correlates with relatively greater EEG amplitudes in the right hemisphere (Goldstein *et al.*, 1972).

Since the left-brain:right body/right-brain:left body alternation is presumably regulated directly by competing sympathetic-parasympathetic influences it is possible that the hypothalamus is the center for integration and regulation of this phenomenon. Therefore, the hypothalamus may play a very important role in the regulation of mental processes and behavior.

Others also attempted to identify an ultradian interhemispheric shift in EEG dominance (Manseau and Broughton, 1983). Instead of using a continuous measurement of the EEG as used in the Werntz *et al.* study (1983), they took 100-sec samples every 15 min during an 8-h recording and used cross-spectral analysis. Seven subjects visually fixated on a dot in front of them during the 100-sec sampling period. The results indicate the presence of a significant 72- to 120-min ultradian EEG fluctuation in the frontal cortex mainly in the 4–20 Hz range and the changes were in phase between the two hemispheres. They conclude "it remains possible that the phenomenon exists but that the technique used was insufficiently sensitive to document it." The dot focusing, which may equalize hemispheres, and the lack of continuous measurements may diminish the chances of finding subtle EEG asymmetries. One other study also found ultradian rhythms of EEG activity during waking in the range of 80–120 min, however, these EEG measures were studied during extended task performance and not during a resting state (Armitage, 1986). The results are stated "Females showed 80 min cycles in absolute difference measures of Beta and Sigma power during task performance. Males showed ultradian variations in relative ratios of Delta power."

Another study showed a broad variety of ultradian periods among EEG electrode placements and frequency bands that varied from a 6-h morning session to a 6-h afternoon session (Ortega and Cabrera, 1990). In this study, 1 min of EEG activity was sampled every 15 min from six female subjects and subjected to time series analysis. The authors also instructed the subjects to look at a spot in front of them. After 1 min of EEG sampling the subjects were tested on two cognitive tasks to probe possible rhythms of alternating cognitive efficiency using verbal and spatial tasks. Seven minutes were used for cognitive testing. The cognitive results exhibited wide fluctuations throughout both sessions but yielded no significant peaks when the data of all subjects were combined. However, concerning the EEG records they remarked "All parameters evaluated showed important ultradian variations. There were broad inter- and intra-individual differences in the period of oscillation from morning to afternoon sessions, from one cortical area to another and from one band to another. Despite this variability, when the group was considered as a whole, some peaks reached the significance level." The negative group finding for cognitive rhythms may have been the result of masking due to the wide inter- and intraindividual variability. However Ortega and Cabrera found significant EEG peaks in relative power at 60 min, 90 min, 2 h, 3 h, 6 h, and for interhemispheric correlation at 30 min, 72 min, and 90 min and 3 h and 6 h. They reported the 3-h period to be the most prominent:

> The interhemispheric correlations showed significant peaks that were more consistent than those for relative power since they appeared in the morning as well as in the afternoon sessions for three and six hour periods

> supporting the idea of ultradian fluctuations in the level of functional relationship between both hemispheres although not at the same frequency as the REM-NREM sleep alternation.

It must be noted here that they assume the REM–NREM period is fixed at 90 min when actually this is only an approximate average of the various different periods over the night. This has always been a confusing point in the analysis of ultradian studies comparing inter- and intranight variations with inter- and intraday variations. These findings of interhemispheric correlations are indicative of periods of similarity between the two hemispheres. This may be another way of looking at the phenomenon of alternating cerebral hemispheric dominance, that is, when the hemispheres are dissimilar in their relative contributions. They do not report left minus right differences, and, in addition, their subjects are occupied performing cognitive tasks for 7 min of the 15-min periods. However, the observed periods of coherence are similar to the observed periods of alternating dominance observed by Werntz *et al.* (1983).

4. *Ultradian Rhythm Studies of Alternating Hemispheric Activity Exhibited by Cognitive Performance Efficiency*

The first report directly supporting the existence in humans of alternating cerebral hemispheric activity during the waking state was a seminal study (Klein and Armitage, 1979). They found significant peaks at 37 min, 96 min, and 4 h. They tested eight subjects (five females and three males, all right-handed) with a verbal and a spatial task every 15 min for 8 h. The best performances on one task occurred during the minimum performances on the other. They concluded that "This finding is consistent with the hypothesis that in humans the BRAC is characterized by oscillations in the relative activation or efficiency of the two cerebral hemispheres, which are specialized for the performance of verbal and spatial tasks."

In a diurnal study of memory, one researcher found evidence supporting cerebral rhythms using two separate memory tasks (Folkard, 1979) and found that the acoustic similarity effect on short-term memory was greater at 10:00 a.m. than at 7:00 p.m. and that the semantic similarity effect on long-term memory was greater at 7:30 p.m. than at 10:30 a.m. He thought "the time-of-day effects in performance reflected a shift in the degree of cerebral dominance during the day, such that the dominant left hemisphere becomes rather less so during the evening." He concluded after looking at only two time points "It is, however, unclear as to what adaptive function such a circadian rhythm might serve, although it has been suggested that an ultradian (approx. 90 min) rhythm exists with such dominance."

We also assessed cognitive performance during different phases of the nasal cycle (Klein *et al.*, 1986). We observed significant relationships between the pattern of nasal airflow and spatial and verbal performance. Right nostril dominance correlated with enhanced verbal performance, or left brain activity, and left nostril dominance correlated with enhanced spatial performance, again indicating that the hemispheres alternate in phase with the nasal cycle.

Researchers in France demonstrated that subjects who undergo a test of immediate memory every 25 min with two modalities (semantic and graphic) present a fluctuation in performance with a periodicity of about 100 min (Leconte and Lambert, 1988). The two modalities were in opposite phase.

Two researchers who contributed to the cognitive testing performance studies on awakening from REM and NREM sleep also tested 12 right-handed male subjects on three separate tests: verbal fluency (word production test), spatial localization, and symbol digit modalities (thought to require both verbal and spatial skills) (Gordon and Stoffer, 1989). The word production test produced two peaks in performance, a major one at 68 min and a minor one at 120 min. The localization test had one peak at 96 min with two other nonsignificant peaks. The symbol digit test had two significant peaks, one that coincided with the 120 min period of the word production test and a second at 48 min which is half the 96 min period of the spatial test. As in many ultradian studies, they reported "that individuals had cycles with peaks at different frequencies, some subjects had no reliable peaks." They concluded that "It is not clear, therefore, what the true phase relationship was, if any, of the two tasks"

(Gordon and Stoffer, 1989). However, they also stated that their results are consistent with those of Klein and Armitage (1979) in which "90-min" shifts in performance were found.

The use of dichotic listening (DL) performance was employed to assess the existence of alternating cerebral hemispheric activity in six males and six females (Meier-Koll, 1989b). He found very distinct and convincing periodicities of 3–4 h in 10 subjects. "Such periodicities were obvious in both right and left ear DL performance and oscillated in counter phase. This suggests that competitive processing of dichotic verbal stimuli mediated by the cerebral hemispheres could be modulated by an endogenous oscillatory system." This same researcher studied a severely mentally handicapped woman by recording the stereotyped hand waving activity in both hands separately using consecutive time-sample intervals of 5 min and he studied her over 10 consecutive days and nights (Meier-Koll, 1989a). "Right and left-handed stereotyped activities were found to be modulated periodically with intervals of about two hours. During the morning and the early afternoon periodicities of both right and left-hand activities occurred predominantly in bilateral synchrony. By contrast, rhythmic variations of both activities developed a counter-phase course during the late afternoon and evening." He concludes that the lateralized hand waving reflects motor arousal levels of the contralateral hemisphere and suggests that independent oscillators are responsible for the alternating pattern. In an earlier paper he reports the results of several days of observation of six severely mentally handicapped children that demonstrated a 2.5-h rhythm in stereotyped behaviors (Meier-Koll and Pohl, 1979). They found that hand (waving and finger movements) and oral (repetitive licking and vocalizations) stereotypes were synchronous and head and whole-body (including autoregressive head banging) stereotypes were 180° out of phase with the hand movements. They viewed these behaviors as primitive expressions of Kleitman's BRAC.

Others studied two populations, a group of right-handed males between 18 and 27 years old who were habitual hashish smokers and a control group of 24 right-handed males of similar age who had never used drugs (Leon-Carrion and Vela-Bueno, 1991). The subjects were administered right- and left-hemisphere-related tests every 15 min for 8 h. For the nonsmokers, the right-hemisphere test yielded the greatest spectral power between 85 and 100 min with a maximum peak at 90 min. For the left hemisphere, the maximum spectral power was between 95 to 120 min, with the peak at 110 min. For the drug users, the right-hemisphere-related task showed a maximum range between 90 and 120 min, with the peak at 90 min. On the left-hemisphere-related task, the distribution was the same as the control group, except that the distribution was not as steep and peaked at 105 min. For the control group the hemisphere relations are 193.62° out of phase for the two tests and for the hashish users it was 226.75° out of phase. These findings again support the alternating levels of activation for the two hemispheres and demonstrate how the rhythm can also be disrupted using intoxicants.

Two researchers studied the endogenous rhythm of processing speed (encoding and recognition) of stimuli presented to the left and right brain hemisphere for 30 subjects during a 24-h constant-routine experiment. However, the memory performance task was only measured eight times, starting at 06:30 h. "Parallel sets of words and pictures were shown to subjects in a random order in either the left or the right visual field on a computer screen. The participants pressed one of two buttons in response to the picture or word, or when answering a question concerning the meaning of a presented stimulus" (Iskra-Golec and Smith, 2006). "Two significant ultradian components were found in a majority of the time series. The results showed an asymmetry between both hemispheres in the frequency of ultradian rhythms in encoding speed" (Iskra-Golec and Smith, 2006).

The spiral aftereffect (SAE) is a visual illusion of a rotating disk that once stopped appears to continue rotating. When subjects are tested over hours, there is a rhythmic variation for the length of time the disk appears to take to stop moving. Its periodicity ranges from 33 to 200 min/cycle with about half of the spectral power in the 100 min range (Lavie *et al.*, 1975). Others studied the SAE using regional cerebral blood flow and found that this phenomenon is correlated primarily with an increase in right cerebral blood flow (Risberg and Prohovnik, 1983). This suggests that the SAE illusion periodicity may reflect relative levels of right cerebral activation. In addition to the SAE as a perceptual illusion, there is also the phenomenon called the "beta movement" described by Max Wertheimer in his 1912 "Experimental Studies on the Seeing of Motion," whereby two or more still images are combined by the brain into surmised motion. The classic beta phenomenon experiment involves a viewer watching a screen where two images are projected in succession. The first image could be a ball on the left side of the screen and the second could be a ball on the right side where the images may be shown quickly, in rapid succession, or with a short delay of several seconds. Once both images have been projected, a viewer will claim that they saw a ball move from left to right, thus the illusion. In one study "14 young adults were tested on the SAE every five min and on the beta movement (another perceptual illusion) every 20 min for eight continuous hrs. Time series analysis revealed significant 100-min rhythms in the perception of the two illusions, which also appeared to be synchronized across the experimental periods" (Lavie, 1976). In another study of the beta-movement, 10 young adults that were awakened from REM sleep and from NREM sleep on two nonconsecutive nights and were tested to determine their upper and lower beta-movement thresholds (Lavie and Sutter, 1975). They stated that:

> The ranges of the illusion were found to be significantly wider after waking from REM sleep than after waking from NREM sleep or before sleep. The differential responding to the beta movement supports the experimental hypothesis that apparent motion may provide sensitive detectors of the operation during wakefulness of the Basic Rest-Activity Cycle, of which REM and NREM sleep are opposite phases that carry over into wakefulness.

Another group found similar spectral peaks for two behavioral tasks in seven adult males (Bossom *et al.*, 1983). Their study consisted of 15 min epochs over 6 h. With a visual-motor coordination and attention task they found a major spectral peak at 86 min (range 68–107 min) and with a short-term memory nonverbal recall task a major peak at 88 min (range 50–107 min). They did not suggest that the two tasks are lateralized to contralateral hemispheres, but that the results are supportive of the BRAC hypothesis.

Hypothalamic releasing factors and pituitary hormones exhibit ultradian rhythms in the same frequency range as the REM–NREM cycle and the cognitive rhythms. Interestingly, it has been shown in men (but not women) that injections of LH releasing hormone prevented improvement in a spatial orientation task (right-hemisphere skill), but enhanced performance on a fluency task (left-hemisphere skill) (Gordon *et al.*, 1986). The resulting increase in LH and correlated enhancement of left-hemispheric skills is consistent with elevated LH during REM sleep, also a correlate of an activated left hemisphere [reviewed in Shannahoff-Khalsa (1991a)].

### C. Ultradian Rhythms of the Cardiovascular, Neuroendocrine, Fuel-Regulatory, Gastrointestinal, and Immune Systems

The cardiovascular, neuroendocrine, and fuel-regulatory (INS and glucose) systems are characterized by multiple periodic or pseudoperiodic (nonlinear) processes, and a major one is the "hourly" ultradian rhythm (Shannahoff-Khalsa *et al.*, 1996, 1997). The immune (Bouayad-Amine *et al.*, 1993) and gastrointestinal systems (Wada, 1922) also exhibit the same "hourly" ultradian rhythms. These "90 min to 120 min" rhythms were found in gastric contractility for humans examined under isolated fasting conditions that help supplement our understanding of the behavioral observations of "oral" drives (Hiatt and Kripke, 1975). "A clear ultradian rhythm was observed, indicating inherent physiologic oscillation in stomach contractions" (Hiatt and Kripke, 1975).

A more recent paper also makes the important point that the activity of the upper gastrointestinal tract is rhythmic (Zabielski, 2004). Zabielski states, "It concerns the gastrointestinal and gallbladder motility, gastrointestinal blood flow, gastric, intestinal, pancreatic and biliary secretions, rate of nutrient absorption, and many other physiological events. Nowadays, the periodic activity of the gastrointestinal tract is considered as a basic physiological pattern in conscious animals and humans." Zabielski recognizes one of the problems that have troubled ultradian chronobiologists for decades and that have led to confusion in the field. "Unfortunately, there are considerable species- and age-related as well as individual differences," and that "A lot of confusion may appear with data interpretation if the periodic activity is neglected" (Zabielski, 2004). Others have reviewed the ultradian and circadian rhythms of gastrointestinal motor and secretory function on the action of orally administered drugs (Sanders and Moore, 1992).

While the circadian (~24 h) rhythm is also common to these five systems, the causal and temporal ultradian relationships within these systems have been questions of long-standing interest and were the focus of a multivariate physiological study (Shannahoff-Khalsa *et al.*, 1996, 1997).

Kleitman first proposed the BRAC hypothesis (Kleitman, 1961) to account for ultradian rhythms in behavior and physiology, and he called them "90 min rhythms" and proposed that they were correlates of the REM and NREM sleep cycles (Kleitman, 1967d, 1982). However, proof of the existence of the BRAC as an integrated multisystem phenomenon had been complicated by the differences in observed periods within and across systems and species and the lack of multivariate studies. The question had not yet been resolved for whether a single oscillator or a multioscillator system controlled the BRAC (Lavie and Kripke, 1981).

An "hourly" variation has long been described in the neuroendocrine system as being "episodic" or "pulsatile", and exhibits as a burst of hormone release. This hourly "rhythm" has been labeled both as the "low-frequency" (Veldhuis *et al.*, 1984) and as the "high-frequency" (Van Cauter, 1990) high-amplitude period in contrast to the "high-frequency" (Veldhuis *et al.*, 1984) or "ultrafast" (Van Cauter, 1990) low-amplitude oscillations that range from 5 to 15 min. One study showed spectra for prolactin in men with periods of 30–32, 51–59, 90–98, and 234 min and cross-spectral analysis demonstrated significantly correlated prolactin and LH cycles with periodicities of 33–37, 47–52, and 84–106 min (Veldhuis and Johnson, 1988).

Although a great deal of progress has been made in the study of the neuroendocrine rhythms, the comparison of results have been complicated because experiments differ in species, sex, age, health status, site of sampling, sampling rates, methods of assay and time history analysis, and experimental conditions. These varied protocols have led to different results for the same hormone. This is the same problem that has been recognized for the gastrointestinal system (Zabielski, 2004). Van Cauter's review of human endocrine function avoided a detailed discussion of pulsatile secretion, but she states that it "generally recurs at intervals in the range of hours" (Van Cauter, 1990). Studies of the autonomic and cardiovascular systems have similar complications. However, the number of hourly rhythm studies in the neuroendocrine system far exceeds those for the autonomic and cardiovascular systems.

The cardiovascular system is also modulated by hourly ultradian rhythms. Heart rate has been reported to have an ultradian periodicity of approximately 90 min in bed-resting normal human males (Orr and Hoffman, 1974), and 1–2 h in unrestrained dogs in a closed environment (Livnat *et al.*, 1984). A period of about 160 min was found in one experiment for mean arterial pressure in unrestrained dogs in a closed environment (Blinowska and Marsh, 1985) and at 90 min in another (Shimada and Marsh, 1979). The ultradian rhythms of mean arterial pressure are also coupled to heart rate (Blinowska and Marsh, 1985; Livnat *et al.*, 1984; Shimada and Marsh, 1979). Some researchers conclude that the SNS drives the ultradian rhythms of the heart (Broten and Zehr, 1989; Shimada and Marsh, 1979).

Also, a study in humans relating REM sleep to systolic blood pressure showed that pressure changes correlate with the cyclical changes of REM EEG patterns, where pressure increases with REM sleep (Snyder *et al.*, 1963). It therefore appears that laterality of ANS function and rhythms of cardiac function are related in a manner consistent with the relationship found in other organs. Since REM sleep seems to be the sleeping analogue of left-hemisphere dominance, we might expect to find that right nostril activity is associated with increased heart rate and blood pressure.

And again, in addition to the neuroendocrine rhythms, ultradians in humans have also been observed in plasma catecholamines (Levin *et al.*, 1979), with a median period of 107 min and a range of 75–188 min, and in monkeys at 90 min (Levin *et al.*, 1978). These researchers concluded that "The observation that plasma norepinephrine has a 90-min ultradian rhythm suggests that it, like several hormones, is subject to some centrally mediated modulator of a BRAC." And we know that norepinephrine is a reliable marker of sympathetic activity, so intuitively, we know there must be a strong coupling with ultradian rhythms of heart rate and neuroendocrine activity.

The similarities in ultradian rhythmicity in the autonomic, cardiovascular, neuroendocrine, and fuel-regulatory systems and their likely common oscillator, the hypothalamus, prompted us to do a multisystem study to investigate these relationships in humans under well-controlled conditions (Shannahoff-Khalsa *et al.*, 1996, 1997). To my knowledge, only one other similar multivariate chronobiological study has been conducted and they studied visceral and behavioral processes measuring blood glucose, growth hormone, cortisol, epinephrine, norepinephrine, mean arterial pressure, heart rate, and testing for hand-eye coordination and recall (Bossom *et al.*, 1983). They concluded that "relations between visceral and behavioral data were not striking" and "that relatively poor relations were found between short-term fluctuations in human performance and human visceral function."

Our multivariate study in 10 healthy humans (8 males, 2 females), ages from 20 to 42 years (mean 31.9 years), included measures of the NC at 4 Hz, 6 cardiac impedance measures averaged over every 12 successive beats [cardiac output (CO), thoracic fluid index (TFI), heart rate (HR), ejection velocity index (EVI), stroke volume (SV), and ventricular ejection time (VET)], blood pressures [systolic blood pressure (SBP), diastolic blood pressure (DBP), mean arterial pressure (MAP)] using an automated ambulatory cuff every 7.5 min, along with six factors from peripheral blood: two pituitary hormones (LH and ACTH), INS, and three catecholamines [norepinephrine (NE), epinephrine (E), dopamine (D)] sampled simultaneously from both arms under strict resting conditions every 7.5 min. All subjects were within normal weight ranges, were nonsmokers, and had only light meals on the morning of the study and abstained from caffeine for 12 h prior to the study. All subjects had experience in donating blood. The subjects relaxed in an adjustable recliner chair with their legs elevated and supported about 6 in. below head level. Both arms remained immobile. No distractions (radio, reading, unnecessary conversation) were allowed. Indwelling intravenous catheters were used in each arm in near identical veins, and all sampling was done simultaneously from both arms. Recordings lasted 5–6 h, and a typical 5-h record of the NC had 72,000 measurements and these measures were converted to means at every 7.5 min using 1800 measurements. The averaging mode for the impedance cardiodynamic monitor was used which gave approximately 1500–1800 measurements per 5-h record for CO, TFI, HR, EVI, SV, and VET and means were calculated for each 7.5 min interval for later comparison with the NC and the blood samples and blood pressure readings that were from single measurements at 7.5 min intervals.

The FOS method (Korenberg, 1988, 1989; Korenberg and Paarmann, 1989a,b) was applied to the time series data. FOS can model time series data as a series of sine features, which unlike the standard Fourier series, is not necessarily harmonic (commensurate frequencies). FOS selects features in the decreasing order of their ability to account for fractions of total variance and the number of features selected is based on a selection criterion consisting of a preset number, or a cutoff error reduction level. The FOS algorithm represents a time history as a linear combination of sine waves and searches a time history by using a list of a priori, candidate periods. In this study we nominated 77 candidate periods ranging from 6 to 720 min. A mean square error reduction (MSER) is calculated for each candidate period and the period that produces the largest error reduction is removed from the time history. The process of selecting and removing periods is repeated until a chosen number of periods

(10 chosen) is identified or further percent error reduction (MSER/total error × 100) is less than a preselected percentage (2% chosen) of the initial total error. Only periods of 40 min or greater were included in the analysis. This choice allowed for a minimum of five time points to define a single period, a conservative value, given the Nyquist theorem which requires at least two time points to define a cycle in the absence of noise. Periods longer than the experimental epochs (300–360 min) are extrapolated by FOS. Periods 10% greater than the recording period were detrended by adding a sine wave with equal period and amplitude but at 180° difference in phase. This detrending eliminated any circadian components from the record, and thus maximized the ultradian features.

The data set for each subject includes measures for the following 21 variables: NC, LH, ACTH, SBP, DBP, MAP, total peripheral resistance (TPR), left epinephrine (LE), left norepinephrine (LNE), right epinephrine (RE), right norepinephrine (RNE), mean of left and right epinephrine values (ME), mean of left and right norepinephrine values (MNE), left/right epinephrines (LRE), left/right norepinephrines (LRNE), CO, TFI, HR, EVI, SV, and VET. The dopamine values were frequently indistinguishable from background values and are not reported here. The left and right values of the catecholamines were analyzed independently since our past studies show that major rhythmic differences can exist on the two sides during rest in normal humans (Kennedy *et al.*, 1986). The left/right ratio for NE was also observed to parallel the NC (Kennedy *et al.*, 1986). Thus, these left/right NE and E ratios are another measure of lateralized autonomic activity. The means of the left and right catecholamines are also included since they give other important information for describing the general autonomic state.

Using the same method used for the sleep studies (see Figs. 9, 12, and 13) (Shannahoff-Khalsa and Yates, 2000; Shannahoff-Khalsa *et al.*, 2001), the dominant periods were determined by lumping the spectral power from all 21 variables as %TMSE for all 10 subjects (Fig. 18), and the mean power for the individual peaks was also plotted (Fig. 19). Visual identification suggests five prominent ranges for consideration: 40–65, 70–100, 115–145, 170–215, and

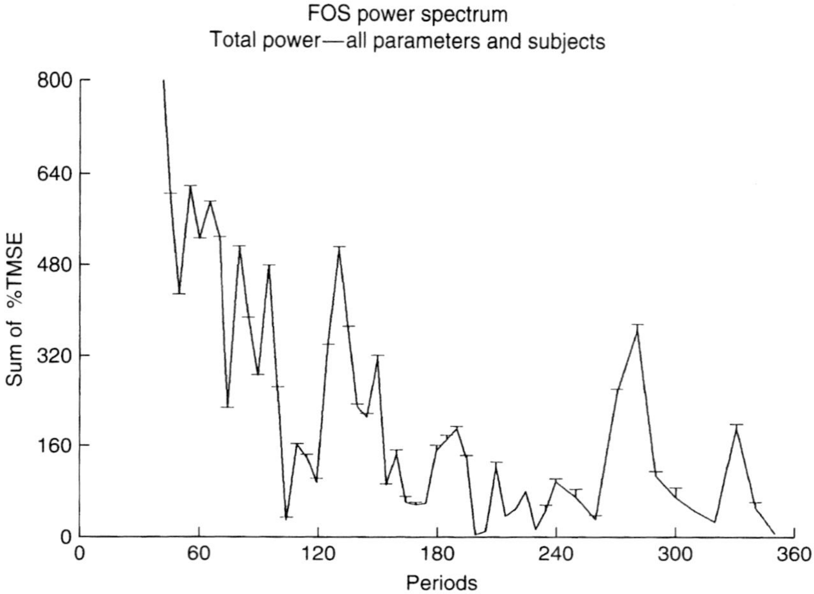


FIG. 18. This spectral density plot shows the FOS time history analysis power distribution, or %TMSE, independent of subject and parameter. This spectral plot is additive for %TMSE at each time period and combines 10 subjects and 21 parameters per subject, except subject 3 with only 14 parameters (impedance measures were lost). Therefore, 203 power spectrums are summed to produce one profile. The horizontal hatch marks represent one-sided standard deviation bars at each time point. Reprinted from Shannahoff-Khalsa, Kennedy, Yates, and Ziegler; copyright (1996), with permission from American Physiological Society.

220–340 min. These are the same ranges consistently reported by others for many of these variables.

### 1. *Interindividual FOS Analysis*

The composite spectral plots of the FOS analysis for all 10 subjects are shown in Fig. 20 for the NC, LH, ACTH, TPR, CO, TFI, HR, EVI, SV, and VET (subject MR's cardiac impedance parameters are not included due to a computer failure during the experiment). The FOS spectral plots for all subjects are shown in Fig. 21 for the catecholamine parameters LE, LNE, RE, RNE, ME, MNE, LRE, and LRNE. The plasma catecholamine levels fluctuate more rapidly than LH and ACTH. The catecholamine assays also

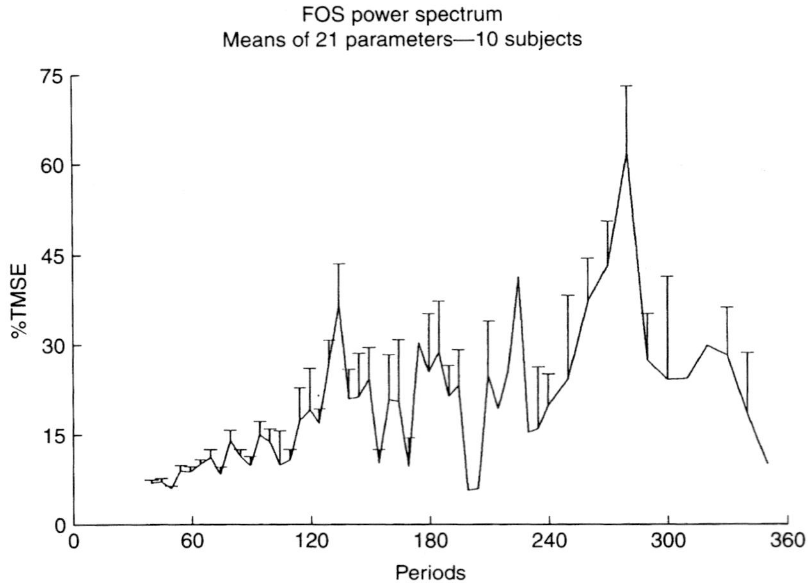


FIG. 19. This spectral density plot shows the FOS time history analysis power distribution as a mean %TMSE for all parameters at any given time period, independent of subject and parameter. This spectral plot combines 10 subjects and 21 parameters per subject, except subject 3 with only 14 parameters (impedance measures are lost). Therefore, 203 power spectrums are consolidated to produce one profile. The horizontal hatch marks represent one-sided standard deviation bars at each time point. Reprinted from Shannahoff-Khalsa, Kennedy, Yates, and Ziegler; copyright (1996), with permission from American Physiological Society.

have more intra- and interassay variance compared to the assays for LH and ACTH. Figure 22 groups the spectral plots for SBP, DBP, MAP, and TPR.

Table V gives the prevalence of a significant peak for the 30-min period range from 115–145 min, the 30-min period range of 70–100 min, and the 25-min period range of 40–65 min for the parameters in Fig. 19 (NC, LH, ACTH, TPR, CO, TFI, HR, EVI, SV, and VET). The broad 120-min period range of 220–340 min had significance for the NC at 10% TMSE in 6 of 10 subjects, $p \leq 0.01$. LH also had significance for the range of 220–340 min at 10% TMSE in 5 of 10 subjects, $p \leq 0.05$. The 45-min period range from 170 to 215 min only had significance for ACTH at 10%

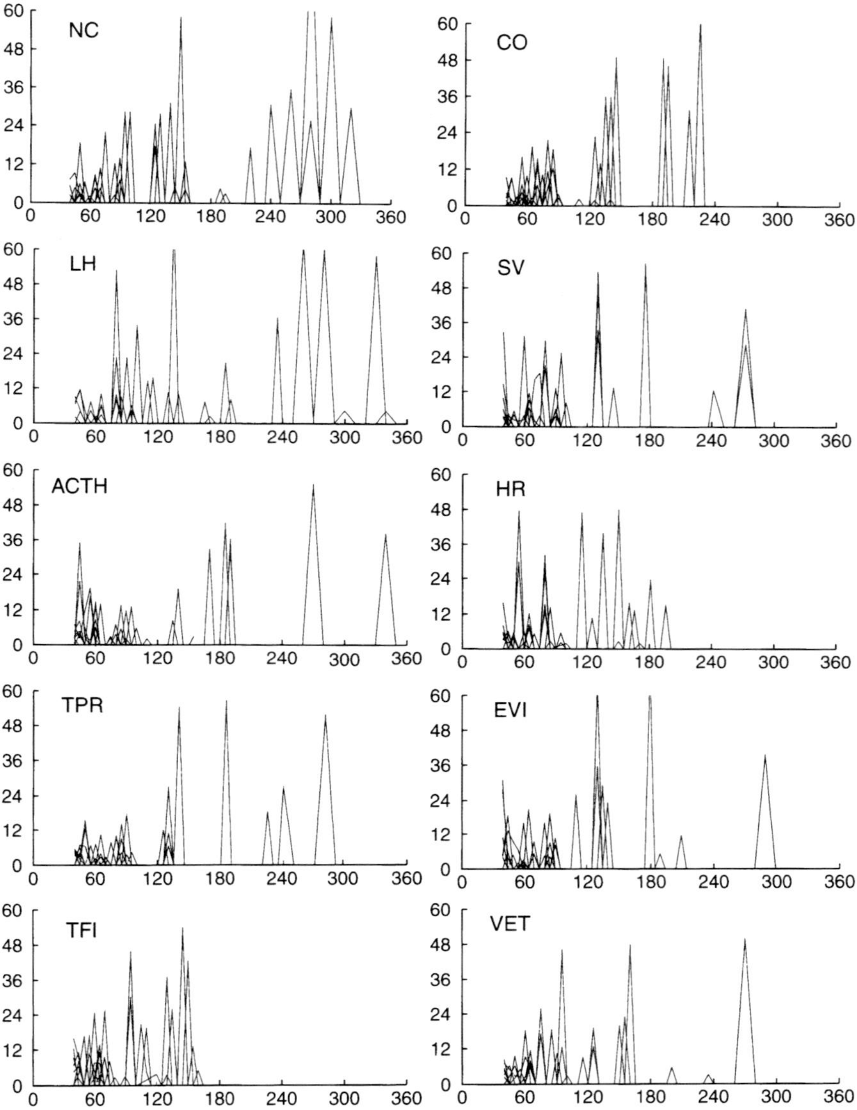


FIG. 20. Spectral density plots of 10 subjects from FOS time history analysis of the nasal cycle (NC), luteinizing hormone (LH), adrenocorticotropin hormone (ACTH), total peripheral resistance (TPR), thoracic fluid index (TFI), cardiac output (CO), stroke volume (SV), heart rate (HR), ejection velocity index (EVI), and ventricular ejection time (VET). The *x*-axis is 0–360 min with data of 0–40 min not included. The *y*-axis is in 0–60% TMSE. Plots of CO, TPR, SV, HR, VET, EVI, and TFI are from nine subjects, subject MR's impedance data were lost. Reprinted from Shannahoff-Khalsa, Kennedy, Yates, and Ziegler; copyright (1996), with permission from American Physiological Society.

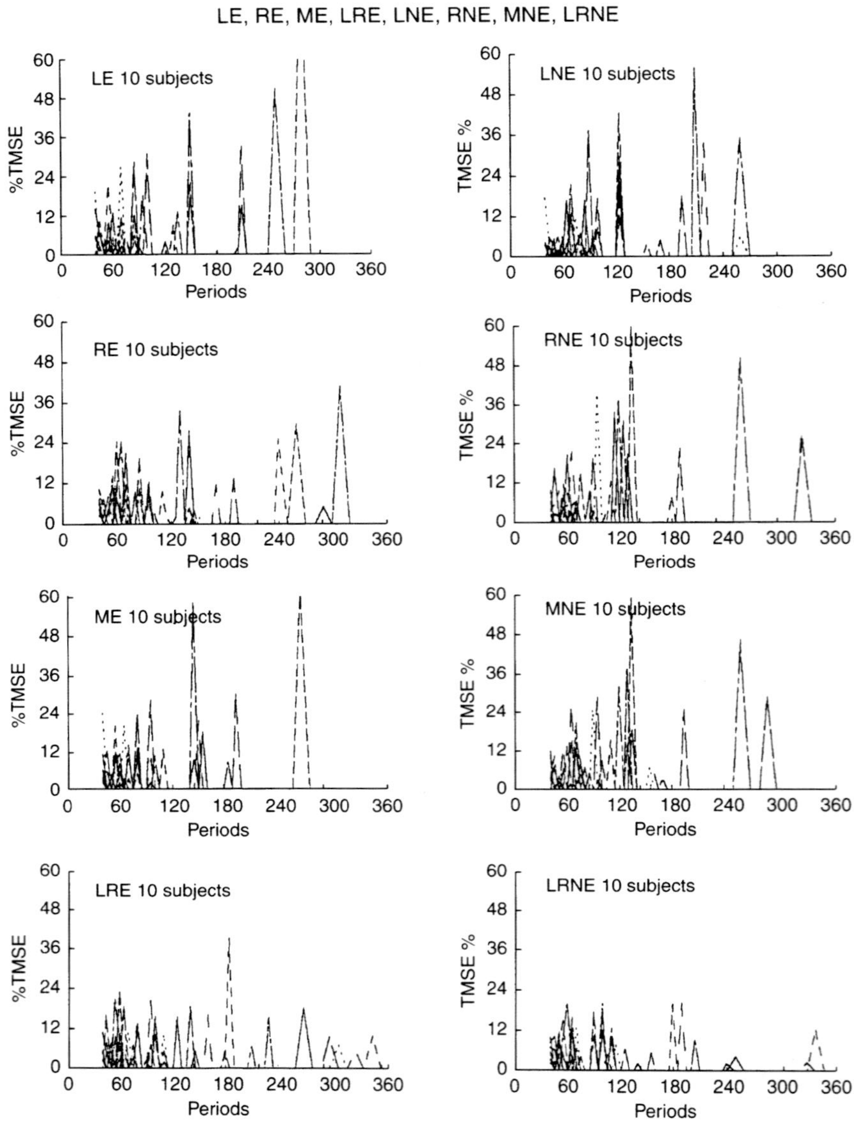


FIG. 21. Spectral density plots of 10 subjects from FOS time history analysis of the left arm epinephrine (LE), right arm epinephrine (RE), mean of left + right arm epinephrine (ME), left/right arm epinephrine (LRE), left arm norepinephrine (LNE), right arm norepinephrine (RNE), mean of left + right arm norepinephrine (MNE), left/right arm norepinephrine (LRNE). The $x$-axis is 0–360 min with data of 0–40 min not included. The $y$-axis is in 0–60% TMSE. Reprinted from Shannahoff-Khalsa, Kennedy, Yates, and Ziegler; copyright (1996), with permission from American Physiological Society.

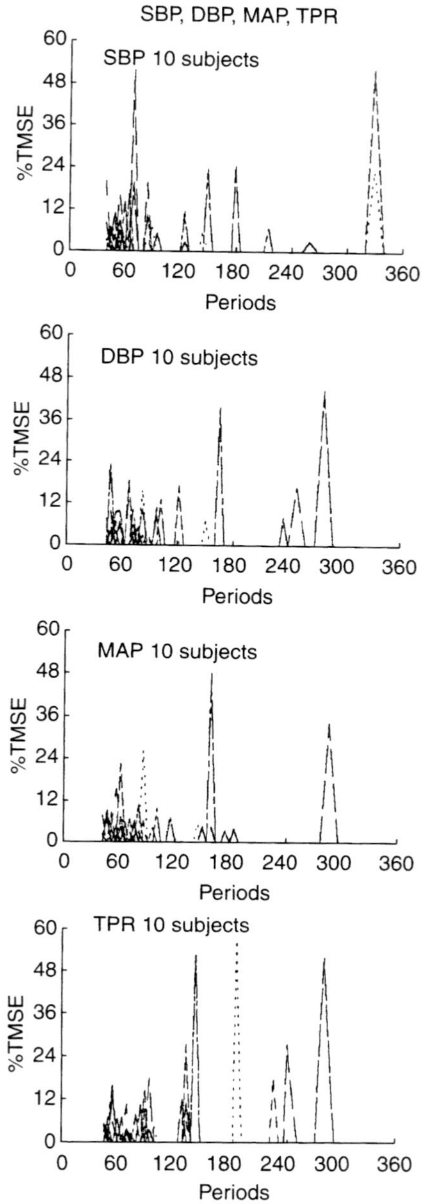


FIG. 22. Spectral density plots of 10 subjects from FOS time history analysis of systolic blood pressure (SBP), diastolic blood pressure (DBP), mean arterial pressure (MAP), and total peripheral resistance (TPR). The $x$-axis is 0–360 min with data of 0–40 min not included. The $y$-axis is in 0–60% TMSE. Reprinted from Shannahoff-Khalsa, Kennedy, Yates, and Ziegler; copyright (1996), with permission from American Physiological Society.

TABLE V
PREVALENCE OF THE MAJOR PERIODS FOR 10 SUBJECTS FOR THE NASAL CYCLE, PITUITARY HORMONES, AND CARDIAC IMPEDANCE PARAMETERS[a,+]

| | NC | LH | ACTH | TPR | CO | TFI | HR | EVI | SV | VET |
|---|---|---|---|---|---|---|---|---|---|---|
| | | | | | 115–145 min period | | | | | |
| 7% | 4* | 5* | 2 | 4* | 5* | 3# | 3# | 4* | 4* | 3# |
| 10% | 4* | 4* | 1 | 4* | 5* | 3# | 3# | 4* | 4* | 2 |
| Mean | 10.6 | 12.4 | 2.8 | 12.6 | 18.1 | 14.2 | 11.1 | 17.0 | 14.9 | 4.6 |
| | | | | | 70–100 min period | | | | | |
| 7% | 6* | 7* | 4* | 6* | 8* | 5* | 6* | 5* | 5* | 7* |
| 10% | 5* | 3# | 3# | 3# | 7* | 4* | 6* | 3# | 5* | 7* |
| Mean | 11.9 | 14.9 | 6.9 | 9.2 | 12.3 | 14.0 | 15.7 | 8.8 | 14.0 | 17.0 |
| | | | | | 40–65 min period | | | | | |
| 7% | 4* | 4* | 7* | 6* | 5* | 8* | 7* | 6* | 6* | 7* |
| 10% | 2 | 2 | 6* | 3# | 3# | 6* | 4* | 6* | 4* | 3# |
| Mean | 6.6 | 6.2 | 12.1 | 7.9 | 8.2 | 12.9 | 15.6 | 15.1 | 13.9 | 9.9 |

[a]7% and 10% are cutoff levels for %TMSE; the number tells how many subjects have peaks at that level, and the "Mean" = the mean for TMSE (maximums) calculated for all 10 (or 9) subjects. Asterisk (*) indicates $p \leq 0.01$, #$p \leq 0.05$; [+]the maximum possible is 10 for the NC, LH, and ACTH, and 9 for others, since subject MR's impedance is missing. Reprinted from Shannahoff-Khalsa, Kennedy, Yates, and Ziegler; copyright (1996), with permission from American Physiological Society.

TMSE in 4 of 10 subjects, $p \leq 0.05$. Table VI gives the peak prevalence for the eight catecholamine parameters (LE, LNE, RE, RNE, ME, MNE, LRE, and LRNE). The 220–340 min and 170–215 min period ranges did not show significance for any catecholamine parameter. Table VII gives the peak prevalence for the four blood pressure-related parameters (SBP, DBP, MAP, and TPR). Chi-square analyses were used to determine if the frequency of occurrence of different peaks was significant across subjects for each parameter. The 220–340 min and 170–215 min period ranges did not show statistical significance for blood pressures. However, our sleep study capturing beat-to-beat blood pressure measures detected periods at 280–300, 215–275, 165–210, 145–160, 105–140, 70–100, and 40–65 min bins with the greatest spectral power in longer periods (Shannahoff-Khalsa and Yates, 2000). The absence during the waking study of significant power in the lower frequency bands (220–340 and 170–215 min) for blood pressures may be due to the single sampling rate of one measure per 7.5-min interval instead of the beat-to-beat sampling rate. Ultradian blood pressure

TABLE VI
PREVALENCE OF THE MAJOR PERIODS FOR 10 SUBJECTS FOR THE CATECHOLAMINE PARAMETERS[a,+]

| | LE | LNE | RE | RNE | ME | MNE | LRE | LRNE |
|---|---|---|---|---|---|---|---|---|
| | | | | 115–145 min period | | | | |
| 7% | 2 | 5* | 2 | 6* | 2 | 5* | 2 | 1 |
| 10% | 1 | 5* | 2 | 6* | 1 | 5* | 2 | 0 |
| Mean | 2.8 | 14.8 | 7.3 | 20.4 | 6.8 | 16.4 | 3.9 | 1.7 |
| | | | | 70–100 min period | | | | |
| 7% | 6* | 10* | 6* | 4* | 7* | 7* | 8* | 5* |
| 10% | 6* | 7* | 4* | 3# | 6* | 4* | 6* | 5* |
| Mean | 14.8 | 15.4 | 8.8 | 10.1 | 11.7 | 12.9 | 10.1 | 8.7 |
| | | | | 40–65 min period | | | | |
| 7% | 5* | 3# | 9* | 7* | 6* | 5* | 7* | 8* |
| 10% | 5* | 3# | 7* | 3# | 5* | 4* | 4* | 5* |
| Mean | 10.0 | 9.0 | 13.3 | 10.3 | 11.0 | 9.7 | 11.1 | 10.7 |

[a]7% and 10% are cutoff levels for %TMSE for each parameter. Mean, mean value for TMSE (maximums) across subjects. Asterisk (*) indicates $p \leq 0.01$, $^{\#}p \leq 0.05$; $^{+}$the maximum number possible is 10 (10 subjects). Reprinted from Shannahoff-Khalsa, Kennedy, Yates, and Ziegler; copyright (1996), with permission from American Physiological Society.

TABLE VII
PREVALENCE OF THE MAJOR PERIODS FOR 10 SUBJECTS FOR THE BLOOD PRESSURE PARAMETERS[a,+]

| | SBP | DBP | MAP | TPR |
|---|---|---|---|---|
| | | 115–145 min Period | | |
| 7% | 1 | 1 | 1 | 4* |
| 10% | 1 | 1 | 0 | 4* |
| Mean | 2.0 | 1.7 | 1.4 | 12.6 |
| | | 70–100 min Period | | |
| 7% | 5* | 6* | 4* | 6* |
| 10% | 4* | 5* | 3# | 3# |
| Mean | 11.7 | 8.7 | 8.1 | 9.2 |
| | | 40–65 min Period | | |
| 7% | 8* | 6* | 7* | 6* |
| 10% | 4* | 4* | 3# | 3# |
| Mean | 10.5 | 10.5 | 9.7 | 7.9 |

[a]7% and 10% are cutoff levels for %TMSE for each parameter. Mean, mean value for TMSE (maximums) across subjects. Asterisk (*) indicates $p \leq 0.01$, $^{\#}p \leq 0.05$; $^{+}$the maximum number possible is 10 (10 subjects). TPR is missing from subject MR. Reprinted from Shannahoff-Khalsa, Kennedy, Yates, and Ziegler; copyright (1996), with permission from American Physiological Society.

rhythms during resting (or sleep) states are subject to a wide variance when measured on a beat-to-beat basis, since they are strongly influenced by Mayer wave frequency activity rhythms (0.008–0.1 Hz) (Mayer, 1876; Penaz, 1978; Polosa, 1984; Preiss and Polosa, 1974; Shannahoff-Khalsa *et al.*, 2004) that impose short-term bursts in power that can obscure some lower frequencies.

Tables V–VII list the number of subjects who exhibit a significant (7% or 10%) %TMSE in the period ranges 115–145, 70–100, and 40–65. The 7% level is a value that is statistically above the background noise level ($p \leq 0.05$). The 10% cut off is more a level of "physiological significance." The TMSE of 7% or 10% is based on measures at 5-min intervals, for example, on any one of the possible 15 peak values that can be identified between 220, 225, 230, 235, 240, 250, 260, . . . , 340 (or 10 values between 170 and 215, 7 values between 115 and 145 min, 7 values between 70 and 100 min, and 6 values between 40 and 65 min). It is not based on the sum of neighboring peaks. Therefore, the cutoff value of 7% or 10% is conservative, since frequently there is significant activity at several neighboring values that are "shoulders" of the major peak. But here only the maximum value was chosen instead of an additive value from neighbors within the same range.

Figure 20 shows a striking similarity between the power spectral plots of the NC and LH. While all 21 parameters, except TFI and HR, show some activity in the 220–340 min range, only the NC and LH are statistically significant at the 10% level for TMSE. The NC, LH, TPR, CO, TFI, HR, EVI, SV, LNE, RNE, and MNE all show significance in the 115–145 min range at 10% TMSE. This excludes significance for ACTH, VET, LE, RE, ME, LRE, LRNE, SBP, DBP, and MAP, although all but LRNE and MAP have some activity. All 21 parameters show statistical significance at the 10% level for TMSE in the 70–100 min range. And all parameters, except the NC and LH, show statistical significance in the 40–65 min range.

The mean values of %TMSE or relative power for each parameter for the five selected period ranges are listed in Tables V–VII. Independent of parameter and subject, the mean for all observed

%TMSE measures in the 220–340, 170–215, 115–145, 70–100, and 40–65 min ranges are 8.88% (SE = 1.31), 4.69% (SE = 0.85), 9.27% (SE = 1.10), 11.66% (SE = 0.72), and 10.63% (SE = 0.51), respectively. The lower frequency periods tend to show greater maximum values for power, or %TMSE, for any single parameter. This pattern is also clearly evident in Fig. 18. The decreasing power with increasing frequency (sometimes called $1/f$ spectral background) is ubiquitous in physical and biological systems.

2. *Interindividual Linear Regression Analyses*

Although a period(s) may predominate within and/or across subjects for different parameters, it is not clear if there is a single oscillator or if mutually entrained oscillators are involved in the regulation of these periods. One approach to gaining further insight here is to perform a linear regression of the values of one parameter against another. A high regression value suggests that the two parameters are phase coupled, but low regression values do not rule out the possibility of coupling when lagging or phase shifting occurs between parameters with similar periods. Additionally, linear regressions violate the requirements that each datum be independent of the next. Therefore, linear regressions have limitations.

A matrix of 20 parameters × 20 parameters was created for each subject that included the NC, LH, ACTH, CO, HR, EVI, SV, VET, SBP, DBP, MAP, TPR, LE, LNE, RE, RNE, ME, MNE, LRE, and LRNE. The dopamine parameters (left and right arm dopamine, mean dopamine, and left/right dopamine) and TFI were excluded from the initial 25 parameters. Each parameter was regressed against the other 19. All regressions were performed on the raw data and not on any of the detrended data that was analyzed by FOS. One subject (MR) had only 14 parameters due to lost impedance data. A regression value of $R = 0.3$ was considered significant based on the statistics which gives a $p \leq 0.05$ for $R = 0.3$, for $n = 41$ (the number of data points per record; two subjects, 1 and 2, with 42 and 48 points each, respectively).

Table VIII gives the mean percent correlation for all 10 subjects for each parameter regressed against the other 19 parameters when

TABLE VIII

LINEAR REGRESSION ANALYSES OF PARAMETER BY PARAMETERS

| | Correlation with 19 parameters (%) (Means for 10 subjects) | Variability in subjects (%) |
|---|---|---|
| NC* | 44.25% | 0–61.53 |
| LH | 38.05 | 0–73.68 |
| ACTH | 43.22 | 5.56–69.23 |
| CO | 45.06 | 16.66–77.77 |
| HR | 48.52 | 21.05–68.42 |
| EVI | 48.53 | 26.31–84.21 |
| SV | 49.70 | 21.05–84.21 |
| VET | 47.36 | 5.26–84.21 |
| SBP | 33.88 | 5.55–66.66 |
| DBP | 38.61 | 11.11–66.66 |
| MAP | 40.68 | 2.50–81.81 |
| TPR | 43.12 | 17.64–70.58 |
| LE | 36.95 | 0–88.23 |
| LNE | 36.86 | 11.76–70.78 |
| RE | 32.83 | 088.23 |
| RNE | 40.96 | 17.64–76.47 |
| ME | 29.70 | 088.23 |
| MNE | 37.11 | 11.76–64.70 |
| LRE | 18.05 | 5.88–41.17 |
| LRNE | 23.90 | 082.35 |
| Mean across 20 Parameters = 38.87% | | 18.05–49.70% (range) |

*44.25% is the mean for all subjects for the linear regressions of the NC against the other 19 parameters when $R \geq 0.30$. LE and RE, and LNE and RNE were not regressed against their means or ratios (or vice versa), but rights and lefts were regressed against each other, and means were regressed against ratios. The mean percentage for the NC did not include subject KW who had a deviated septum. Reprinted from Shannahoff-Khalsa, Kennedy, Yates, and Ziegler; copyright (1996), with permission from American Physiological Society.

there is a significant *R* value along with the percent variability across subjects for each parameter. The left and right arm catecholamines were considered as separate parameters, however, they were not regressed against their means or left/right ratios. TPR was not regressed against CO or MAP. Subject KW had a severe left nostril occlusion and his NC value (0%) was not included in the group mean. Subject CC's (female, age 20) LH did not correlate with any other parameter but her 0% value was calculated in the mean percent. She reported having an irregular menstrual cycle. The other female (FR) had a 31.57% correlation of LH with the other parameters. The mean of means across all 20 parameters was 38.87%, and the range was 18.05–49.70%. The parameter with the highest percent correlation with other parameters was SV (49.70%). The decreasing order of percent correlation for all 20 parameters is SV > EVI > HR > VET > CO > NC > ACTH > TPR > RNE > MAP > DBP > LH > MNE > LE > LNE > SBP > RE > ME > LRNE > LRE.

3. *Profiles of Individual Parameters Within Subjects*

The primary time series (raw data) for the NC, LH, ACTH, SV, HR, and MNE are shown for subjects, 6 males (Figs. 23–28) and 2 females (Figs. 29–30), respectively. Phase relations of the different parameters are readily observed here and help answer important questions. For example, does ACTH secrete during the left or right nostril-dominant phase of the NC? Does ACTH have a positive or negative correlation with LH, SV, HR, and MNE, etc.? With 21 parameters per subject, there are 231 possible interparameter comparisons that can be made for each subject, resulting in either a positive, negative, or nonsignificant relationship. The subject KW in Fig. 28 had a severe left nostril occlusion and only shows one spike of activity in the left nostril-dominant mode that appears to last for about 20 min and it appears that his nasal cycle and LH profile are negatively coupled. These parameters were selected to give a less inclusive array but still be representative of the different systems.

Examples of the primary time series are presented in Figs. 23–30 for eight subjects for selected parameters and several correlations of parameters are discussed here among the groupings. In Figs. 24–30, ACTH is higher during the relative right nostril-dominant mode. Subject 1 (JWB) is the exception where ACTH increases during the left nostril-dominant mode, $R = 0.49$, $p = 0.002$. Subject 2 (DSK) has a negative correlation for NC to ACTH, $R = -0.53$, $p < 0.0001$, subject 3 (MR) $R = -0.89$, $p < 0.0001$, and for subject 8 (FR) $R = -0.19$, $p > 0.05$. Table IX shows the average $R$ value (independent of sign) and significance for the interactions of the NC, LH, ACTH, MNE, SV, and HR for the four subjects JWB, DSK, MR, and FR. Figure 23 shows that the NC and LH for subject JWB is

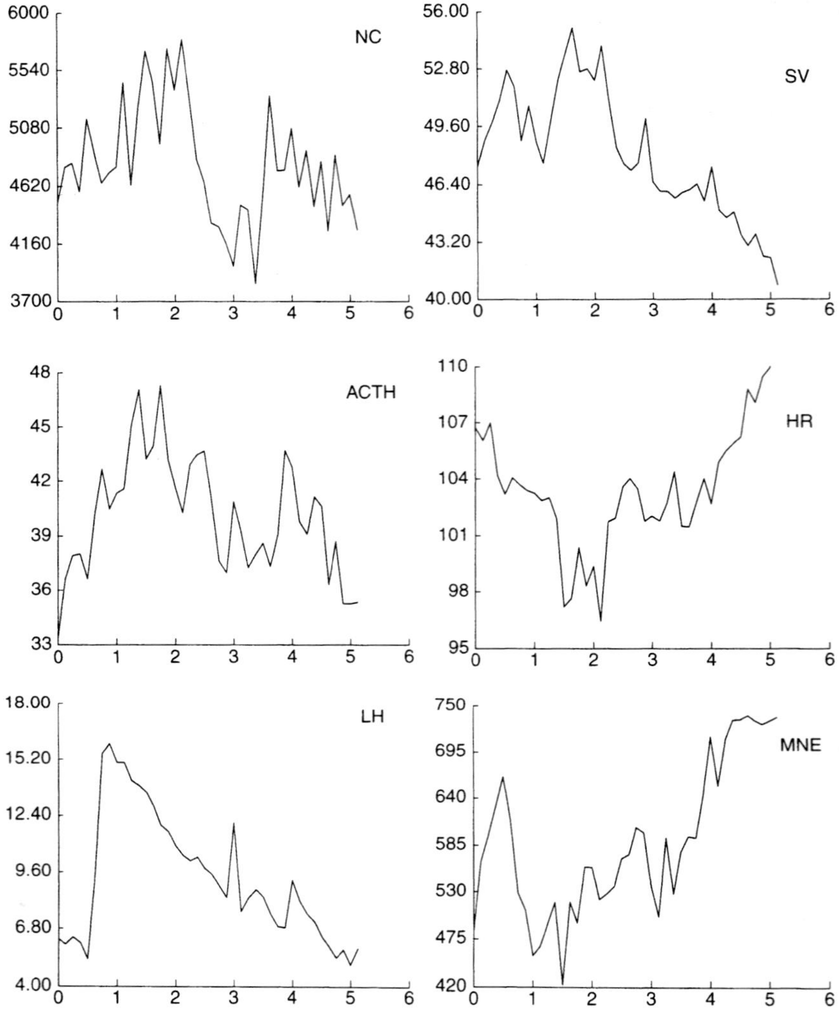


FIG. 23. Subject JWB's primary data are plotted for the nasal cycle (NC), luteinizing hormone (LH), adrenocorticotropin hormone (ACTH), stroke volume (SV), heart rate (HR), and mean norepinephrine (MNE). The *x*-axis for all plots is 0–6 h; for the NC plot the *y*-axis is left minus right nostril values (arbitrary values) with all values greater than 0, therefore all shifts occur while in the left nostril-dominant mode; ACTH, LH, and MNE are in pg/ml; SV is in ml/beat; and HR is in beats/min. Reprinted from Shannahoff-Khalsa, Kennedy, Yates, and Ziegler; copyright (1996), with permission from American Physiological Society.

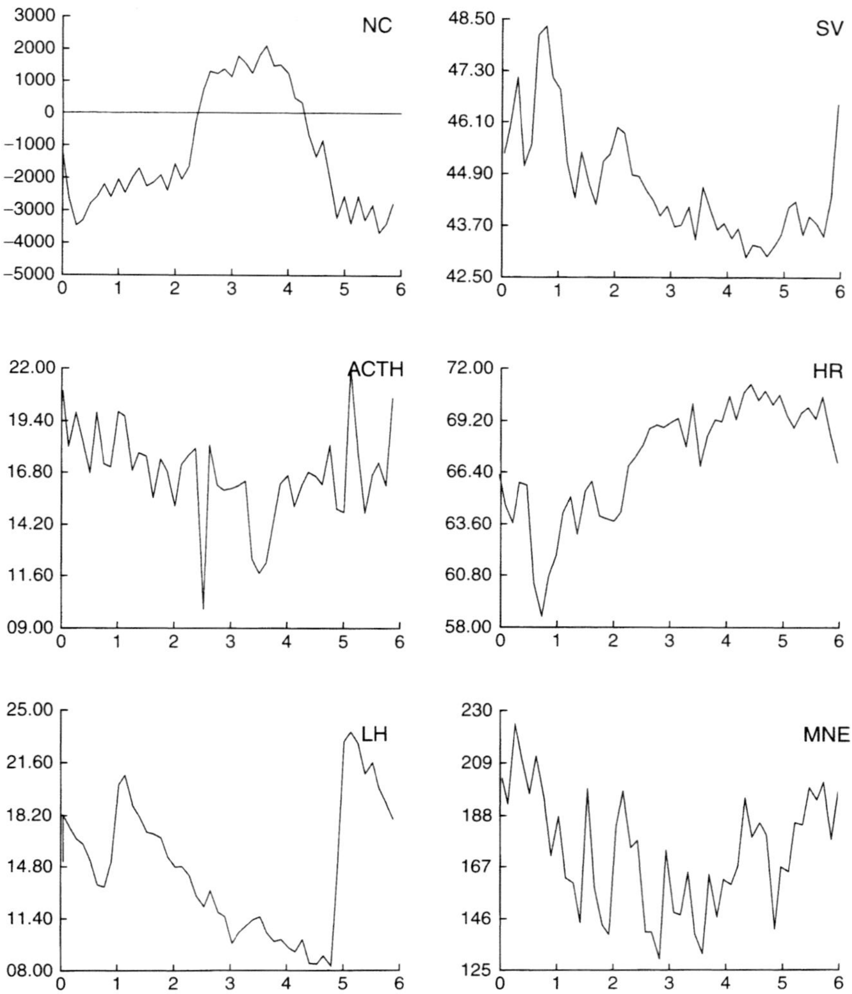


FIG. 24. Subject DSK's primary data are plotted for the nasal cycle (NC), luteinizing hormone (LH), adrenocorticotropin hormone (ACTH), stroke volume (SV), heart rate (HR), and mean norepinephrine (MNE). The *x*-axis for all plots is 0–6 h; for the NC plot, the *y*-axis is left minus right nostril values (arbitrary values), values greater than 0 show left nostril dominance and values less than 0 show right nostril dominance; ACTH, LH, and MNE are in pg/ml; SV is in ml/beat; and HR is in beats/min. Reprinted from Shannahoff-Khalsa, Kennedy, Yates, and Ziegler; copyright (1996), with permission from American Physiological Society.

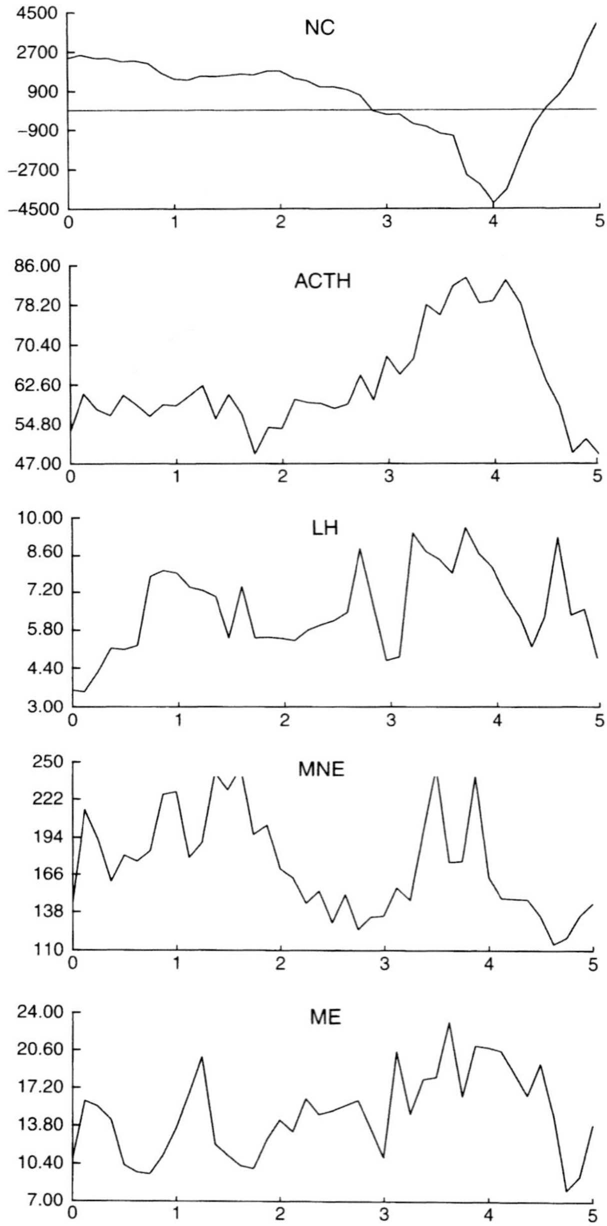


FIG. 25. Subject MR's primary data are plotted for the nasal cycle (NC), luteinizing hormone (LH), adrenocorticotropin hormone (ACTH), mean epinephrine (ME), and mean norepinephrine (MNE). The *x*-axis for all plots is 0–5 h; for the NC plot, the *y*-axis is left minus right nostril values

positively correlated, that is, appears to have LH surges during the left nostril mode ($R = 0.36$, $p = 0.023$) while subjects DSK, MR, and FR have negative correlations, with LH surges during the right nostril-dominant mode: $R = -0.72$, $p < 0.0001$; $R = -.547$, $p < 0.0001$; and $R = -0.48$, $p = 0.007$, respectively. Therefore, subject 1 (JWB) shows inverse correlations for pituitary hormones with the NC. The NC is negatively correlated with MNE in the same four subjects, but only significantly in DSK ($R = -0.600$, $p < 0.0001$), and marginally with JWB ($R = -0.296$, $p = 0.06$). Subject JWB shows a reverse correlation of the NC with SV and HR compared to subjects DSK and FR. LH has a positive correlation with SV for JWB, DSK, and FR (MR has no SV). LH and ACTH have positive correlations in all four subjects here. These interactions are again selected out of the 15 possible different combinations in this subgroup of six parameters.

The time series history analysis for the NC, LH, ACTH, SBP, DBP, MAP, TPR, LE, LNE, RE, RNE, ME, MNE, LRE, LRNE, CO, TFI, HR, EVI, SV, and VET, using the FOS method (Korenberg, 1988, 1989; Korenberg and Paarmann, 1989a,b), clearly demonstrates for most parameters the predominance of major peaks in the ranges of 115–145, 70–100, and 40–65 min. The exceptions are seen in the absence of statistical significance for ACTH at 115–145 min; NC and LH at 40–65 min; the epinephrines at 115–145 min; and SBP, DBP, and MAP at 115–145 min. While all parameters (except TFI and HR) have some activity at 220–340 min, only the NC and LH show significant chi-square values along with their greatest spectral power in the 220–340 min range.

The broad range of 70–140 min is the range of periodicity most commonly reported for the "hourly" ultradian rhythms (Bossom *et al.*, 1983; Broten and Zehr, 1989; Kennedy *et al.*, 1986; Kleitman,

(arbitrary values), values greater than 0 show left nostril dominance, and values less than 0 show right nostril dominance; ACTH, LH, and MNE are in pg/ml. Reprinted from Shannahoff-Khalsa, Kennedy, Yates, and Ziegler; copyright (1996), with permission from American Physiological Society.

1982; Lavie and Kripke, 1981; Levin *et al.*, 1978, 1979; Livnat *et al.*, 1984; Orr and Hoffman, 1974; Shimada and Marsh, 1979; Van Cauter, 1990; Veldhuis and Johnson, 1988; Veldhuis *et al.*, 1984). Here this "hourly" range was expanded and analyzed as three components, the 40–65, the 70–100, and the 115–145 min ranges. These three ranges represent the three largest of the five in respect to %TMSE.

At least one other report (Veldhuis and Johnson, 1988) finds a significant ultradian period at 242 min for a pituitary hormone (prolactin), similar to our peak of 220–340 min, and with smoothing of spectral data the 242 min peak becomes 234 min. In addition, their major peak occurs approximately every 95 min (Veldhuis and Johnson, 1988). Additionally, in that study, although a coupling of prolactin and LH occurs, cross-spectral analysis of the two fails to exhibit a period coupling at larger than 106 min. In the data presented here, LH and NC have the majority of their power at 220–340 min, with smaller peaks in the three highest frequency ranges.

We state "These data provide new insight to the relationship of the autonomic, cardiovascular, and neuroendocrine systems. Our results suggest that a single oscillator or that mutually entrained oscillators are regulating the 'hourly' ultradian rhythms, at least under the conditions of this study (strict rest in a reclined position)" (Shannahoff-Khalsa *et al.*, 1996). Also:

> The linear regression data, although of questionable statistical value, indicates a high degree of coupling within subjects and across variables (39%). This high level of correlation would not be expected by chance alone. The earlier studies of the NC [multi-study reviews (Keuning, 1968; Hasegawa and Kern, 1978)] report major periods at 3–4 hr and 2.9 hr, respectively. The periods of 3–4 hr and 2.9 hr are closer to the 220–340 min period range observed here compared to most other neuroendocrine, autonomic, and cardiovascular studies. However, these NC studies (Hasegawa and Kern, 1978; Keuning, 1968) are not based on spectral analysis of the time series data, but are averages visually identified from peak-to-peak measures (Shannahoff-Khalsa *et al.*, 1996).

Prior to these multivariate studies (Shannahoff-Khalsa *et al.*, 1996, 1997), the regulatory mechanisms of INS ultradian secretory

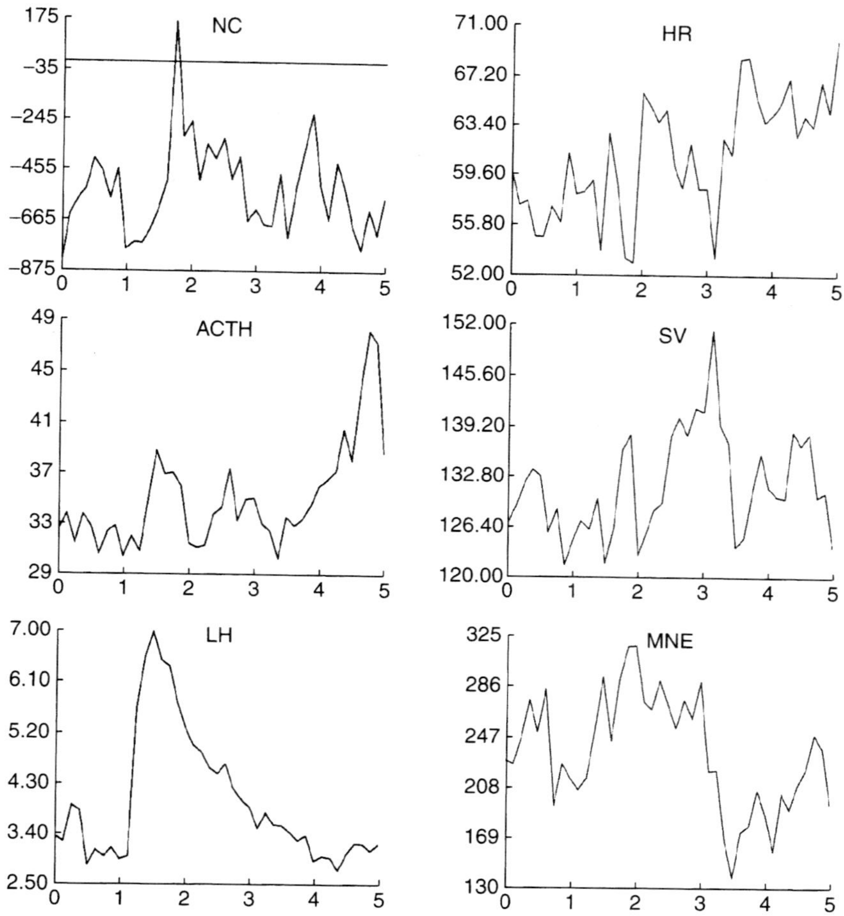


FIG. 26. Subject JB's primary data are plotted for the nasal cycle (NC), adrenocorticotropin hormone (ACTH), luteinizing hormone (LH), heart rate (HR), stroke volume (SV), and mean norepinephrine (MNE). The *x*-axis for all plots is 0–5 h; for the NC plot, the *y*-axis is left minus right nostril values (arbitrary values), values greater than 0 show left nostril dominance, and values less than 0 show right nostril dominance; ACTH, LH, and MNE are in pg/ml; SV is in ml/beat; and HR is in beats/min.

rhythms remained to be fully elucidated. Both high (5–15 min) and low (50–150 min) oscillatory frequency ranges have been observed. The high-frequency range was observed in fasting humans (Hansen *et al.*, 1982; Lang *et al.*, 1981; Sonnenberg *et al.*, 1992), rats (Chou *et al.*, 1991), monkeys (Goodner *et al.*, 1977), dogs (Jaspan *et al.*,

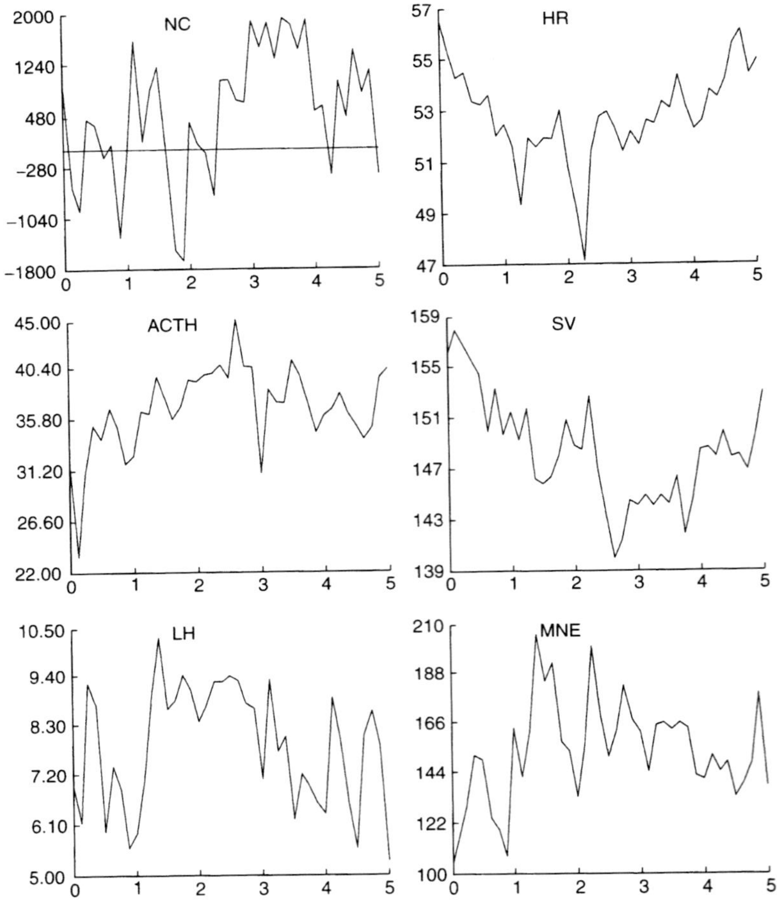


FIG. 27. Subject PM's primary data are plotted for the nasal cycle (NC), adrenocorticotropin hormone (ACTH), luteinizing hormone (LH), heart rate (HR), stroke volume (SV), and mean norepinephrine (MNE). The *x*-axis for all plots is 0–5 h; for the NC plot, the *y*-axis is left minus right nostril values (arbitrary values), values greater than 0 show left nostril dominance, and values less than 0 show right nostril dominance; ACTH, LH, and MNE are in pg/ml; SV is in ml/beat; and HR is in beats/min.

1986), and is presumed to be controlled by the intrapancreatic ganglia that may function as a pacemaker or integration center for the generation of periodic islet secretion (Sonnenberg *et al.*, 1992). The high-frequency rhythms have been shown to persist in an *in vitro* pancreas preparation (Stagner and Samols, 1985) and in pancreas transplant recipients (Sonnenberg *et al.*, 1992). However, the

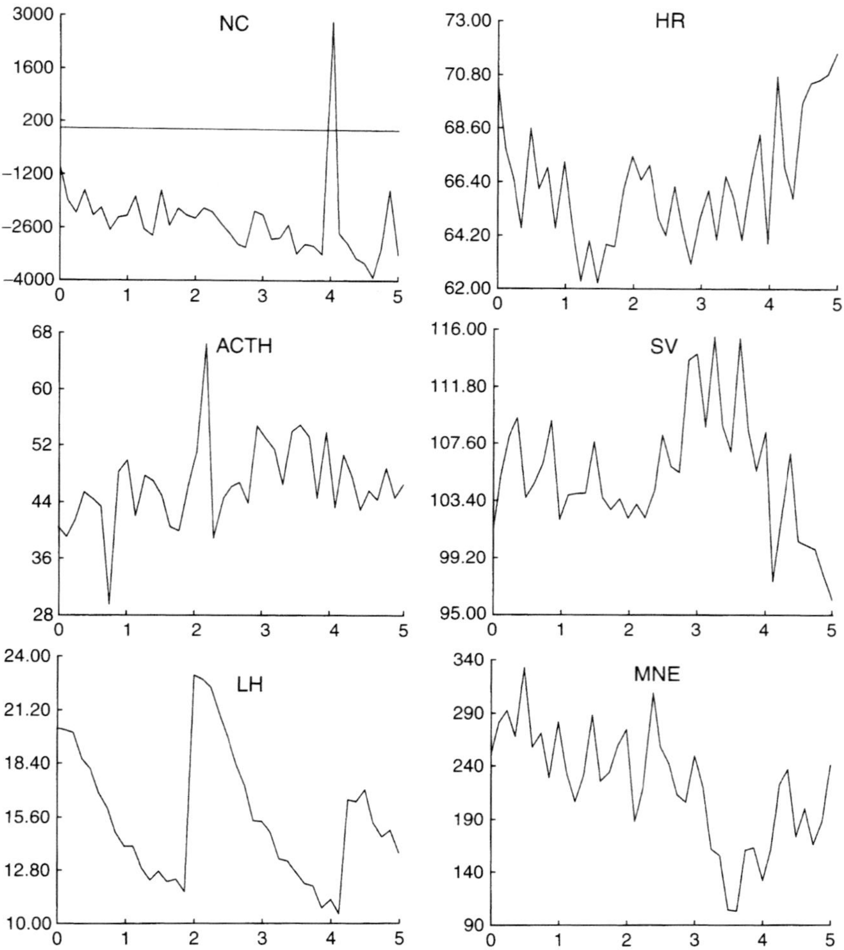


FIG. 28. Subject KW's primary data are plotted for the nasal cycle (NC), adrenocorticotropin hormone (ACTH), luteinizing hormone (LH), heart rate (HR), stroke volume (SV), and mean norepinephrine (MNE). The *x*-axis for all plots is 0–5 h; for the NC plot, the *y*-axis is left minus right nostril values (arbitrary values), values greater than 0 show left nostril dominance and values less than 0 show right nostril dominance; ACTH, LH, and MNE are in pg/ml; SV is in ml/beat; and HR is in beats/min.

intrapancreatic ganglia also receive extrapancreatic innervation from adrenergic, cholinergic, and peptidergic nerves (Larsson, 1980; Stagner and Samols, 1985). The low-frequency ultradian rhythms have been reported during 24-h sampling protocols in

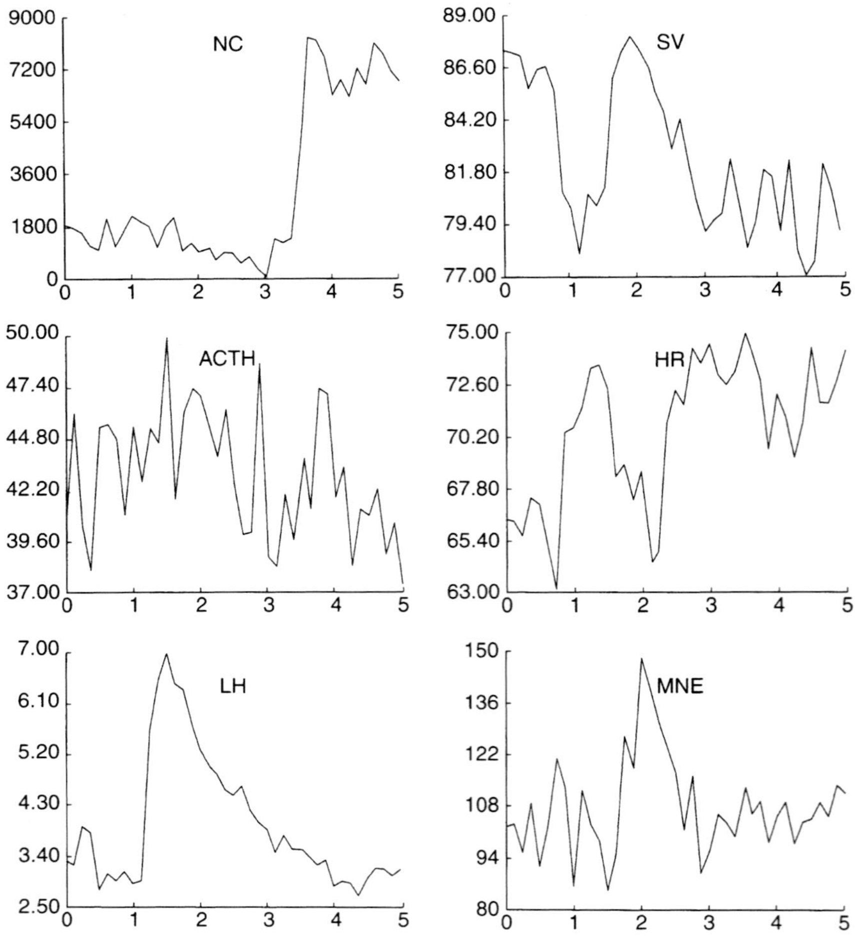


FIG. 29. Subject FR's primary data are plotted for the nasal cycle (NC), adrenocorticotropin hormone (ACTH), luteinizing hormone (LH), stroke volume (SV), heart rate (HR), and mean norepinephrine (MNE). The *x*-axis for all plots is 0–5 h; for the NC plot, the *y*-axis is left minus right nostril values (arbitrary values) and the left nostril is dominant throughout the recording with a much greater left nostril-dominant mode in the last 2 h, values greater than 0 show left nostril dominance and values less than 0 show right nostril dominance; ACTH, LH, and MNE are in pg/ml; SV is in ml/beat; and HR is in beats/min. Reprinted from Shannahoff-Khalsa, Kennedy, Yates, and Ziegler; copyright (1996), with permission from American Physiological Society.

normal humans with three meals (Polonsky *et al.*, 1988), during continuous enteral nutrition (Simon *et al.*, 1987) and during intravenous glucose (Shapiro *et al.*, 1988), but also in transplanted humans

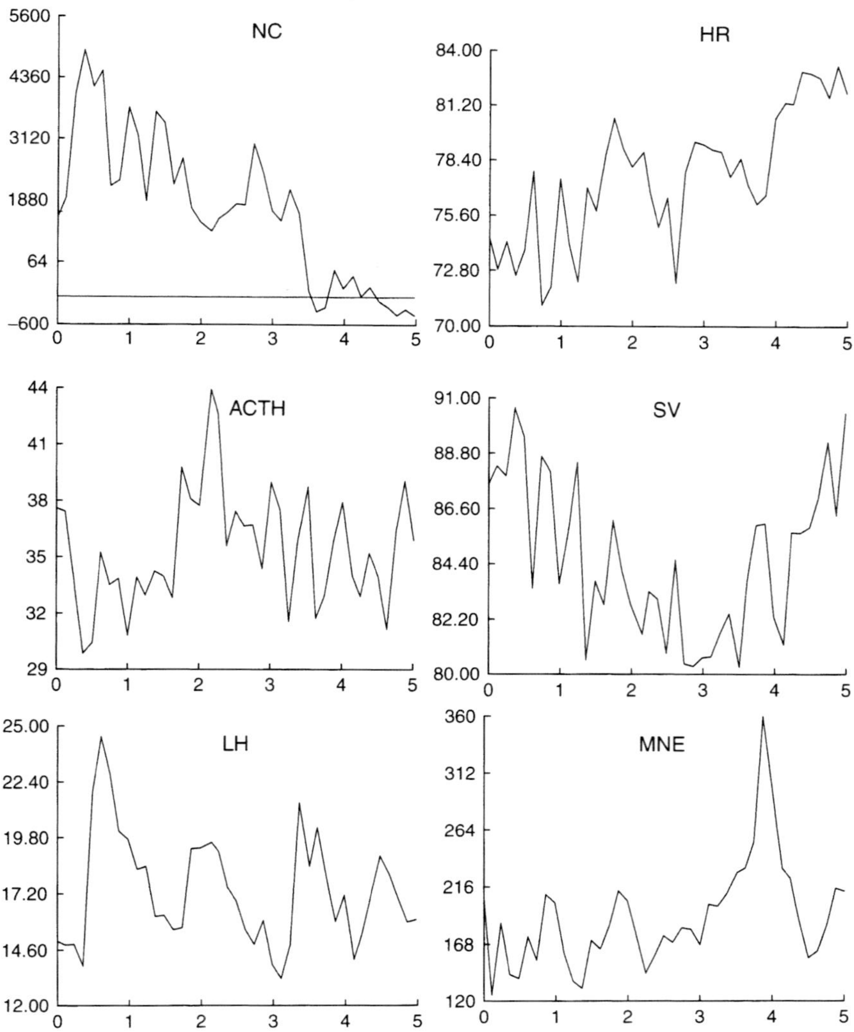


FIG. 30. Subject CC's primary data are plotted for the nasal cycle (NC), adrenocorticotropin hormone (ACTH), luteinizing hormone (LH), heart rate (HR), stroke volume (SV), and mean norepinephrine (MNE). The $x$-axis for all plots is 0–5 h; for the NC plot, the $y$-axis is left minus right nostril values (arbitrary values) with almost all values greater than 0, therefore all shifts occur while primarily in the left nostril; ACTH, LH, and MNE are in pg/ml; SV is in ml/beat, HR is in beats/min.

TABLE IX
AVERAGE LINEAR REGRESSION RELATIONS FOR FOUR SUBJECTS FOR THE NC, LH, ACTH, MNE, SV, AND HR[a,#]

| | NC | LH | ACTH | MNE | SV | HR |
|---|---|---|---|---|---|---|
| NC | | 0.528 | 0.521 | 0.252* | 0.518 | 0.428 |
| LH | | | 0.497 | 0.343 | 0.389 | 0.301* |
| ACTH | | | | 0.277 | 0.388 | 0.383 |
| MNE | | | | | 0.449 | 0.390 |
| SV | | | | | | 0.833 |

[a]Subjects JWB, DSK, MR, and FR (see Figs. 21–24 for the time series of the raw data for each subject for these six parameters). [#]Linear regressions are performed on the raw data (not detrended data). *A one-tailed *t*-test was used to test whether the average from the individual subject's *R* values (independent of sign) was significant. All *R* values were significant except NC-MNE and LH-HR with $p \leq 0.05$. Reprinted from Shannahoff-Khalsa, Kennedy, Yates, and Ziegler; copyright (1996), with permission from American Physiological Society.

(Sonnenberg *et al.*, 1992). One group (Sonnenberg *et al.*, 1992) suggests that the extrapancreatic autonomic influences only modulate INS amplitudes by exerting a dampening effect. And one researcher suggests in his review of the fuel-regulatory hormones that INS is under "autonomous oscillatory secretion" via the pancreas while the other fuel-regulatory hormones are organized by the CNS (Weigle, 1987). However, Kleitman had earlier proposed a general integrated view of how systems are coordinated, including the possible regulation of INS and other fuel-regulatory hormones and that all low-frequency (hourly) ultradian endocrine, physiological, and behavioral rhythms could be accounted for by the BRAC, and that these rhythms were also correlated to the REM NREM sleep cycle (Kleitman, 1961, 1982). The Sonnenberg autonomic "dampening effect" theory (Sonnenberg *et al.*, 1992) and the Weigle "autonomous" control theory (Weigle, 1987) versus the BRAC theory of INS were investigated by comparing the time series analysis relationships of INS with the autonomic, cardiovascular, and neuroendocrine rhythms (Shannahoff-Khalsa *et al.*, 1997).

Figure 31 profiles the FOS plots of INS sampled at 7.5 min intervals and collected simultaneously with the reported data above for 9 of the 21 variables that include here MNE, SV, NC, HR, LH, VET, ME, TPR, and ACTH. INS was significant at the

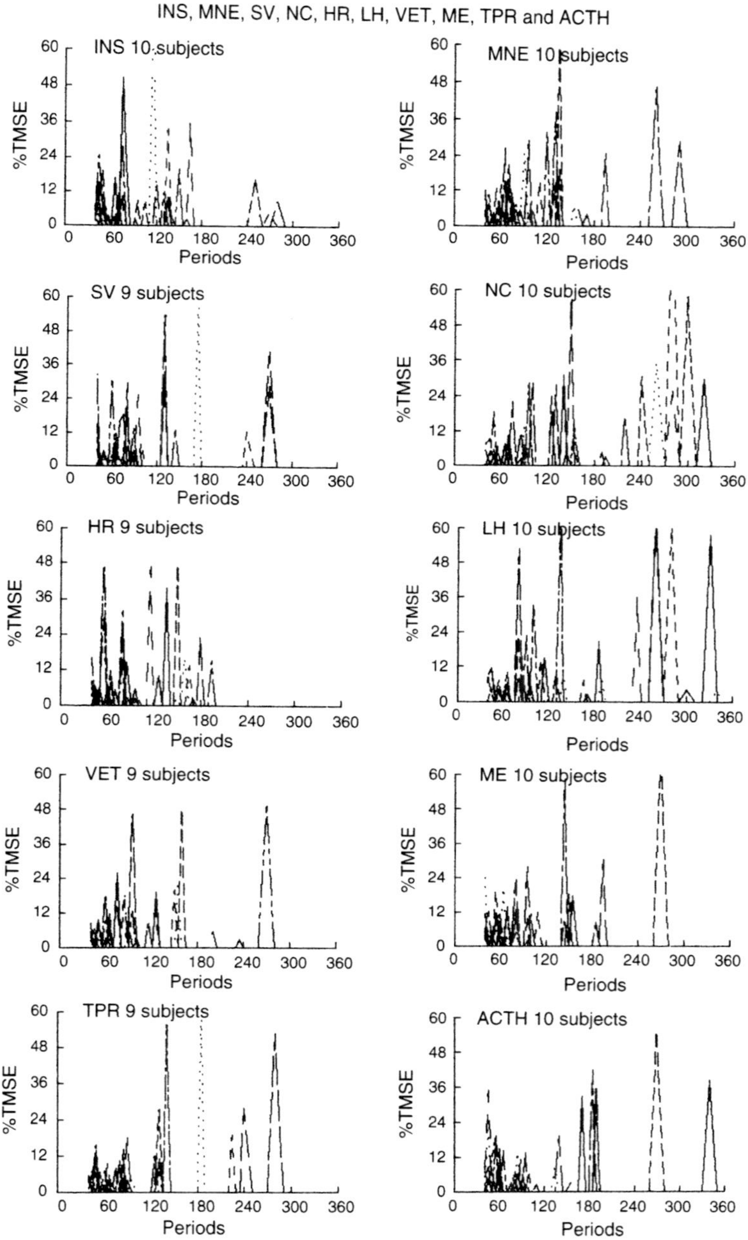


FIG. 31. Spectral density plots of 10 subjects from FOS time history analysis of insulin, the nasal cycle (NC), luteinizing hormone (LH), adrenocorticotropin hormone (ACTH), total peripheral resistance (TPR), stroke volume (SV), heart rate (HR), ventricular ejection time (VET), mean

10% level for the 115–145, the 70–100, and the 40–65 min range, with the respective mean values for TMSE for all 10 subjects at 16.0, 11.8, and 10.2. Figure 31 shows the striking similarity between the power spectral plots of INS and the other nine parameters.

4. *Profiles of Individual Parameters*

The observed time series for INS for all 10 subjects is shown in Fig. 32. Figure 33 shows the observed time series for INS, SV, ACTH, MAP, MNE, and NC for male subject JB. Phase relations of the different parameters are readily apparent here and help answer important questions. For example, INS increases with increases of SV, ACTH, MAP, MNE, and during the left nostril-dominant phase of the NC. When INS is included there are 22 parameters per subject in this experiment, and there are 252 possible interparameter comparisons that can be made for each subject, resulting in either a positive, negative, or nonsignificant relationship. These parameters were selected to give an example of how INS and the other three systems can compare as linear time series for one subject.

This work shows that INS has a similar power spectral profile when compared to the other 21 parameters previously measured (NC, LH, ACTH, SBP, DBP, MAP, TPR, LE, LNE, RE, RNE, ME, MNE, LRE, LRNE, CO, TFI, HR, EVI, SV, VET) with a predominance of major peaks in the ranges of 115–145, 70–100, and 40–65 min. These data provide new insight to how one fuel-regulatory hormone (INS) is coupled to the autonomic, cardiovascular, and neuroendocrine systems and suggests that a single pacemaker or mutually entrained pacemakers are regulating the "hourly" ultradian rhythms that include INS under a strict resting condition.

Since the NC is tightly coupled to the ultradian rhythm of alternating cerebral hemispheric activity (Werntz *et al.*, 1983), this ANS–CNS linkage implies that INS, a fuel-regulatory hormone, like

norepinephrine (MNE), and mean epinephrine (ME). The $x$-axis is 0–360 min with data of 0–40 min not included, and the $y$-axis is in 0–60% TMSE accounted for by that period. Plots of TPR, SV, HR, and VET are from nine subjects, subject MR's data were lost. Reprinted from Shannahoff-Khalsa, Kennedy, Yates, and Ziegler; copyright (1997), with permission from American Physiological Society.

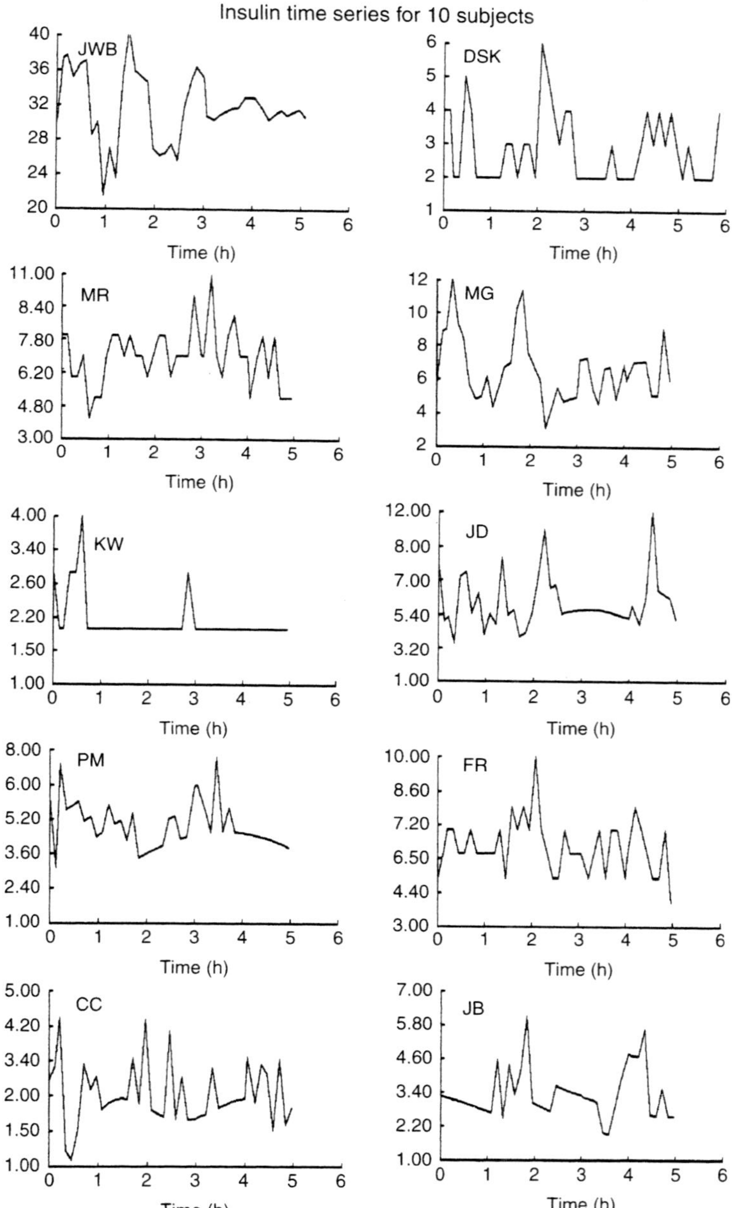


FIG. 32. The primary time series data for insulin is plotted for each subject individually. The time series for JWB, MG, KW, JD, PM, CC, and JB were all detrended to eliminate circadian components. The $x$-axis is from 0–6 h, and the $y$-axis is in micro units of insulin and varies for each subject. Reprinted from Shannahoff-Khalsa, Kennedy, Yates, and Ziegler; copyright (1997), with permission from American Physiological Society.

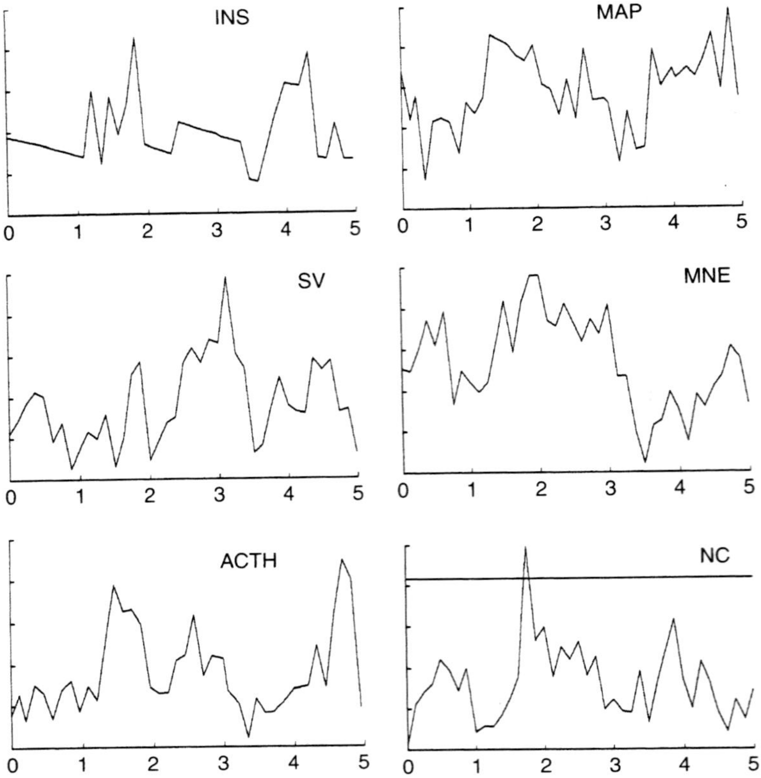


FIG. 33. Subject JB's primary data are plotted for insulin (INS), stroke volume (SV), adrenocorticotropin hormone (ACTH), mean arterial pressure (MAP), mean norepinephrine (MNE), and the nasal cycle (NC) as representatives of the different systems. The $x$-axis for all plots is 0–5 h; for the NC plot, the $y$-axis is left minus right nostril values (arbitrary values) with most values showing negative values and relative shifts during right nostril dominance. The actual values for INS, SV, ACTH, MAP, and MNE are not provided but are shown only as relative values. Reprinted from Shannahoff-Khalsa, Kennedy, Yates, and Ziegler; copyright (1996), with permission from American Physiological Society.

the cardiovascular and neuroendocrine rhythms, may also be coupled to the ANS–CNS rhythm of alternating cerebral hemispheric activity. We reported that:

> This result with INS is further evidence to suggest that all ultradian rhythms may be related via the proposed ANS-CNS rhythm and that the hypothalamus itself is "the pacemaker." The confusion between

> the "single" vs. "multiple" ultradian pacemaker theories arises from the (erroneous, we believe) assumption that there is no coordinated relationship among the various systems, and therefore, individual pacemakers would be needed for each rhythm. This view is equivalent to saying that the fuel regulatory hormones, the neuroendocrine system, the cardiovascular system, and behavioral phenomena are not coupled to autonomic phenomena or under hypothalamic control (Shannahoff-Khalsa *et al.*, 1997).

Another result also supports this hypothalamic model of control (Kern *et al.*, 1996). The Kern *et al.* study shows that INS secretion is positively coupled to the NREM phase of the NREM–REM sleep cycle. They conclude that the hourly ultradian oscillations of INS are modulated by CNS mechanisms entraining this pancreatic function to the NREM–REM sleep cycle (Kern *et al.*, 1996).

We concluded that:

> This coupling may have evolved to help maintain a coordination among systems and to allow for transitions between two distinct polar physiological states, that of rest and activity, that occur during both wakefullness and sleep. Our results also suggest that the two phases (left or right dominance) of the waking cerebral rhythm are best served by two polar physiological states. This waking rhythm is analogous to the REM/NREM rhythm during sleep that is presumed to be the nighttime correlate of alternating cerebral hemispheric dominance (Shannahoff-Khalsa *et al.*, 1997).

In addition, we stated that "the ultradian rhythms of pituitary hormone and catecholamine secretion, cardiovascular function, and fuel regulation are also tightly coupled to the nasal cycle. This work as a whole demonstrates a lack of autonomy for different systems and suggests that the hypothalamus and the ANS play the primary regulatory and integrative role for mind-body states."

Furthermore, it is important to point out that others demonstrated ultradian rhythms in humans for cytokines (interleukine-1beta and interferon-gamma) ranging from 80–240 min, with the most frequent period found of 160 min, when sampling at 20-min intervals for 8 h (Bouayad-Amine *et al.*, 1993). Their result which is temporally coincident with ours suggests that the immune system is also coupled to the other major bodily systems. Another study relevant to immune function showed a simultaneous coupling of EEG activity and histamine release where:

> ultradian rhythms in the delta and theta frequency bands are negatively correlated to the release rate of histamine; periods of high neuronal activity, which might reflect synchronization of firing, coincide temporally with low release rate of histamine, while periods of low neuronal activity coincide with high histamine release rate. The alpha and beta frequency bands did not correlate with histamine release. The ultradian rhythm of EEG power and histamine release might be of importance for regulatory mechanisms, such as the secretion of hormones (Prast *et al.*, 1997).

We suggested that:

> the left nostril dominant state is coupled to the rest phase of the BRAC, NREM sleep, and to increased immune function. Together these results expand upon the BRAC phenomenon and provide a structural basis for Kleitman's temporal hypothesis. The lateralized rhythm of CNS–ANS function apparently involves most of the major physiological systems, with the hypothalamus playing the central role as pacemaker. This pacemaker integrates subsystems participating in the rest-activity cycle. If these subsystems diverge from a "dynamical equilibrium" with each other, a new and fascinating basis for disease states may arise (Shannahoff-Khalsa *et al.*, 1997).

## D. Hypothalamic Regulation and Integration of the ANS–CNS Rhythm and the BRAC

Shannahoff-Khalsa first reported a model for the hypothalamic control and integration of various ultradian rhythms (Shannahoff-Khalsa, 1991b). The same model was again later described in a multivariate physiological ultradian study of the autonomic, neuroendocrine, cardiovascular, and fuel-regulatory systems (Shannahoff-Khalsa *et al.*, 1996). That same model is again reported here.

In Swanson's comprehensive overview and review of the hypothalamus he states:

> It has been accepted for many years on the basis of physiological and behavioral evidence that the essential role of the hypothalamus is to integrate endocrine, autonomic, and behavioral responses that are

> essential for survival of the individual (homeostasis) and the species as a whole (reproduction). It may very well be that gram for gram the hypothalamus is the most important piece of tissue in any organism (Swanson, 1987).

Swanson also states "the outstanding question has always been, what is the organization and neurotransmitter specificity of hypothalamic circuitry underlying this integration and mediating these responses?" A simplistic view is discussed here for how the hypothalamus may integrate and regulate this ANS–CNS rhythm which may account for many endocrine, autonomic, cardiovascular, and behavioral rhythms.

Others (Van Cauter and Honinckx, 1985) have discussed the issues of "single" or "multiple ultradian pacemakers" having hypothalamic origins, or a "central ultradian clock" possibly outside the hypothalamus, or the "extra-hypothalamic modulation" hypothesis with a hypothalamic ultradian pacemaker(s) influenced by ultradian rhythms outside the hypothalamus, or in general, a "uni- versus multioscillatory phenomena" for the various ultradian rhythms (Lavie and Kripke, 1981). There are two major questions: first, are all ultradian rhythms related? And if so, are they regulated and integrated by the same central pacemaker? Our results suggest that these ultradians are related and are probably primarily regulated by the same central pacemaker (Kennedy *et al.*, 1986; Shannahoff-Khalsa and Yates, 2000; Shannahoff-Khalsa *et al.*, 1996, 1997, 2001; Werntz *et al.*, 1983).

The model presented here explains how all ultradian rhythms may be related via the proposed ANS–CNS rhythm and second, that the hypothalamus itself is "the pacemaker." The confusion, in part, with the "single" versus "multiple" ultradian pacemaker theories comes first by assuming there is no coordinated relationship between the various rhythms, and therefore individual pacemakers would be needed for each rhythm. This is equivalent to saying that neuroendocrine, cardiovascular, and behavioral phenomena are not coupled to autonomic phenomena or under hypothalamic control. Part of this confusion may also come from viewing the individual hypothalamic nuclei as independent of each other. This confusion of multi- versus single-pacemaker theories may in part stem from regulation of circadian rhythms by the suprachiasmatic nucleus (Watanabe and Hiroshige, 1981). It is likely, however, that this nucleus also helps couple circadian activities with the ultradian.

In the model proposed here, the hypothalamus is envisioned as a single organ in which the various nuclei, like organs, are functional parts of "a" body. Everything works together and has some relationship even with distant parts. The hypothalamus works much like a clock or pacemaker in a classical sense in which different regions, at different times, are more active. In this model that views the hypothalamus as a circle (see Fig. 34), the two sides and their respective fiber systems are directly related to the ipsilateral sides of the body and the ipsilateral cortex.

This neuroanatomical relationship is supported by the fact that the vast majority of autonomic fibers run ipsilaterally without the crossing-over seen in most other fiber systems running in and out of the brain (Saper *et al.*, 1976). The hypothalamus is, therefore, first bisected with respect to the two sides and the homologous nuclei are then divided between the two halves of the circle. Second, a division is made between the rostral and caudal halves. The rostral parts are predominantly concerned with parasympathetic mechanisms while the caudal parts are predominantly concerned with sympathetic mechanisms. This rostral-parasympathetic versus caudal-sympathetic axis is based on the early seminal work on the hypothalamus (Hess, 1947, 1954; Ranson and Magoun, 1939). We now envision our circle as a clock with four quadrants. The midline posterior point is 12 o'clock, the line bisecting the posterior and anterior regions runs from 3 o'clock on the right side to 9 o'clock on the left, and so on.

This hypothalamic clock has only one hand that runs as a rigid diameter of the circle rotating about its midpoint. This hand specifies both the "time" of the ANS–CNS rhythm and the nuclei that are most active. The nuclei closest to the hand determine what would be an increase in or a "metabolic gradient of activity" in the expression of their respective functions. This organizing principle makes the model useful for considering the possible relations of

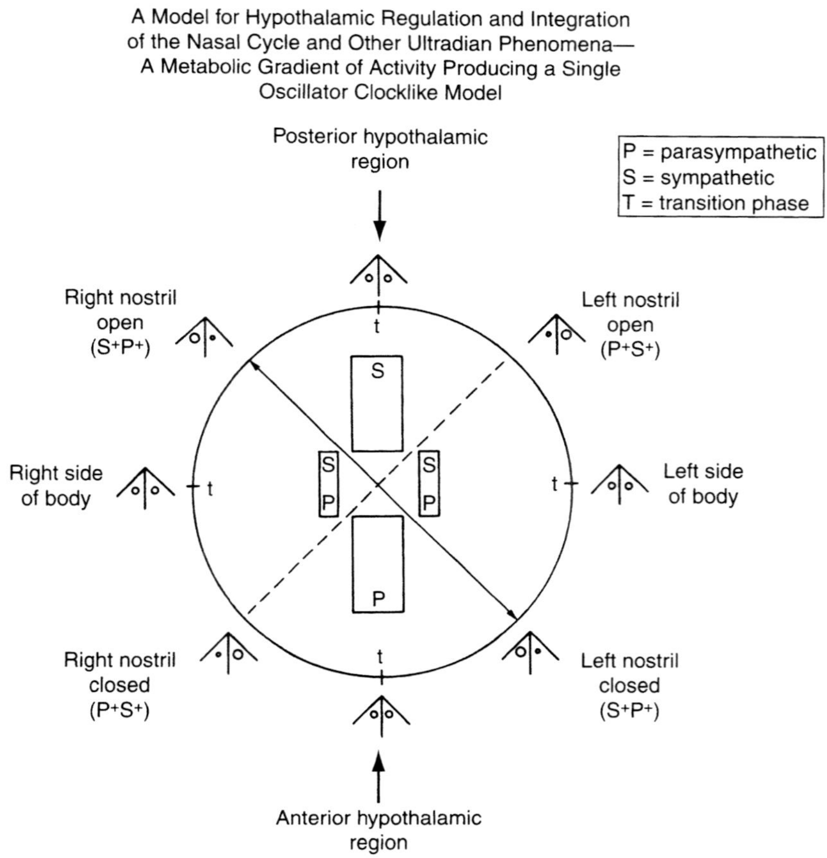


FIG. 34. This is a model for the hypothalamic regulation of the hourly ultradian rhythms. The circle represents the hypothalamus as one organ composed of the individual nuclei without differentiating beyond four hypothetical quadrants. A midline bisection (not drawn in) of posterior to anterior regions or 12 to 6 o'clock divides the hypothalamus into right and left mirror images, separating homologous nuclei. A perpendicular bisection separating the anterior and posterior regions on both right and left sides (not drawn in) indicates a division between parasympathetic and sympathetic regions, respectively. The hatched line from 1:30 to 7:30 indicates a hypothetical clock time for the proposed metabolic gradient of activity within the hypothalamus with its expression in the periphery where the left nostril is open and the right nostril is congested. The unbroken line represents another hypothetical time in this clock where the "hand" indicates the phase of the metabolic gradient of activity, here with dominance in the right posterior quadrant producing sympathetic dominance on the right side of the body, and right nostril open, and dominance in the left anterior quadrant producing parasympathetic dominance and congestion in the left nostril. Reprinted from Shannahoff-Khalsa; copyright (1991), with permission from Taylor & Francis.

various functions and their respective nuclei. In a physical sense, the "time" is also told by the phase of the nasal cycle. If the hand extends from 12 to 6, then equal activity is expected along this midline region where equal right and left sympathetic and parasympathetic function is expected on the two sides of the body, thus producing equal vasoconstriction-vasodilation in both nostrils and equal airflow in both nostrils. This represents a transition point in nasal dominance. A transition point also occurs when the hand is at 3 and 9 o'clock, where the left body will have half sympathetic and half parasympathetic influence, as would be the case for the right side of the body. When the hand is at 1:30 and 7:30, the first quadrant (left side of body) shows dominant sympathetic function (open left nostril) and the third quadrant (right side of body) shows dominant parasympathetic function (congested nostril). The complete reverse event occurs again at 4:30 and 10:30.

The proposed dynamics of the hand are as follows: the clock starts with the hand straight up (12 and 6) and then turns either clockwise to 3 and 9 o'clock or counterclockwise to 9 and 3. After it goes from 12 and 6 to 3 and 9, it resets back to 12 and 6 then reverses to 9 and 3, and again back to 12 and 6. This operation gives equal time to the functions of each quadrant and accounts in principle for a clocklike ANS–CNS rhythm. This clock could be the regulator and integrator for physiological and psychological phenomena. It does not presume a separation between the two, a distinction that is usually perceived for mental and physical systems.

Is there additional evidence to support this hypothesis? Here, only a few of the many pieces of supportive evidence are included. First, several studies show a direct neural connection between one side of the hypothalamus and an ipsilateral organ. Studies show a direct ipsilateral neural link to the ovaries (Gerendai, 1980; Gerendai and Halasz, 1997; Nance *et al.*, 1984), testes (Mizunuma *et al.*, 1983), and adrenal glands (Halasz and Szentagothai, 1959). Another study shows an asymmetrical lutenizing hormone releasing hormone (LHRH) distribution in the rat hypothalamus, with Wistar rats exhibiting higher LHRH content in the right hypothalamus and albino rats exhibiting higher LHRH content on the left

(Bakalkin *et al.*, 1984). These researchers state that LHRH content changes from side to side over a 24-h period and that unilateral castration or cold stress lead to a shift in LHRH distribution in the hypothalamus. When total hypothalamic dopamine and norepinephrine are measured in the rat over time, ultradian rhythms appear (Eriksson *et al.*, 1980) and resemble those found in the periphery (Kennedy *et al.*, 1986; Shannahoff-Khalsa *et al.*, 1996). Knobil states "the hypothalamus of mammals contains an oscillator or pulse generator that in the unmodulated state has a period of approximately 1 h in monkeys and humans. The activation of this system initiates a cascade of neuroendocrine events that are required for normal gonadal function in both sexes. Deviation from the physiological frequency of the pulse generator leads to profound disturbances of the reproductive process" (Knobil, 1987). Sometimes pulse-related neuronal activity was found only on one side of the hypothalamus (Knobil, personal communication).

Another relevant finding is that the hypothalamic paraventricular nucleus seems to play a modulating role in the production of REM sleep and in the generation of its rhythm (Piepenbrock *et al.*, 1985). Electrical stimulation of specific regions within the hypothalamus in cats can induce bilateral and unilateral nasal constriction, retraction of the nictitating membranes, and a rise in arterial blood pressure (Eccles and Lee, 1981). These responses occur on stimulation of regions previously described as the defense area. Many other studies support the concept of defense areas being located in the posterior region of the hypothalamus and parasympathetic functions being located in the anterior regions. For example, lesions placed in the anterior hypothalamic region led to a decrease in immune responses, suggesting that this region is related to resting or parasympathetic functions (Roszman and Brooks, 1985; Roszman *et al.*, 1985).

The model presented here provides only a very simplified view, but may accurately describe a mechanism for how autonomic, neuroendocrine, cardiovascular, immune, and behavioral activities may be regulated in concert. Knobil (1987) emphasizes the importance of not deviating from the normal pulse generator frequency, lest profound disturbances in reproductive processes occur. It may be that health is determined by the proposed metabolic gradient of activity in the various hypothalamic nuclei and that the consequent integration of these nuclei is a direct correlate of health where some rhythmic regularity is required. It may be that stress directly affects this hypothalamic clock and determines the balance of activity in the four quadrants. Different forms of stress would likely impact the clocks timing differently. Fight-or-flight stress, catastrophic depression, and anxiety are all likely to affect different quadrants:

> The wobble nature of these hourly ultradian rhythms may reflect in part a loosely integrated, or degenerative condition in specific hypothalamic nuclei, and/or a "flexibility" in the hypothalamic neural network that regulates and integrates this clock-like relationship of the individual nuclei. "Flexibility" may have evolved to help account for the adaptive requirements of variable conditions, especially external to the system. However, this "wobble," aperiodic, or nonlinear dynamical quality is inherent in all biological systems and is likely to have evolved to enable changes that are both internal (including developmental) and external (Shannahoff-Khalsa *et al.*, 1996).

Some subjects in our study show exception to the general phase coupling relationship between certain parameters (see Figs. 23–30), suggesting that "wobble" and "flexibility" may be a way of allowing for different physiological intersystem relationships. Studying the multivariate physiology of subjects at different ages, environmental conditions, and states of health and disease may help us to better understand the observed nonlinear features of ultradian rhythms and their relationship to health.

## E. Laterality and the BRAC

The evolutionary emergence of the lateralized rhythms of neural activity reflects an advancement in the integration of the structural and temporal aspects of an organism's metabolic activities, no doubt to help enhance survival in an ever-changing environment. While lateralized neural rhythms are not incorporated in Kleitman's

BRAC hypothesis, the BRAC reflects one of the most elementary needs of any organism—expending energy and resting. The ultradian rhythms have been viewed as an "economic principle not to spend energy continuously at a relative high level (as demanded at times) but to alternate between expenditure and restoration of energy" (Aschoff and Gerkema, 1985). Any remaining controversy over the existence of the general phenomenon defined by the BRAC hypothesis, and sometimes for ultradian rhythms per se is based on two issues. First is the variability and wobble quality in the frequency with these rhythms, and second is whether there is a single or multiple oscillators driving them. Furthermore, the functional significance of ultradian rhythms has been much debated. For example, two prominent researchers state that "In considering the functional significance of ultradian rhythms, one should first keep in mind that a rhythmic organization (of whatever frequency) is one of the means to keep temporal order within the organism. Where many processes have to be maintained which to some degree are mutually exclusive, but nevertheless cooperate, a temporal compartmentalization by rhythmic alternation is an obvious solution" (Aschoff and Gerkema, 1985). They also state that "it is impossible to postulate one common mechanism for all ultradian rhythms" (Aschoff and Gerkema, 1985). However, when the phenomenon of the lateralized neural rhythms of the CNS and ANS and their coupling with the cardiovascular, neuroendocrine, and fuel-regulatory systems are included, a broader perspective can be conceived for the functional significance of these numerous ultradian rhythms and a structure–function model becomes more apparent. And a single oscillator model for hypothalamic regulation and integration of these various rhythms becomes a logical candidate given the data to date. This model that includes the hypothalamus as the central integrating, coordinating, and regulating agent is thus an extension to the BRAC hypothesis with a new spatial–temporal framework and thus adds to our understanding for how systems at large are organized. It has been proposed that this phenomenon has also evolved as "a neural matrix for coupling mind and metabolism" (Shannahoff-Khalsa, 1991b). I argue that these lateralized rhythms manifest as a pendulum of ANS–CNS activity to help maintain homeostasis, "not as a single homeostatic state, but as a continuous alternation between two polar conditions for both mind and metabolism" (Shannahoff-Khalsa, 1991b). The alternating dominance of two polar states of mind would be advantageous compared to a static and rigid state of cerebral activity. Rhythms of alternating cerebral hemispheric efficiency can be used to accommodate different and specific tasks. This alternation can be coupled to metabolic states such as the ergotrophic and trophotropic states that may more readily support their respective activities. This alternation may thus be one of nature's ways of maximizing economic efficiency and increasing competence under specific conditions.

What follows is a further history and explanation of various studies of how the BRAC and lateralized rhythms are coupled. Although numerous ultradian rhythms have been discovered, it may be that all physiological and psychological phenomena exhibit ultradian dynamics. However, few researchers have sought to study the multivariate relations among the discovered ultradian phenomena. This lack of effort has impeded the development of an integrated view of the interactions among the various systems, a view that can provide a new understanding of the structural and temporal organization of biological processes, and thus also a better understanding of psychophysiological states.

Tables X–XIII (X, autonomic physiology; XI, cerebral relations; XII, neuroendocrine relations; and XIII, behavioral relations) list the proposed relationships among known ultradian rhythms and lateralized autonomic dominance. This autonomic dominance is either right sympathetic dominance coupled with left parasympathetic dominance, or the converse, left sympathetic dominance coupled with right parasympathetic dominance. Question marks in the tables indicate that correlations are uncertain. In Table XI, various correlations are proposed for the severity of syndromes linked to the psychopathologies discussed in Section VI.

Kleitman's BRAC hypothesis of interacting systems had its origins in the discovery that EEG and eye movement patterns change in concert during sleep, giving rise to the concept of REM and NREM

TABLE X

PROPOSED ORGANIZATION OF ULTRADIAN RHYTHMS: AUTONOMIC PHYSIOLOGY[a]

| R. sympath./L. parasympath. dominance | L. sympath./R. parasympath. dominance |
|---|---|
| Right nostril dominance | Left nostril dominance |
| Right lung dominant | Left lung dominant |
| Right adrenal more active | Left adrenal more active |
| Right-side increased perspiration | Left-side increased perspiration |
| Right-side increased catecholamines | Left-side increased catecholamines |
| Ergotrophic state | Trophotropic state |
| Active phase-BRAC-blood glucose up | Resting phase-BRAC-blood glucose lower |
| Generalized sympathetic tonus | Generalized parasympathetic tonus |
| Locomotor activity increased | Locomotor activity reduced |
| Right pupil more dilated than left | Left pupil more dilated than right |
| Heart rate increased (stroke volume reduced) | Heart rate reduced (stroke volume increased) |
| Blood pressure increased | Blood pressure reduced |
| Respiration rate increased | Respiration rate reduced |
| Oxygen consumption increased | Oxygen consumption reduced |
| Body temperature increased | Body temperature reduced |
| Involuntary eyeblink rate reduced | Involuntary eyeblink rate increased |
| Intraocular pressure reduced | Intraocular pressure increased |

[a]This table lists the relationship of various ultradian phenomena that are part of autonomic physiology and are proposed to correlate with two polar and separate states of lateralized autonomic balance, described as (1) right sympathetic dominance with simultaneous left parasympathetic dominance; and (2) left parasympathetic dominance with simultaneous left sympathetic dominance. Reprinted from Shannahoff-Khalsa; copyright (1991), with permission from Elsevier.

TABLE XI

PROPOSED ORGANIZATION OF ULTRADIAN RHYTHMS: CEREBRAL RELATIONS[a]

| R. sympath./L. parasympath. dominance | L. sympath./R. parasympath. dominance |
|---|---|
| Left-hemisphere dominance | Right-hemisphere dominance |
| Verbal performance increased | Spatial performance increased |
| Left-hemisphere EEG power greater | Right-hemisphere EEG power greater |
| REM sleep | NREM sleep |
| Cerebral metabolic rate increased | Cerebral metabolic rate reduced |
| Lateralized immune functions? | Lateralized immune functions? |
| Daydreaming reduced? | Daydreaming increased? |
| EEG alpha minimum? | EEG alpha maximum? |
| Spiral aftereffect shorter? | Spiral aftereffect longer? |
| Depression/anxiety minimum? | Depression/anxiety maximum? |
| Euphoric-manic state maximum? | Euphoric-manic state minimal? |
| Hysteria reduced? | Hysteria increased? |
| Catatonia reduced? | Catatonia increased? |
| Schizoid active positive syndrome? | Schizoid withdrawn negative syndrome? |

[a]This table lists ultradian phenomena that exhibit as cerebral activities and how they correlate with the two polar autonomic states. Reprinted from Shannahoff-Khalsa; copyright (1991), with permission from Elsevier.

TABLE XII

PROPOSED ORGANIZATION OF ULTRADIAN RHYTHMS: NEUROENDOCRINE RELATIONS[a]

| R. sympath./L. parasympath. dominance | L. sympath./R. parasympath. dominance |
|---|---|
| Cortisol increased | Cortisol reduced |
| Growth hormone reduced | Growth hormone increased |
| Luteinizing hormone increased | Luteinizing hormone reduced |
| LHRH enhances verbal fluency (males) | LHRH reduces spatial (males) |
| Prolactin secretion reduced | Prolactin secretion increased |
| Testosterone increased | Testosterone reduced |
| Penile tumescence increased/sleep | Penile tumescence reduced/sleep |
| Parathyroid hormone reduced | Parathyroid hormone increased |
| Calcium (+2) increased | Calcium (+2) reduced |
| Endorphins increased | Endorphins reduced |
| Corticotrophin releasing hormone increased? | Corticotrophin releasing hormone reduced? |

[a]This table lists the ultradian phenomena of neuroendocrine activity with their correlations. Reprinted from Shannahoff-Khalsa; copyright (1991), with permission from Elsevier.

TABLE XIII

PROPOSED ORGANIZATION OF ULTRADIAN RHYTHMS: BEHAVIORAL RELATIONS[a]

| R. sympath./L. parasympath. dominance | L. sympath./R. parasympath. dominance |
|---|---|
| Oral drive increased | Oral drive reduced |
| Hunger sensations increased | Hunger sensations reduced |
| Stomach contractions increased | Stomach contractions reduced |
| Gastric acid secretion increased | Gastric acid secretion reduced |
| Salavation increased | Salavation reduced |
| Grip strength increased | Grip strength reduced |
| Thorndike intelligence exam improved | Thorndike intelligence exam reduced |
| Urine flow reduced? | Urine flow increased? |
| Urine osmolarity increased? | Urine osmolarity reduced? |

[a]This table lists the behavioral relations and their proposed correlations. Phenomena that are listed with question marks have proposed relationships as discussed in the text. Reprinted from Shannahoff-Khalsa; copyright (1991), with permission from Elsevier.

sleeps stages where there are cyclic variations in EEG patterns, they are tightly coupled to eye movements, body motility, and dreaming (Dement and Kleitman, 1957a,b; Kleitman, 1961, 1967d, 1982). The BRAC formulation was supposed to explain why some psychological and physiological activities are integrated and account for the obvious patterns of intermixed locomotor activity and quiescent states during sleep. Kleitman proposed the BRAC to include a waking correlate of the sleep pattern with a variation of integrated events during the 24-h period (Kleitman, 1967d), and that "the BRAC is probably a fundamental variation in the functioning of the central nervous system, increasing in duration with phylogenetic progression" where "in each species of mammal studied, the BRAC also lengthens during ontogenetic development."

One of the first seminal studies on ultradian rhythms goes back to 1922 with work on hunger and its relationship to activity, and how these results give us insight to endogenous rhythms and homeostasis (Wada, 1922). Wada proposed that food was the first form of property for primitive man; the value of things supposedly first came to be measured in terms of food, and primitive migration was primarily motivated by food. Wada, therefore, surmised that basic homeostatic mechanisms are coupled to hunger. Investigations of the relationship of the hunger rhythm with bodily movements, dreaming, motor activity, salivation, and mental activity led Wada to discover a rhythm of salivary flow that parallels the gastric hunger contraction rhythm (Wada, 1922). But surprisingly, Wada also found that men dream more at the hunger contraction periods than during quiescence. Motor activity during waking, as judged by a hand-dynamomotor, showed that at hunger contraction periods the power of grip is greater than at the quiescent or after-dinner periods. Hunger contractions also correlated with scores on the Thorndike Intelligence Examination. These seminal studies on the relationship of activity to hunger predate Kleitman's concept of the BRAC. Wada recognized that "with the onset of hunger the sleeping baby awakes to feed," and in general, "when the effort to satisfy hunger is thwarted, the whole organism reacts to the situation, or thwarting agent, with such hypertension of all organs and muscles and fibers that the excitement may lead to various types of defensive behavior." Therefore, Wada saw the hunger mechanism as one of the most primitive, and as certainly a central regulating aspect of physiology. This primitive rhythm and mechanism is another way of viewing the BRAC: hunt and eat, then rest. An important question is how is this homeostatic rhythm of hunger coupled with those such as the secretion of pituitary hormones and other ultradian rhythms.

One study in 1980 showed that "in rats, lengths of cycles of growth hormone (GH) secretion and of cycles of feeding are 3.6–4.0 h" and that they are phase coupled (Richter, 1980). Richter also suggested that "these two cyclic phenomena may be manifestations of the same timing mechanism in the brain or they could function entirely independently." GH is known to be secreted predominantly during NREM sleep in humans (Parker and Rossman, 1973; Pawel *et al.*, 1972). Even though GH secretion does not exhibit an apparent rhythm during much of the 24-h cycle, this link with NREM is an important clue to an association between hypothalamic and cortical rhythms. Since pituitary rhythms vary with age, sex, and species, this variance has complicated attempts to establish relationships among the various rhythmic phenomena.

The first discovery of the pulsatile or episodic nature of pituitary hormone secretion was in 1966 with the observation that discrete pulses of cortisol secretion reflect rhythmic secretion of ACTH (Weitzman *et al.*, 1966). Early work also showed that the pituitary hormones are secreted with an ultradian rhythm (Kripke, 1982; Van Cauter and Honinckx, 1985) and that their secretion patterns are related to REM and NREM sleep. Lutenizing hormone secretion is positively coupled to REM sleep (Boyar *et al.*, 1972a,b). Testosterone secretion was found to be phase linked with cortisol secretion (Van Cauter and Honinckx, 1985) providing evidence for synchronization between the pituitary-adrenal and pituitary-gonadal axis. Testosterone is also known to be secreted in phase with the ultradian cycles of penile tumescent during sleep (Schiavi *et al.*, 1977) that coincide with REM sleep cycles (Karacan *et al.*, 1972). Prolactin secretion was found to increase during NREM periods (Parker *et al.*, 1974; Weitzman, 1976a,b). However, this finding was later refuted (Van Cauter and Honinckx, 1985). In adult rats, the 3-h rhythms of GH and corticosterone secretion are 180° out of phase, with GH being secreted during NREM sleep (Kimura *et al.*, 1985). These phase relations between GH and corticosterone secretion are similar to those found in adult humans (Takahashi *et al.*, 1968). Plasma parathyroid hormone and calcium levels are also related to sleep stages (Kripke *et al.*, 1978) so that peaks in parathyroid hormone secretion are significantly related to NREM sleep stages 3 and 4 while elevated calcium levels are significantly related to REM sleep. Cross-correlation analysis between "humoral endorphin," an endogenous opioid, and sleep stages confirmed a relationship with REM sleep (Sarne *et al.*, 1981).

One study of the secretion of corticotrophin-releasing factor (CRF), the hypothalamic hormone that initiates and integrates the stress response, revealed a diurnal rhythm in human males when sampled with only four samples per day (Watabe *et al.*, 1987). However, continuous monitoring of CRF in the cerebrospinal fluid of adult male monkeys by contrast produced profiles characteristic of an ultradian rhythm (Kalin *et al.*, 1987). And in an effort to measure the temporal release of CRF directly, one group of researchers established an *in vitro* perifusion system using the isolated hypothalamus from the macaque where perifusate samples were collected at 10-min intervals for 20 h (Mershon *et al.*, 1992). They found a very regular, pulsatile pattern of hormone release with a pulse interval of 90 + 11 min. CRF, like other hypothalamic-pituitary factors, thus appears to have variations in levels of secretion that also exhibit ultradian rhythms of the "hourly" domain. Even though it is considered a "stress" peptide, CRF secretion may also covary with locomotor activity under normal unstressed conditions. Plasma levels of LH, for example, show a direct relationship to rhythmic motor activity or the ultradian rest–activity cycle in ovariectomized sheep (Rasmussen and Malven, 1981). Rats who have lost their circadian rhythm due to lesions in the suprachiasmatic nuclei show an ultradian phase-locked relationship between locomotor activity and plasma corticosterone (Watanabe and Hiroshige, 1981). Most authors do not ascribe any particular significance to the ultradian nature of pituitary hormone secretion, suggesting that the cause of this rhythmic phenomenon is unknown. However, in light of the available evidence, it is reasonable to propose that such rhythms help modulate and reflect the coupling of the CNS with the ANS. This coupling underlies the BRAC and the accompanying coupling of psychological phenomena with rhythms of the hypothalamic-pituitary-adrenal-gonadal axes. Interestingly, it has been shown in men (but not women) that injections of LHRH prevent improvement in a spatial orientation task (right-hemisphere skill), but enhanced performance on a fluency task (left-hemisphere skill) (Gordon *et al.*, 1986). The resulting increase in LH and correlated enhancement of left-hemispheric skills is consistent with elevated LH during REM sleep, also a correlate of an activated left hemisphere.

In addition to the earlier work (Wada, 1922) on the relationship of stomach contractions to dreaming and body movement, there are other studies showing that "REM periods are related to a cyclic waxing and waning of instinctual drive activity mediated through the limbic system," particularly in eating behavior (Friedman and Fisher, 1967). They report a statistically significant waking state oral activity cycle of 80–120 min based on the subject's use of drink, food, and tobacco. Another study of human ingestive activity shows a similar activity cycle of about 90 min (Oswald *et al.*, 1970). Although both studies show considerable variability in the cycles, the range is similar to that of other ultradian phenomena. Ultradian rhythms of gastric pH in humans during night show a range of 1.07–5.5 h, clustering around 2–3 h (Tarouini *et al.*, 1986). A nocturnal study of gastric secretion in fasting subjects, showed "a wide individual variation and a considerable spontaneous variation of the gastric secretion in the same individual from hour to hour and also from night to night" (Levin *et al.*, 1948, 1950). In another study, gastric motility and pH were recorded during night sleep and showed a consistent pattern of motility decreasing and acidity increasing in deep sleep relative to waking levels (Baust and Rohrwasser, 1969). Motility was markedly enhanced during REM sleep, but there was not a constant relation between the occurrence of peristaltic waves and the outbursts of REMs. Others demonstrated 100-min cycles in gastric motility during sleep and found only minimal relations to REM periods (which may be due to the lack of adaptation nights, and/or a nasogastric tube sometimes with or without a balloon) (Lavie *et al.*, 1978). They conclude, "since hunger and feeding behaviors may be weakly related to stomach contractions, it is still to be determined if appetitive behaviors have any mechanism in common with stage REM." Also, periodic interdigestive secretion of the pancreas, liver, and stomach were found in canines with a peak interval of 100 min and a range of 80–130 min (Magee and Naruse, 1983).

Others demonstrated an ultradian rhythm in human respiration rates when looking for a correlate of the BRAC (Horne and Whitehead, 1976). Most subjects showed a periodicity of 90 min (±15). Oscillations in oxygen consumption in resting humans with periods of 1–2 h, with changes in amplitudes of 7–20% of the mean, have also been discovered (Bailey *et al.*, 1973). They conclude "that the oxygen consumption of men and women resting comfortably in the postabsorptive state is not constant, but subject to cyclic variations." Also, "We have no direct experimental or theoretical explanation for cycles of 1–2 h. They may be examples of 'hunting reactions' about a set point in the control system for body temperature." Aspects of the BRAC have been studied in rats where an ultradian rhythm in body temperature was found that is coupled to the rhythms of locomotor activity (Honma and Honma, 1985). They state "Generally, a locomotor burst preceded a rise in abdominal temperature, but occasionally the rise in body temperature preceded the burst of locomotor activity. This reversed pattern seems to preclude the possibility that there is a causal relationship between the two parameters." Therefore, it is likely that these relations are centrally mediated and are two ways of measuring a more general phenomenon. In a study of lateralized relations of handgrip strength and body temperature in 48 male subjects (testing only at four to five times per day, intervals which are not adequate to elicit ultradian periods), researchers found a circadian period in oral temperature in humans that was correlated with the grip strength of the dominant hand, but not with the nondominant hand (Reinberg *et al.*, 1988). They conclude "Thus, circadian rhythms in oral temperature and dominant handgrip strength may be driven by the same oscillator while that of the non-dominant hand may be governed by a different one. . . . A coherent body of indirect evidence thus emerges supporting the idea that circadian oscillators may well be located in the human brain cortex and not only (or mainly) in the archaic brain as has been shown in animal rodent models." This suggests that the active phase of the BRAC in humans correlates with left cerebral hemisphere dominance. Other results on sleep and hemisphericity are presented (see Section II.B.1 and II.B.2).

Taken together, the available evidence suggests that the ultradian rhythms of the BRAC, eating-oral-gastric rhythms, pituitary rhythms, sleep stages, and other cerebral rhythms have a central common regulator. This conclusion helps to reshape how we think about the cerebral-hypothalamic-pituitary-adrenal-gonadal axes and the role that this CNS–ANS rhythm, modulated by the hypothalamus, plays in the regulation of psychophysiological states.

### 1. *Ultradian Rhythms in Arousal, Performance, and Behavior*

The discovery of the REM and NREM sleep cycle has inspired many studies looking for the waking correlates of the sleep rhythm. While this topic is not reviewed here in any depth due to the large number of studies over the years, I will only discuss a few representative papers to provide a chronobiological perspective on arousal, performance, and behavior. These rhythmic phenomena are likely to reflect the waking rhythm of alternating cerebral hemispheric activity.

First it is important to note that the REM–NREM cycle duration is species-specific and dependent on age, body size, and metabolism. The REM–NREM sleep cycle is typically and perhaps confusingly been called "the 90-min rhythm" as if it were without significant variability. The cycle length of REM and NREM sleep in humans has been reviewed (Kobayashi *et al.*, 1985). The range in one study is 38–170 min in young adults (mean age 23 years) and in another 31–171 min (mean age 22 years), and between 27 and 138 min in older subjects (mean age 58 years). They state that cycles greater than 140 min in young adults are composed of very long NREM stage 4 sleep, which usually occurs as the first NREM event. In addition, it is important to note that NREM periods are much longer and REM periods shorter at the beginning of the night. And then NREM periods almost disappear and REM periods increase in length as the night progresses. This same group also studied ultradian components of daytime arousal in nine subjects between 11:00 a.m. and 7:30 p.m. by administering the multiple sleep latency tests every 20 min an objective index of sleepiness (Tsuji and Kobayashi, 1988). They also analyzed long-duration wideband EEG by using principal components analysis (PCA) constructed from the percentage-power values of 16 frequency bands (2–18 Hz) to extract the features of ultradian rhythmicities. They state:

> The diurnal rhythm of the arousal EEG was made up of 2 ultradian components with periods of about 100 min and 3–8 h. The shorter component is thought to represent the oscillation of vigilance level between mental "rest" and "activity" states in the BRAC. The longer component is thought to represent variations in levels of consciousness between "wakefulness" and "drowsiness" states. Our interpretation of the data suggests that the shorter component is superimposed upon the longer one, and that the specific arousal state involved in the shorter ultradian rhythmicity changes to another state at around the "breaking point" in mid-afternoon (Tsuji and Kobayashi, 1988).

They also found a significant correlation and visually convincing relationship between the multiple sleep latency tests and the PCA in five of nine subjects. In the subjects that did not show a tight coupling, they note these subjects did not show any cyclical change in their multiple sleep latency tests.

One group studied ultradians of performance in 25 subjects (16 males and 9 females) aged 18–27 using the Rosvold-Mirsky Continuous Performance Test (12 letters are flashed in sequence and every time A–K appears a lever press response is required) (Globus *et al.*, 1971). The data from 19 usuable 6-h records indicate a broadband around 100 min (range 21.7–266.7 min).

In a study of heart rate and the performance of a complex vigilance task (monitoring of three panel meters with scored responses), one group planned to observe 11 young male adults for 48 h or until they felt they could no longer continue (Orr *et al.*, 1974). All subjects completed at least 21 h and two went to 44 h. The data were subjected to complex demodulation to determine the characteristics and presence of a period in the range of 90 min. The primary finding in 75% of the analyses was a marked increase in the amplitude of the 90-min rhythm in both heart rate and performance measures.

The social and solitary behavior of four pairs of subadult to adult male monkeys was observed for 8.5 h (Maxim *et al.*, 1976). The social activity occurred at a regular rate for a given pair but differed among pairs. The youngest pair had a rhythm of 40–45 min, the two middle pairs showed cycle lengths of 65 and 85–90 min, and the oldest pair had a cycle of 125 min for interactive versus solitary behavior. The solitary activities of ingestion, self-grooming, exploration, and locomotion all had periodicities of 40–45, 85–95, 125–140, and 155–170 min in length.

One of the pioneers of ultradian rhythms studied alertness by measuring pupillary motility, size, and light reflexes every 15 min for 10 h in eight young adults and found a 75–120 min rhythm in pupillary motility that was out of phase with the diameter and light reflex response (Lavie, 1979). He concludes, these rhythms "reflect underlying rhythms in CNS arousal that also modulate perceptual, cognitive, and EEG processes, a conclusion which supports Kleitman's BRAC model."

Ten years later, due to the confusion in the field of ultradian rhythm research over the exact "periodicity," he addresses the variability in ultradian rhythms of arousal and how they can be easily masked (Lavie, 1989). Lavie states "The ultradian cycles in arousal are of relatively low amplitude compared with the large changes in the state of the brain associated with the sleep–wake circadian cycles. The ultradian cycles are unstable and frequently cannot be detected without sophisticated mathematical and statistical techniques. Furthermore, attempts to explain their origin relied on a single hypothesis (Kleitman's BRAC model) which appeared to be too ambiguous and parsimonious." He further elaborates on the difficulties of linking the REM–NREM cycle with waking rhythms of arousal due to masking and the variability of the morning (1.5 h) and afternoon (2.5–3 h) arousal rhythms.

### 2. *A Neural Matrix for Coupling Mind and Metabolism*

Earlier I described how the lateralized rhythms of the ANS and the regulatory role of the hypothalamus affect the lateralized CNS rhythms. This relationship provides compelling evidence that the ANS via its sympathetic, parasympathetic, and enteric branches acts as a "neural matrix for coupling states of mind and metabolism"

(Shannahoff-Khalsa, 1991b). States of lateralized cerebral activation, whether during waking or sleep, are clearly rhythmic and have a direct relation to other important physiological and psychological phenomena, and without exception the BRAC. Looking at these individual ultradian rhythms, without being aware of the generalized rhythm of the ANS–CNS as the integrating phenomenon, evokes the tale of the blind men and the elephant. As a single physical phenomenon, the nasal cycle as a marker of ANS activity, allows us to assess other ultradian ANS-dependent phenomena, since the nasal cycle can be easily and noninvasively measured and apparently provides direct access for the assessment of other ANS–CNS phenomena. In this way, the nasal cycle becomes a marker of state.

Besides the humoral effects of the nervous system on the immune system, the ANS serves as neural matrix for regulation of the immune system. It has been shown that the ANS innervates virtually all lymphoid tissues (Bulloch, 1985). For example, the thymus, a dual-lobed organ, receives independent innervation from sympathetic and parasympathetic nerves for each lobe. Therefore, in light of the lateralized rhythms of the ANS, it is possible that the functions of the two thymic lobes are rhythmic, one being active while the other is resting and regenerating as is the case with the kidneys (Beickert, 1951) and the adrenals (Benton and Yates, 1990). An important question is whether the two thymic lobes are identical in their functions. Do the functions of one lobe and its immune parameters correlate with one mode of cerebral intelligence and its respective neuroendocrine state, etc.? Thymic hormones are known to have an influence on the hypothalamic-pituitary axis (Hall and Goldstein, 1983). There are also connections in the other direction. Bilateral electrolytic lesions in the anterior hypothalamus influence an animal's immune potential, causing a marked decrease in the number of nucleated spleen cells and thymocytes as compared to normal animals or frontal cortex lesioned animals (Roszman *et al.*, 1985). Also, bilateral lesions produced in either the anterior or posterior basal hypothalamus of guinea pigs have differential effects, where anterior lesions result in protection to anaphylactic shock, compared to posterior lesions or sham-operated controls (Macris *et al.*, 1970). If the two thymic lobes are dissimilar, it may be that different pituitary hormones help facilitate one lobe of thymic function over the other.

The evidence reviewed here also suggests that there are lateralized ultradian rhythms of the lymph nodes and bone marrow activity on the two sides of the body, and that certain spleen functions may also correlate with different modes of cerebral intelligence. Therefore, "the ANS is also a neural matrix for coupling mind and immunity" (Shannahoff-Khalsa, 1991b). Various studies indicate that lateralized cerebral states may correlate with lateralized expression in the immune system. Bereavement, depression, and stress, for example, all affect immunity (Stein, 1985). It has also been shown in mice that lesions of the left frontoparietal cortex lead to depression of T lymphocyte functions while lesions of the right cortex augment T cell functions (Renoux *et al.*, 1983). Others find the same results with T cell functions (Neveu *et al.*, 1986), and that mitogenesis of B cells induced by lipopolysaccarides was modified by cortical lesions in the same way as T cells. They found that left-lesioned animals showed B cell proliferation decreased by 60% compared to controls, whereas right-lesioned animals showed B cell mitogenesis enhanced by 120% as compared to controls. The results for B cells were not found by Renoux *et al.*, who used pokeweed as a mitogen instead of lipopolysaccarides.

Studies of depression in humans show greater right cerebral dysfunction by EEG (Flor-Henry, 1987). This result, in the light of the animal cortex lesion studies, may help explain how immunity is suppressed by abnormal right-hemispheric activities in humans. Studies of hemispheric laterality and immune function have shown that left-handedness is associated with increased risk of autoimmune disease (Marx, 1982). Our understanding of psychoneuroimmunology may be increased by considering how the ANS acts as the neural matrix for coupling mind and immunity, especially with regard to lateralized rhythms. If we constantly shift between two separate modes of intelligence, modes of consciousness, or psychophysiological states, we may find that this rhythm is coupled to rhythms of T cell activity and other immune factors such as cytokine secretion.

Rhythms of immune function are an important but overlooked area both in immunology and chronobiology. However, we do know that there are ultradian rhythms in cytokines that have near identical chronobiological features with all the other ultradian phenomena so far discussed (Bouayad-Amine *et al.*, 1993).

Laterality also plays an important role in the neuroendocrine system which has many significant functional asymmetries that are manifested in gonadal control, thyroid control, differential prolactin responses to right- and left-sided mastectomies in mice, differential grooming responses to right- and left-sided vagotomy in mice, and mortality rates after unilateral brain lesions in mice; for review see Gerendai (1984, 1986), Gerendai and Halasz (1997). And clearly, all glands in the body have a dual representation or have two independently innervated lobes. This suggests that each side may play a different role in the BRAC, if not only one where one gland or lobe rests while the other secretes at greater levels.

Since sudden cardiac death is the leading cause of death in the industrialized world, it captures the attention of anyone interested in stress since the pathophysiological mechanisms of the phenomenon are rather mysterious and poorly understood. Although we know death is triggered by an abnormal electrical event to the heart that leads to ventricular tachycardia. This is supported by the fact that strong emotions play a primary role in sudden cardiac death, where they first affect the CNS which then affects the ANS causing ventricular fibrillation. Recently, one group showed an interesting result that has direct bearing on stress and lateralized brain stem mechanisms related to sudden cardiac death. They comment "From a cardiological perspective, the likelihood of arrhythmia is strongly associated with abnormalities in electrical repolarization (recovery) of the heart muscle after each contraction. Inhomogeneous and asymmetric repolarization, reflected in ECG T-wave abnormalities, is associated with a greatly increased risk of arrhythmia, that is a proarrhythmic state" (Critchley *et al.*, 2005). They studied the potential brain mechanisms by which stress can induce cardiac arrhythmia through efferent autonomic drive using 10 typical cardiac outpatients. They used $H_2O^{15}$ PET and ECG during mental and physical stress challenges and compared against control conditions. They state:

> Proarrhythmic changes in the heart were quantified from two ECG-derived measures of repolarization inhomogeneity and were related to changes in magnitude and lateralization of regional brain activity reflected in regional cerebral blood flow. Across the patient group, we observed a robust positive relationship between right-lateralized asymmetry in midbrain activity and proarrhythmic abnormalities of cardiac repolarization (apparent in two independent ECG measures) during stress. This association between stress-induced lateralization of midbrain activity and enhanced arrhythmic vulnerability provides empirical support for a putative mechanism for stress-induced sudden death, wherein lateralization of central autonomic drive during stress results in imbalanced activity in right and left cardiac sympathetic nerves. A right-left asymmetry in sympathetic drive across the surface of the heart disrupts the electrophysiological homogeneity of ventricular repolarization, predisposing to arrhythmia (Critchley *et al.*, 2005).

Interestingly, an earlier study employed a yogic breathing technique that is supposedly useful for helping to prevent and eliminate sudden cardiac death that would originate through abnormal electrical events to the heart. We showed a result that suggests the possibility of resetting the cardiopulmonary brain stem pacemaker that is likely to be implicated in the abnormal stress-related effects on the heart (Shannahoff-Khalsa *et al.*, 2004). This brain stem cardiopulmonary pacemaker is likely the same brain center that shows a lateral imbalance that is induced by stress (Critchley *et al.*, 2005).

A number of studies show that the ANS input to the heart is lateralized, with control of heart rate being more affected by the right sympathetic system, and heart rhythm or arrhythomogenesis being more affected by the left (Natelson, 1985). Laterality also exists in parasympathetically induced arrhythmias, with left vagus stimulation producing an A–V block via the atrioventricular node, and right vagus stimulation producing sinus arrest via the sinoatrial node. It appears therefore that activation or interference with specific sites in either the CNS or ANS may selectively affect heart rate and rhythm (Natelson, 1985). For further discussion on the differential and lateralized ANS influences and effects of selective unilateral activation of the left and right stellate ganglion and vagus nerves on the heart, see Section V.

### 3. *A Pendulum of ANS–CNS Activities and Homeostasis: A New Paradigm for Stress and Disease*

Knowledge of a pendulum-like activity of alternating lateral dominance in autonomic and CNS activity provides a new approach and perspective for the study of stress and stress mechanisms. The concept of a pendulum implies movement not within a single homeostatic state, but a continuous alternation between two polar states for both mind and metabolism. The lateralized rhythm of ANS–CNS activity is an integrative temporal and structural paradigm. This pendulum-like activity is the key to understanding how many apparently independent physiological and psychological phenomena are in fact coupled together. The pendulum of autonomic activity sets the frequency at which various activities are entrained and the autonomic fibers are the regulating circuitry. Stress may thus be defined by how long or how frequently a particular position of the pendulum is maintained. Too much left brain activity and right sympathetic dominance may indeed be what we normally think of as stress or "overwork and overactivity." It is easy to envision both acute swings and prolonged shifts toward one position of this pendulum, where either can lead to a disequilibrium or imbalance in system–system interactions.

As discussed earlier, the terms ergotrophic and trophotropic were coined by Hess to describe ANS functions. Again, ergotrophic reactions are coupled with energy expenditure and an endophylactic–trophotropic system provides for protection and restitution (Hess, 1954). These concepts have also been discussed at length in discourses on ANS-somatic integration (Gellhorn, 1967). The key concept here is the antagonistic relationship of the sympathetic and parasympathetic systems in maintaining these two polar states.

Left nostril/right brain dominance, or left sympathetic/right parasympathectic dominance, is unlikely to underlay the fight-or-flight response as it appears to represent the resting state of a generalized increase of parasympathetic tone which is antithetical to the stress response. It is also likely that peaks of immune function, regeneration, and healing occur during the increased parasympathetic state that appears to correlate with right brain/left nostril-dominant states as judged by the coupling of cerebral rhythms, sleep stages, and the BRAC. It may also be that dramatic increases in CRF release are coupled to right nostril/left brain dominance during the fight-or-flight response, as the apparent ultradian rhythms of CRF are likely to have their peaks during the active phase of the BRAC.

Certain observations in two case studies of multiple personality disorder (MPD), or as now referred to as dissociative identity disorder, are suggestive of this lateralized ANS relationship. In 1955, a physician reported significant lateralized findings during a neurological examination of two different patients with similar personality traits where each patient had two diametrically opposed personality types (Ischlondsky, 1955):

> One was an impulsive, irresponsible, mischevious and vindictive personality, full of rebellion against authority and of hate towards the people around her, the patient in this phase was extremely aggressive, using abusive language and scaring other patients with lurid tales of state hospitals, sex relations, etc., in the opposed behavioral pattern to which the first personality would suddenly switch, the patient appeared dependent, submissive, shy, self-effacing, affectionate, and obedient. In a very timid way she expressed friendliness, sought affection, acceptance, and approval from the same personnel she had reviled and abused. There was no trace left of any inappropriate word or expression, no manifestation of hostility to her surroundings, and not the slightest reference to sex. In fact, any sex thought or word would induce in her extreme fears of perdition, feelings of guilt and anxiety, depression, and shame (Ischlondsky, 1955).

In each of these two opposed mental states there was amnesia to the other, which is characteristic of this disorder. A strong stimulus was capable of evoking the antipode of the existing mental condition:

> During the *aggressive or active phase* (emphasis added) of the patient's behavior examination revealed that the left and right sides of her body responded differently to sensory stimulus: while the right side was hyposensitive the left side displayed hyper-sensitivity. Thus vision and hearing were unclear and far away on the right side but very clear and close on the left side. Her response to touch and pain showed a high threshold on the

> right, and a low threshold on the left side. Characteristically, with regard to the olfactory sense the patient in this mental state manifested a diametrically opposed attitude: she was hyper-sensitive to smell on the right side and her *right nostril was clear*, while on the *left side* her sense of smell was absent and *the nostril congested and closed* (emphasis added). With regard to the other neurological signs such as the size of pupils, reflexes, salivation, sweating, there was a similar difference in the response of the two sides of the body: the aggressive personality type displayed on the right side, a small pupil, a hypo-secretion of saliva, absence of sweating on sole and palm and lack of abdominal reflexes, while on the left side there was a large pupil, hypersecretion of saliva, very strong sweating on palm and sole and extremely strong abdominal reflexes. (It is difficult to account for the observation of pupil size etc. being inconsistent with nasal congestion and pain sensitivity.) And just as fast as the psyche switched to the *shy, passive, and permissive* personality (emphasis added) all neurological manifestations also switched to reverse dominance, where the olfactory sense proved now to be very sharp on the left side while completely absent and with *nostril congested and closed on the right side* (emphasis added) (Ischlondsky, 1955).

These extraordinary case studies showing that lateralized ANS phenomena switch instantaneously with the psyche in two patients also suggest that right nostril dominance or sympathetic dominance on the right side of the body correlates with the active phase of the BRAC and the fight-or-flight response pattern.

Other examples of laterality and the neurology of emotion and psychological profiles have been reviewed (Bear, 1983). Bear states that the patient with right-hemisphere damage may be severely impaired by unconcern, unrealistic assessment of emotional priorities, and failures in emotional communication while left-hemisphere damage more often results in aphasia. Others compared left versus right temporal lobe epileptics showing that right-hemisphere foci produce an impulsive aggressive pattern compared with a controlled reflective profile of those with left-hemisphere foci (McIntyre *et al.*, 1976). This finding is further supported by studies in humans with one hemisphere anesthetized by barbiturates. Left-hemisphere anesthesia usually produces a depressive-catastrophic reaction while a euphoric-maniacal reaction occurs when the right hemisphere is anesthetized (Rossi and Rosadini, 1967). In summary, it seems that left brain function produces an active or aggressive state if not checked by normal right brain activity and vice versa. This pendulum of cerebral activity provides a simple view of how stress may arise in the nervous system. Certainly the fight-or-flight status is an extreme swing to the left brain. An "active state" coincident with work-related stress may alternate with a passive-depressive state in which the right brain mode dominates and causes different physical sequelae. One personality in the MPD patients represented completely passive, receptive victims in a state of helplessness. The neurology of this adaptive mechanism represents an interesting trait from an evolutionary perspective. It may be that this passive state has its correlate in other species that react by playing dead in certain situations in which escape or attack seems impossible, and a similar shift in physiology occurs exhibiting extremes of the resting mode of the BRAC.

These rhythmic pendulum shifts in ANS–CNS activity present a novel concept for studying disease that now provides us with novel ways of conceiving how stress as a relational factor may precipitate a wide range of events and disorders that may include brain stem-based imbalances leading to sudden cardiac death, potential imbalances in the regulation of the immune system, and potential abnormalities in the neuroendocrine system. These imbalances, or states of disequilibrium, may thus eventually lead to, or represent, a cascade of other effects on the various systems of the body that under normal unstressed conditions will otherwise help us to maintain a state of health and equilibrium.

## III. Implications of Lateralized Rhythms for Adaptation and Homeostasis

Adaptation is defined here as the adjustment of the organism to environmental conditions. The only certainty in nature is change, and survival of the fittest implies the ability to adapt to change when necessary. This requires both skill and flexibility. The lateralized rhythms of the CNS and ANS may be one of the clearest examples of how higher vertebrates have developed the flexibility to adapt to change. These rhythms are an economic means of organizing the temporal and structural elements of biological systems for both adaptation and the maintenance of "homeostasis." In any living system it is not possible to maximize all "housekeeping" functions simultaneously, just as the ergotrophic and trophotropic states cannot coexist. The lateralized specialization of the cerebral cortex makes it possible to have two diverse repertoires of mental skills to provide solutions to problems. The cerebral rhythm, in part, creates the opportunity to cope with changes by alternating between two views or skill sets for dealing with reality. In addition, when emergency situations exist, survival is increased by maximizing a mental and metabolic relationship that has evolved to cope best with a threat. The lateralized switching in the MPD patients is an excellent example of the neurology of this adaptive mechanism. However, the switching between these two states in the MPD patients are extreme examples in shifts of the pendulum. Although the fight-or-flight mechanism is a well-studied example of adaptive mechanisms, the example of adaptation by the passive mode in the subjects with MPD is also important. The apparent right-brain left-sided sympathetic dominant mode is the polarity of the fight-or-flight state. This passive state may have its correlate in other species which "play dead" in certain situations to avoid attack. It may be that humans become more prone to depression (a right cerebral disorder, see Section IV.B) when they are forced to accomodate a passive state for prolonged periods or are forced to cope with situations where they have no control and the outward fight-or-flight response is not an option. Any environmental condition which demands the overuse of one cerebral state may in the long run have a negative impact both psychologically and physiologically, since imbalanced metabolic shifts may occur. As discussed above, this time inequality in lateralized activities may be a primary determinant of disease.

The relationship of lateralized neural rhythms to the BRAC suggests that the right side of the body would undergo greater sympathetic activity during the active phase of the BRAC. In his famous work on the general adaptation syndrome, Selye (1946) showed that stress is also marked by adrenal enlargement. Therefore, it is likely that the right adrenal gland may be somewhat larger than the left due to greater use. In fact, two researchers studied the right and left adrenal activities in resting dogs and observed not only "90-min" ultradian rhythms in adrenal blood flow that differed on the two sides, but also that the right adrenal gland averaged 1.8 g in weight and the left adrenal gland averaged 1.3 g, a statistically significant difference (Benton and Yates, 1990). This is either a developmental and perhaps necessary difference in size or the hypothesis that more work (stress) yields a larger gland could account for this difference. In humans the right suprarenal vein drains into the inferior vena cava while the left side empties into the renal vein. This anatomical arrangement indicates that right adrenal activity may have quicker metabolic impact due to its more direct influence on circulation. Not only is the right adrenal gland larger, but the right lung is also larger. Developmentally, it may be more important to have the larger lung on the right side as enhanced sympathetic activity in the lung induces vasodialation in contrast to vasoconstriction in most other tissues. This would provide for greater blood gas exchange during the active phase of the BRAC. Classically it is reasoned that the left lung is smaller to accomodate for the position of the heart. These relations reflect nature's economic considerations.

Selye described stress-induced diseases or "diseases of adaptation" (ulcers, hypertension, cardiac infarct, psychiatric disturbances, immune diseases) to in part come from an excess of corticoids and catecholamines (Selye, 1946). He also saw this as an imbalance in the proportion of the prophlogistic and antiphlogistic hormones secreted from the adrenals. In Selye's thesis the prophlogistic corticoids stimulate the proliferative ability and reactivity of connective tissue, thus inhancing their "inflammatory potential" while the antiphlogistic corticoids apparently depress the "inflammatory potential." Selye also recognized that changes in the activity of the ANS played an important role in diverse stress-induced diseases. He and others called this a "vegetative total reorientation" which is in essence a modification of the relative predominance of sympathetic or parasympathetic nervous impulses. Selye's "diseases of adaptation" may also be accounted for by an imbalance in the lateralized neural rhythms that organize the BRAC. Greater right-sided sympathetic tone correlates with the active phase of the BRAC and in general a greater sympathetic state of arousal, or the ergotrophic energy expenditure state.

An interesting study of how lateralized changes in hypothalamic activity occur under stress adaptation comes from some interesting work by the Russians (Bakalkin *et al.*, 1984). Their study shows an asymmetrical LHRH distribution in the rat under normal conditions. Wistar rats exhibit higher LHRH content in the right hypothalamus and albino rats exhibit higher LHRH content on the left. They state that LHRH content changes from side to side over a 24-h period and that unilateral castration or cold stress leads to a shift in the LHRH distribution in the hypothalamus (Bakalkin *et al.*, 1984). This may be one example of how lateralized changes in metabolism accomodate changes in the environment.

While Selye's theory of stress is an attempt to relate the whole individual to organ systems, he emphasized the adrenal cortex as a major organizer of nonspecific adaptive responses to environmental demands (Selye, 1950a,b,c; Selye and Fortier, 1950). Responses to stress include both the active and passive styles of avoidance and while both may tax the adrenal system, perhaps to different degrees, it is clear there are individual differences in these two styles in the behavioral, physiological, and endocrine changes that occur in response to stressors in the environment (Bohus *et al.*, 1987). Despite extensive stress research, one group states "the problem still remains to link directly the macro- and microworld," and that "Stress, hormonal states and adaptation (in its broadest sense) need to be fitted into one concept" (Bohus *et al.*, 1987). The lateralized rhythms of the CNS and ANS provide a more integrated view of the "whole individual." This view is that of a balance between two polar states of mind and metabolism in a continuous rhythm to meet the biological needs of the organism. How stress affects the mind–body would now include a consideration of how this pendulum of ANS–CNS activity can be affected by the environment. And as stated earlier, it is likely that this pendulum is generated by an endogenous oscillator system within the hypothalamus that reflects patterns of neural excitation and inhibition organized during development where there is a metabolic gradient of activity operating in a clocklike fashion through the four major zones of the hypothalamus (right and left anterior regions and right and left posterior regions). The shifting and relative activities of the different hypothalamic nuclei adjust to meet the shifting needs and patterns of external activity for the organism. The neural circuitry of the hypothalamus thus appears to compensate for a range of environmental stressors. It is possible that different regions within the hypothalamus are more frequently activated than others in some daily routines and with specific forms of stress. While this theory does not deny the innate neural relations that have evolved between the hypothalamus and other structures, it emphasizes the frequency of routines where the firing of nerve patterns for certain functions becomes preferred. Stress may therefore be defined as an event that attempts to shift established patterns; while in addition, certain patterns are probably more conducive to a balanced pendulum. Given this view of neural systems, that support the lateralized rhythms of mind and body, it may be easier to understand how laterality plays an important role in states of health and disease.

## IV. Implications of Lateralized Rhythms for Psychopathology

During the decades of the 1960s, 1970s, and 1980s, pioneering studies on the basic fundamentals of laterality in brain function in normals and states of psychopathology led to fascinating insights. The first of these studies was the Nobel Prize winning work of Sperry and colleagues with split–brain patients that gave us unique insight to the different modes of intelligence and personality dependent factors in the left and right hemispheres (Gazzaniga *et al.*, 1962; Sperry, 1964). The first studies in the domain of the psychopathologies was the work that showed that left temporal lobe epilepsy is associated with increased risk of schizophrenia-like psychosis while right temporal lobe epilepsy is associated with affective psychoses (Flor-Henry, 1969a,b). Flor-Henry later suggested that the various forms of psychopathology reflect "bilateral but asymmetrical disturbances in hemispheric function" where "cerebral disorganization is least severe in the neurotic forms of depression, increasing in the psychotic depressions, more with manias, and maximal disorganization in schizophrenia. The overlapping nature of the psychotic symptoms in these disorders argues against strick independent categories of disease states, but more for dimensions of disorder" (Flor-Henry, 1987). The pioneering work of Flor-Henry and others led to an understanding of three key principles of interaction that underlay double-brain systems: (1) intrahemispheric activation, (2) interhemispheric coupling, and (3) contralateral inhibition. Flor-Henry concludes that the "Functional disturbance of one or more of these fundamental elements of neurophysiological organization has been demonstrated in all the psychopathological syndromes investigated" and "It is important to note that an abnormal pattern of lateralized hemispheric state can arise either because of ipsilateral activation or through a reduction or loss of normally stabilizing contralateral inhibition" (Flor-Henry, 1987). All three aspects of double-brain interaction would be profoundly affected by rhythms of alternating cerebral hemispheric activity. Undoubtedly, the temporal expression of symptoms with the cerebral psychopathologies is dominated by this ultradian rhythm.

Bear concludes in his review of lateralization of psychological profiles and the neurology of emotion that "the patient with right-hemisphere damage may be severely impaired by unconcern, unrealistic assessment of emotional priorities, and failures in emotional communication, while left-hemisphere damage more often results in aphasia" (Bear, 1983). One group compared left versus right temporal lobe epileptics showing that right-hemisphere foci produce an "impulsive" aggressive pattern compared with a controlled "reflective" profile of those with left-hemisphere foci (McIntyre *et al.*, 1976). As described earlier, this finding is further supported by studies in humans where one hemisphere is anesthetized by barbiturates. Left-hemisphere anesthesia usually produces a "depressive-catastrophic" reaction while a "euphoric-maniacal" reaction occurs when the right hemisphere is anesthetized (Rossi and Rosadini, 1967).

In general, it seems that left brain function produces an active or aggressive state if not checked by the contralateral inhibition of normal right brain activity and vice versa. The endogenous oscillator which governs the pendulum of cerebral rhythms provides a simple concept for understanding what may be one of the most important elements of the dynamics of cerebral psychopathology. The double-brain system is analogous to two separate, different, and interlocked computers in a rhythmic relationship that yields a complementary and supplementary interaction swinging between two separate modes of intelligence. It seems that the pathological character of each "cognitive program" can vary somewhat independently. In 1987, Flor-Henry concluded "that sufficient evidence exists to show that personality dimensions are dependent on hemispheric organization" ... and ... "Obsessional personality is associated with relative activation of the left hemisphere, hysterical personality with relative activation of the right hemisphere. Schizoid introversion is related to dominant temporal lobectomy (i.e., to right-hemisphere preponderance); extraversion to nondominant lobectomy (i.e., to left-hemisphere preponderance)." With these findings it is not difficult to view how rhythms of the two brains that manifest with alternating cognitive content and complementary personalities may or may not lead to a cooperative and effective working relationship. Most chronobiological studies of the major psychopathologies have been primarily limited to the affective disorders, and with the circadian and infradian rhythms (Halaris, 1987). A major drawback to these studies is that of the infrequent sampling of the parameters which leaves the ultradian periodicity (1–4 h range), perhaps the most interesting rhythm, as an overlooked phenomenon. A major exception to this lack of interest in the ultradians is the early study of the REM–NREM sleep rhythm in depression. One interesting result here is with the study of cortisol secretion in normals and patients with endogenous depression that shows a slowing of the frequency from 8.8 episodes per 24 h to 6.5 in the patient group (Halbreich, 1987). This may reflect an inequality or an abnormality in the dynamics of this cerebral pendulum.

In a later study on depression and ultradians, one group sought to assess the quantity and quality of mood variation in depressed patients where they compared mood variation in a group of nine depressed patients and a group of nine nondepressed subjects over 12 consecutive hours from 8 a.m. to 8 p.m. (Hall *et al.*, 1991). "The depressed group demonstrated greater mood score variability over the course of the day. Both groups demonstrated ultradian cycles and circadian trends; however, the depressed group demonstrated ultradian cycles of significantly greater amplitude than the nondepressed group" (Hall *et al.*, 1991). Although the differences were not significant, the periodicity for the depressed patients had a mean = 4.7 h, and the normals had a mean = 5.3 h. However, two patients had 3-h rhythms where the mood variability was much greater than the amplitude of the circadian component. They conclude, in part, "the mechanism of depressive disorders may include a deregulation of a normal oscillatory mood variation pattern." Clearly, larger groups of patients and normal subjects need to be studied, not only with depression, but with all forms of psychopathology. We may find significant variations in the chronicity of mood and related mental correlates, including symptom severity with the various psychopathologies when compared to normal healthy subjects.

While one study did assess patterns of mood regulation among patients with major depression, patients with borderline personality disorder, patients with premenstrual syndrome (PMS), and normal subjects, their assessment only included one morning and one evening rating (Cowdry *et al.*, 1991). They measured the mean and standard deviation of morning and evening ratings over 14 days of mood self-ratings with 10 patients with major depression, 16 with borderline personality disorder, 15 with PMS, and 24 normals. They also measured the mean absolute change in mood from one day to the next, and the change from morning to evening was also determined. They found that:

> the four groups differed significantly on every measure of mood and mood variability except diurnal variation. As expected, the group with major depression had the lowest global ratings and a low degree of variability. The group with borderline personality disorder was less depressed than

> the group with major depression and showed a high degree of mood variability. Autocorrelation analysis suggested that mood ratings in borderline personality disorder vary randomly from one day to the next. The mood variability over the 14 days of the patients with PMS was significantly greater than that of normal subjects (Cowdry *et al.*, 1991).

They concluded "Mood disorders differ not only in the degree of abnormal mood but also in the pattern of mood variability, suggesting that mechanisms regulating mood stability may differ from those regulating overall mood states." The chronobiology and temporal nature of psychiatric disorders is a neglected topic, and in part, perhaps because the ultradian phenomenon of alternating cerebral hemispheric activation has received little overall attention. Below are studies that give us further insight to the disorders of anxiety, depression, and schizophrenia.

### A. Anxiety

Many clinical observations on unilateral brain damage, unilateral carotid injection of barbiturate, and epileptic foci have all indicated lateralized differences in regards to emotional processing, especially in the frontal lobes. These studies have been reviewed (Bear, 1983). In general, it can be concluded that the experience of positive emotions, such as happiness and excitement, indicate greater left-hemispheric involvement and that negative emotions are associated with greater right-hemispheric activity (Ahern and Schwartz, 1979). One group has studied facial asymmetries. They conclude that the right hemisphere is specialized for the expression of negative emotions and that both hemispheres are involved in positive emotions (Borod *et al.*, 1988). Others have studied the neural substrates of emotion and found evidence for cortical asymmetries for aspects of emotion. A recent study used a new imaging method to interrogate facial movement in 3D to assess possible asymmetrical action during expressions of happiness and sadness (Nicholls *et al.*, 2004). Greater left-sided movement, particularly during expressions of sadness, was observed which has implications for understanding the hemispheric differences in emotion and this supports the data that aspects of emotion processing are differentially localized to the two hemispheres.

One group using PET found higher metabolic rates in the right hemisphere in high-anxiety compared to low-anxiety subjects (Reivich *et al.*, 1983). Others observed cerebral blood flow asymmetries in resting subjects with higher activity in the right hemisphere, especially in the superior frontal and frontotemporal areas (Hagstadius and Risberg, 1989). They suggested that these asymmetries are related to the anxiety-producing events of the study. This was later confirmed in resting subjects while comparing low- and high-anxiety subjects (Hagstadius, 1989). The frontal asymmetries showed a clear relationship between activity in the right hemisphere and the level of trait anxiety in normal subjects as a "first-run" effect only. Specific associations were found between the anxiety level and degree of mean flow asymmetry especially in the frontotemporal regions.

These studies suggest that the severity of anxiety, as a lateralized event, is likely to be affected by the phase of the ultradian cerebral rhythm. The acute symptoms of anxiety may be more severe during the right-brain left nostril-dominant mode. It is also possible that during the resting phase of the BRAC, the general metabolic state and cognitive conditions are not as conducive for coping with anxiety-producing events. During this right-brain-dominant mode the apparent increased sensitivity to threats may leave a person feeling more susceptible to dangers, real or imagined. It stands to reason that the active phase of the BRAC, which appears to correlate with the fight-or-flight response, is better suited for coping with threats, as this psychophysiological state is the correlate of the "hunting" mode, or mode suited to combat, a mode less likely to be vulnerable to, or prone to anxiety.

### B. Depression

One of the most important clues to understanding the cerebral dynamics of depression in respect to the ANS–CNS rhythm comes from studies of REM and NREM sleep patterns. There is a perturbation of the endogenous ultradian oscillator regulating REM sleep in depressive psychosis when compared to normal healthy sleep patterns. The first sleep study of depressed patients found more REM sleep in the first third of the night (Gresham *et al.*, 1965). Others also found a decrease of REM sleep latency at sleep onset, and an increased percentage of REM sleep (Green and Stajduhar, 1966; Hartmann *et al.*, 1966). In depressed patients, REM sleep is typically the first sleep stage while NREM sleep usually proceeds REM sleep in normals (Vogel *et al.*, 1980). The first REM periods are generally longer in the beginning of the night and decrease in length as sleep progresses for depressives, whereas in normals the first REM period is the shortest and it later increases in duration. It would be possible to predict this if it is assumed that depression correlates with a greater amount of right-hemisphere activity compared to normals. Therefore, the need to balance out this effect would lead to first engaging the left hemisphere during sleep, the hemisphere which dominates during REM sleep in the beginning of the night. "Today, the reduced latency of REM sleep appearance, which expresses a pressure of this sleep stage, is well established" (Gottesmann and Gottesman, 2007). This same need for a balance of the ANS–CNS pendulum may also exhibit in the more recent findings that show there is also an increase of eye movement density, that is, the number of REMs per period of REM sleep, especially in the first part of night (Rush *et al.*, 1986). This increase of REM density and shortened REM sleep stage latency is also associated with a tendency for plasma cortisol to shift to the beginning of the night (Rao *et al.*, 1996). One would expect that if the "activity" phase of the BRAC were to be rebounding via expression of REM sleep exhibiting with a greater preponderance in depressed patients in the early part of the night that increased cortisol levels would also exhibit early compared to normals. The concept of the cerebral pendulum would imply the need for a compensation for the greater right-hemispheric activity that seems to occur during waking hours in depressed patients. This compensation might occur during sleep and would manifest by initiating sleep with the most needed left brain correlate of

REM sleep. This observation in depressives also implies that sleep may be a time to equilibrate cerebral hemispheric activity.

Also, one group found that NREM sleep correlates with lower levels of cerebral activation as measured by blood glucose utilization "where there is a 23% reduction in metabolic rate across the entire brain" when compared to waking subjects (Buchsbaum *et al.*, 1989). This implies, as Kleitman proposed, that NREM sleep is the correlate of "rest" in the BRAC, and that REM sleep correlates with the activity stage of sleep "as subjects in REM sleep tended to have higher cortical metabolic rates than waking subjects." These correlations argue that depression is primarily a right cerebral disorder, given the proposed relations of left/right autonomic relations with the BRAC as discussed in Section II.E. Thus, it is not surprising to see the first stage of sleep initiated with REM sleep in depressives.

The theory that depression is primarily a right-hemisphere cerebral dysfunction is supported by many other studies, of which only a few are cited here. There is a lateral asymmetry of the electrodermal response amplitudes in depressed patients, with a decrease on the right side of the body and an increase on the left which indicates increased right-hemispheric activity (Gruzelier and Venables, 1974; Myslobodsky and Horesh, 1978). The opposite of this is found in schizophrenia. Abnormal right-hemisphere activation is also found in depressives from studies of the directional bias of saccadic eye movements in which depressives show excessive eye movements to the left (Myslobodsky and Horesh, 1978). Other evidence also comes from studies on the behavioral effects of unilateral hemispheric activation by barbiturates (Rossi and Rosadini, 1967; Terzian, 1964), the relative activation of the hemispheres during different mood states or in different clinical conditions (Tucker, 1981), the neuropsychological performance of depressed patients before and after treatment for depression (Kronfol *et al.*, 1978), and the behavioral indices of hemispheric arousal in negative emotional states (Hatta, 1984).

While many brain imaging and quantitative EEG studies have implicated the right hemisphere and the left prefrontal cortex in depression as sites of abnormality, this has not always been the case (Flor-Henry *et al.*, 2004). In an effort to help further clarify this picture,

Flor-Henry *et al.* (2004) employed a spatial filter known to be effective for elucidating differences between EEG populations when combined with an electrical tomographic approach called low-resolution electromagnetic tomography. They compared the source-current densities with a 43-electrode recording from a group of 25 male subjects with depression (unmedicated) and a group of 65 matched controls to compare resting conditions, and the effects of a verbal and spatial cognitive challenge. "Regions of significantly increased current density in depression compared to controls were generally right hemispheric, while regions of significantly decreased current density were generally frontal and left hemispheric. A within-group comparison of the depressed subjects during the two cognitive challenges suggested a left anterior functional hypoactivation in depression" (Flor-Henry *et al.*, 2004).

Other studies, but not all (Debener *et al.*, 2000), also support this comparatively reduced left frontal activity found in depression. One study compared patients with major depression and controls using PET and found a reduced cerebral blood flow in the left prefrontal cortex and that this left reduction was remedied in remission (Bench *et al.*, 1995). Alpha band EEG asymmetries have also been used to show a pattern of left frontal functional hypoactivation in depressed patients that also exhibits after remission (Henriques and Davidson, 1997). And other studies have also found asymmetries in frontal activation (Knott and Lapierre, 1987; Monakhov and Perris, 1980; Nystrom *et al.*, 1986). Yet others have found contradictory results here (Pollock and Schneider, 1990; Reid *et al.*, 1998).

Even physical pain, whether psychogenic or not, is perceived to be more severe on the left side of the body (Otto *et al.*, 1989). A left-sided bias for somatic complaints and pain and the evidence for the hemispheric lateralization of emotion and depression suggests that "the right hemisphere may play a special role in producing pain, conversion symptoms, and disorders of emotional expression" (Merskey and Watson, 1979).

Depression may be a self-perpetuating condition if the cerebral pendulum can be shifted by moods. That is, if depression is primarily a right cerebral disorder that manifests by excessive activation, and right-brain dominance correlates with the resting phase of the BRAC, it seems likely that depression may be further aggravated by this metabolic state of low energy. The melancholic nature of depression itself leaves little drive to act and alter life's circumstances, thus leading to the possibility of a self-perpetuating condition. In fact, it has been shown that the ultradian rhythms of mood appear longer in melancholic patients compared to controls (Wefelmeyer and Kuhs, 1996). Negative mood in healthy subjects also has larger ultradian amplitudes for those scoring higher on depression and psychological distress (Totterdell, 1995).

Most recently, the ultradian dynamics of depressed patients have been studied by assessing oscillations of dopamine and serotonin measured in cerebrospinal fluid samples collected every 10 min for 24 h in 13 depressed patients (Salomon *et al.*, 2005). These researchers studied patients before and after medication. In respect to the altered profiles of ultradian dynamics with these two neurotransmitters, they state "Periodic neurotransmitter relationships in depressed patients were altered by treatment in this analysis of a small data set. This may represent a baseline abnormality in the regulation of periodic functions involved in the depression pathophysiology, but it could also be due to an unrelated antidepressant effect" (Salomon *et al.*, 2005).

Experiments to correlate the phases of the nasal cycle in depressed patients may find that left nostril dominance prevails during the more severe episodes of depression, and in general that there is a bias toward left nostril dominance. It may also turn out that mania correlates with a predominance of right nostril left brain dominance, as mania is frequently the antipode state, or ergotrophic side of depression in bipolar patients.

### C. Schizophrenia

Hemispheric specializations are seldom all or none, but are more accurately classified as having graded individual differences (Gruzelier, 1983). Schizophrenia also has subtypes as do most other psychopathologies. With schizophrenia, however, understanding the complications of subtypes may be increased by considering the schizophrenic symptoms generated in some epileptic conditions. Regarding the epileptic-related schizophrenias, this "is a disruption of the functions of the left temporal lobe" (Flor-Henry, 1986). And that, "A considerable body of evidence has emerged in the last decade which shows that the endogenous schizophrenias are also related to left temporal disorganization; while psychotic depression relates essentially to disruption of right fronto-temporal limbic systems" (Flor-Henry, 1986). In contrast to the left-hemisphere-related epileptic foci with schizophrenic-like episodes "Evidence from epileptic studies confirms the lateralization to the nondominant hemisphere in depression associated with epilepsy" (Flor-Henry, 1986). With the left temporal lobe epilepsies which progress to a schizophrenic evolution, most do so in the second decade of life, around puberty, which is a critical stage of development. This is also common with the endogenous schizophrenias. Flor-Henry believes that this is in part due to the disruption of hemispheric organization during critical periods of development, but certainly does not imply that all schizophrenias are generated by abnormal "organic developments."

With all the various proposed classes or subtypes, whether it be paranoid versus nonparanoid, organic versus nonorganic, cognitive impairment versus noncognitive impairment, cortical versus subcortical deficits, etc., Gruzelier believes the most enduring classification may now be the positive versus negative symptom distinction (Gruzelier, 1987), and that this postive/negative syndrome model can be cast in terms of imbalances in functional hemispheric activation. He states:

> Results showed that the negative or Withdrawn syndrome reflected greater functional activation of the right hemisphere as measured with electrodermal response asymmetries, EEG activity, event related potentials, lateral eye movements, and attentional biases towards the left ear and the left visual field. The syndrome representing non-Schneiderian positive symptoms, the Active syndrome, included those delusions involving exaggeration of self-concepts (grandiose, religious, fantastic, sexual, hypochondriacal), affective hallucinations, positive affect, and accelerated cognition. The

neuropsychological underpinning of this syndrome was an overactivated left hemisphere coupled with right hemisphere underactivation, the opposite state of hemispheric imbalance to the Withdrawn syndrome (Gruzelier, 1987).

In an earlier review of the literature on lateralization in schizophrenia (Gruzelier, 1983), he concluded that there is additional evidence to suggest that there are two states of hemispheric imbalance in schizophrenia (Gruzelier, 1987). The two descriptions above on negative/withdrawn versus positive symptoms have similarities to the lateralized differences found in MPD patients on the two diametrically opposed personality types (Ischlondsky, 1955) (see Section II.E.3).

Flor-Henry summarized the findings on schizophrenia from a 1986 meeting on cerebral dynamics, laterality, and psychopathology: "Studies strongly implicate the left frontal and/or left temporal regions in schizophrenia" . . . "left hemisphere activation in acute, positive symptomology syndrome and more generally a dislocation of intrahemispheric organization, bilaterally in schizophrenia and mania" . . . "neurometabolic activity is disorganized in the frontal-temporal regions bilaterally asymmetrically (left > right) in most of the studies, with a correlation between intensity of psychopathological symptoms and degree of left hemisphere changes" . . . "thalamo-striate patterns are hypometabolic on the left and hypermetabolic on the right. Correlations are established between left frontal hypometabolic activity and catatonic features, blunted affect and emotional withdrawal. Most of the first rank symptoms are associated with local circulatory changes in the left frontal or temporal region, with the notable exception of delusional mood and persecutory delusions which relate to the right posterior hemisphere." . . . "Shifts of lateral cognitive organization occur not only in schizophrenia but also in depressive psychoses" (Flor-Henry, 1987).

While the psychopathology of schizophrenia is extremely complex with its variety of symptoms and subtypes, it seems that the left hemisphere may play a greater role in this disorder, while the reverse appears true with depression. However, even with depression,

Flor-Henry concludes that "The quantitative EEG, evoked potential and acoustic investigations of major endogenous depressions all demonstrate right-hemispheric perturbation; however, it is possible that the initial disturbance is left frontal" (Flor-Henry, 1987).

In a more recent effort to further explore the idea of a "disruption in left hemispheric activity" in schizophrenia, Koles and colleagues again employed a spatial filter that helps enhance EEG differences in populations with a group of 57 unmedicated chronic severe schizophrenic male subjects and 65 matched controls during rest and during verbal and spatial cognitive challenges again with a 43-electrode system for recordings. "The results confirm that schizophrenia is a left-hemispheric disorder centered in the temporal and frontal lobes" (Koles *et al.*, 2004). The literature is further reviewed supporting the finding of a greater left-hemispheric disorder with schizophrenia (Koles *et al.*, 2004), and for the possible etiological basis and risk factors for developing schizophrenia, including environmental, genetic, neurodevelopmental, brain abnomalities and laterality, immunological, oxidative stress, and the neural diathesis-stressor model (Loganovsky *et al.*, 2005).

Whether the origins for both major forms of psychopathology originate in the left hemisphere or not is debatable, but what seems abundantly clear is the lateralized differences in the over- and underactivation patterns in the two hemispheres which help to characterize these disorders. The severity of symptomologies in the various forms of schizophrenia and how they are expressed are probably coupled to the rhythms of cerebral hemispheric activity. This rhythm and its nasal cycle correlates deserve attention in the study of this disorder both in the classification of symptoms, which like most psychological parameters must have their temporal characteristics, and in the consideration of the possible therapeutic approaches to treatment that can take advantage of endogenous or other ways to affect dominance and cerebral dynamics.

From an evolutionary perspective it is quite conceivable that this double-brain system could have differences in psychopathologies that are more correlated to disorders of one hemisphere than the other. It may be that one side has evolved with sensitivities and weaknesses that reflect a unique difference in susceptibility to dysfunction. In addition, if lateralized dysfunctions can originate in only one hemisphere, then in time it is probable that this dysfunction will affect the other. Although both the disorders of depression and schizophrenia must predate historical accounts, it seems that the "working knowledge" or functional "software" necessary to avoid these conditions remains a mystery. The discovery of the ultradian rhythm of alternating cerebral activity may help lead us to a deeper understanding of rhythms of laterality in mind and metabolism. The nasal cycle may be a useful marker for the study of these rhythms.

In fact, most recently, the nasal cycle has been compared as a measure in left-handed versus right-handed subjects in an attempt to elucidate any potential differences (Searleman *et al.*, 2005). Nostril dominance was studied at 15-min intervals for six continuous hours yielding 24 bilateral serial measures for each subject. Their study included 11 right-handed and 9 left-handed healthy adult male college students between the ages of 18 and 22 years. The subjects were studied using two hot wire anemometers mounted on a fixed bar, and subjects were then positioned at each measure over the bar to test for nostril dominance. During the intervals between measures, the subjects were permitted to watch movies, read, play cards, do homework, and/or other stationary activities. However, "they were not allowed to eat, drink, lie down, or exercise at anytime during the six hours since these are activities that could disrupt the normal nasal cycle" (Searleman *et al.*, 2005). They found that the left-handed males were significantly more likely than chance to have their left nostril dominant (59.3%), rather than their right, and that the right-handed males showed the reverse pattern with the right nostril dominant 59.5% of the time. Also, they found that the average number of minutes to complete a cycle shift was 63.1 min for left-handers and 120 min for right-handers. "This study also provides the first data comparing the nasal cycle patterns of left-handers and right-handers" (Searleman *et al.*, 2005). This is clearly an interesting and important result; however, this study deserves to be repeated under stricter conditions and perhaps with more sophisticated measures of airflow, including continuous sampling under resting conditions. What we do not know is if the two populations for some reason chose to engage in somewhat different behaviors during the intervals between measures that may affect nasal cycle activity.

In addition, the nasal cycle, handedness, and eye dominance have recently been compared in 37 children with autism and 20 controls (Dane and Balci, 2007). The autistic subjects included 27 boys (mean age 9.04 years) and 10 girls (mean age 9.6 years), ages of 5–20 years. The control group included 14 boys (mean age 8.84 years) and 6 girls (mean age 9.2 years) who ranged in age between 5 and 20 years. They assessed hand preference by determining which hand was used to write and throw a ball. Eye preference or dominance was determined by which eye was used to look through the keyhole of a door, and nasal dominance was assessed by measuring the condensation on a glass using a simple but gross method (Gertner *et al.*, 1984). For the autistic subjects, in writing, 56.8% were left-handers, 10.8% were right-handers, and 32.4% were ambiguous. In throwing, 48.65% were left handers, 16.22% were right-handers, and 35.13% were ambiguous. Of the 20 controls, 10% were left-handers by writing and throwing and 90% were right-handers. For the 37 autistic patients, 83.7% had left eye preference and 16.3% had the right eye preference. For the controls, 70% were right-eye dominant and 30% were left-dominant. They assessed nasal dominance 24 times between 8 a.m. and 8 p.m. in all subjects, or at 30-min intervals. They summarize their nasal cycle measures as:

> Seven children with autism had the left nasal dominance for all measurements. Two patients for only one time in 24 measurements and 2 patients only 2 times had the right nasal dominance. Four patients had the right nasal dominance for 12 or more times in 24 measurements. In summary, a majority of patients with autism had the left nasal dominance for major portion of the day-time. However, in controls the rates of right and left nasal dominance were about equal. The mean use number of left nostril in 24 assessments in autistic children (19.59 ± 4.32) was more than controls (11.75 ± 1.97) ($t = 7.67, p = 0.00$) (Dane and Balci, 2007).

They conclude "Autism and early language impairment may be associated with left handedness, eyedness and nasal dominance."

They also note that the rate of left-handedness was higher in patients compared to normal subjects and there is an increased rate of left-handedness in autistic individuals with early language impairment compared to controls but not autistic individuals without early language impairment (Escalante-Mead *et al.*, 2003) and that across all autistic individuals mixed handedness dominance was higher than normal subjects. They also comment "It can be stated that autism and early language impairment may be associated with left-handedness or anomalous dominance" (Dane and Balci, 2007). And, "In this study, the rate of left-eyedness was higher in patients with autism compared to normal population. To our knowledge, there is no literature concerning relations between eyedness and autism." And, "To our knowledge, there is no literature concerning relations between nasal cycle and autism. These results show that the patients with autism had no normal nasal cycle; probably they had almost continuous left."

The results here with autism are indeed unique, important, and may help to explain a great deal about the nature of autism. It appears that the cerebral rhythm is dramatically affected during the waking state in this population. This may help explain why language is so problematic in some subpopulations of autistic individuals. If the left hemisphere has little or less opportunity to function for some reason, the acquisition of language and many other daily working skills and abilities that are left-hemisphere dominant may indeed be severely limited. Section V may help provide some useful approaches to consider for therapy with autistic and other patient populations.

## V. Translational Elements of Psychophysiological States: Selective Regulation of the Lateralized Activities of the ANS and CNS

To date, there are two methods that are known to directly affect the ultradian ANS–CNS rhythm and one that may potentially alter the rhythm. All three methods have therapeutic applications and implications for psychiatry and health. These methods all involve the principle of selective unilateral autonomic activation (SUAA). All three methods have been tested on humans in the laboratory. Two are ancient yogic methods. The first yogic method is called unilateral forced nostril breathing (UFNB) where the practitioner employs forced breathing through only one nostril while closing off the other. This is a technique discovered by yogis to affect changes in the nasal cycle, the cerebral rhythm, and the corresponding psychophysiological states, and it has been studied by a number of independent groups in western laboratories (Shannahoff-Khalsa, 2001, 2006, 2007). UFNB is reviewed below. The second method employs pressure applied against the fifth intercostal space under either the left or right arm pit, using a crutch or stick, called the "yoga danda" stick. This technique can be applied while standing. Yogis found that this autonomic reflex point can alter the phase of the nasal cycle and its psychophysiological correlates. This method has also been studied in a number of independent western laboratories and is reviewed below. The third is a new surgically invasive method that employs unilateral vagal nerve stimulation (VNS). This method requires a procedure where an electrical pacemaker is implanted in the chest with a wire connecting to the mid-inferior cervical branch of the vagus on one side of the body, usually the left side, and the relevant studies are reviewed below.

Since the ANS consists of two separate divisions, the SNS and the PNS, and most organs, including the cerebral cortex, are innervated by fibers from both divisions, and the influence of the two divisions have opposing effects, the potential for SUAA holds great therapeutic promise. UFNB appears to work by a mechanism that selectively activates the ipsilateral branch of the SNS with a possible compensation effect leading to contralateral VNS. Both UFNB and VNS have been employed to treat psychiatric disorders. However, studies with VNS have yet to be conducted to ascertain the potential effects that this therapy may have on the body's natural endogenous rhythms of the ANS–CNS.

First, it is useful to review the physiological effects of SUAA on the left and right stellate ganglion and left and right vagus nerves, and their respective stimulation effects on the heart. Studies have shown that stimulation of the right branch of the vagus can lead to increased cardiac instability, and most studies in humans employ only left VNS (Henry, 2002). Levy and Martin (1979) review studies on the autonomic innervation and control of the heart. They discuss the lateral differences for both the SNS and PNS. There is considerable right-left asymmetry in the distribution of the sympathetic fibers to the heart (Furnival *et al.*, 1973; Levy *et al.*, 1966). In dog studies, researchers have found that stimulation of the right stellate ganglion can increase HR by 85 beats/min while the effects of left-sided stimulation produce a much smaller increase, and that right-sided stimulation can also increase left ventricular systolic pressure (LVSP) by 50 mm Hg while left-sided stimulation increases LVSP $\gg$ 50 mm Hg (Levy *et al.*, 1966). They conclude that right-sided stellate ganglion stimulation has greater chronotropic effects while the left produces greater inotropic effects; right stellate ganglion stimulation decreases systolic duration and left-sided stimulation increases mean arterial pressure. Thus the right sympathetic trunk has relatively greater effects on HR and the left has relatively greater effects on left ventricular function.

The right vagus has a greater cardiac deceleratory effect compared to the left vagus (Hondeghem *et al.*, 1975), and right vagal transection causes a greater cardiac acceleration than left transection, suggesting that the right vagus exerts greater restraint on the sinoatrial node compared to the left vagus (Hamlin and Smith, 1968). Also, the heart period is more prolonged when a stimulus is given to the right vagus compared to the left (Hondeghem *et al.*, 1975). Henry states "The left vagus nerve carries most of the parasympathetic fibers that less densely innervate the ventricles, and the right vagus nerve carries most of the parasympathetic fibers that more densely innervate the cardiac atria. Therefore, vagal anatomy favors left (over right) vagus stimulation to avoid cardiac effects" (Henry, 2002). While SUAA effects on the heart are well known, the potential unilateral ANS stimulation effects on other organs and systems are not as well studied.

## A. Unilateral Forced Nostril Breathing

UFNB has now been studied in western laboratories for more than 25 years (Shannahoff-Khalsa, 2001, 2006, 2007). The CNS rhythm of alternating cerebral hemispheric activity and its coupled physiological and psychological correlates are the reason to employ the natural endogenous method of UFNB (Shannahoff-Khalsa, 1991a,b, 2006, 2007; Werntz *et al.*, 1983). Yogis believed that UFNB has effects not only on the brain but throughout the periphery (Shannahoff-Khalsa, 2001, 2006, 2007), and that UFNB selectively stimulates the contralateral cerebral hemisphere and the ipsilateral branch of the SNS. The first example of using UFNB to selectively stimulate the contralateral hemisphere was demonstrated using EEG in young healthy naive subjects (Werntz *et al.*, 1981, 1983, 1987). This study involved a continuous measurement of EEG activity in the two cerebral hemispheres using a variety of electrode sites to compare homologous left and right power. Subjects naive to the intent of the study were asked to force breathe through the more congested nostril for 11–20 min followed by one, two, or more periods alternating sides with each phase of the experiment (Werntz *et al.*, 1987). Results showed that UFNB increased EEG power in the contralateral hemisphere regardless of the phase of the nasal cycle. Figure 35 shows the results from one subject with six complete periods of UFNB and it is clear how the EEG power drifts toward the contralateral hemisphere regardless of the endogenous phase of the nasal cycle. The profile presents the EEG activity using the occipital–parietal bipolar montage ($O_2$-$P_4$:$O_1$-$P_3$). This phenomenon was observed in five out of five untrained subjects. In two of the five subjects the data are presented as means of seven pairs of bipolar montage in one subject and six pairs in the other subject (see Fig. 36). The power in the total EEG using 2-min artifact free samples during the left nostril breathing period and the right nostril breathing period, with a baseline mean, calculated from the 16 channels of bipolar montage was then averaged for the left minus right difference. Figure 36 shows that for both subjects the left UFNB exercise shifted the EEG power toward greater power in the right hemisphere and

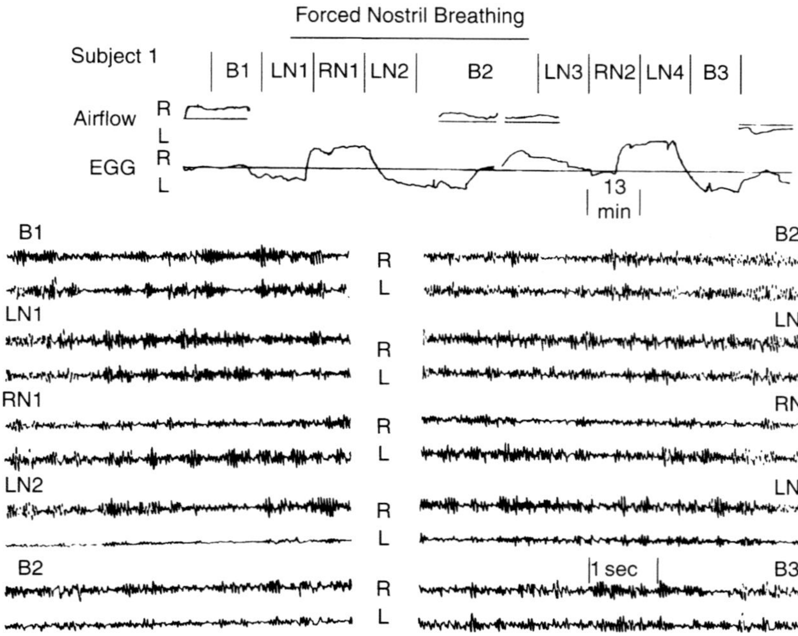


FIG. 35. Effects of UFNB on EEG asymmetry. Subject 1 Trial 2. Top: "Airflow" tracing—points above the baseline indicate greater right nostril airflow and points below greater left nostril airflow. Periods of forced nostril breathing are indicated. "EEG" tracing points above the baseline indicate relatively greater left-hemisphere EEG amplitude: points below relatively greater right-hemisphere amplitude. B, baseline; LN, left nostril breathing; RN, right nostril breathing. Montage ($0_2$-$P_4$:$0_1$-$P_3$). Bottom: representative segments of the primary EEG that were integrated and subtracted to produce the tracings in the top section. For each pair the top tracing is from the right hemisphere and the bottom is from the left hemisphere. Reprinted from *Human Neurobiology*, 6, 1987, 165–171, Selective hemispheric stimulation by unilateral forced nostril breathing, Werntz, D. A., Bickford, R. G., Shannahoff-Khalsa, D. S., Figure 1. With kind permission of Springer Science and Business Media.

vice versa. These differences were significant at $p < 0.01$ for both subjects (Werntz *et al.*, 1987). We concluded "These results suggest the possibility of a noninvasive approach in the treatment of states of psychopathology where lateralized cerebral dysfunction have been shown to occur" (Werntz *et al.*, 1987).

A pilot study with a whole-head 148-channel magnetoencephalography (MEG) instrument located at The Scripps Research Institute (4-D Neuroimaging, San Diego) was used to explore the effects of left and right UFNB at one breath per minute (BPM) for 31 min. This study also showed similar patterns of contralateral hemispheric

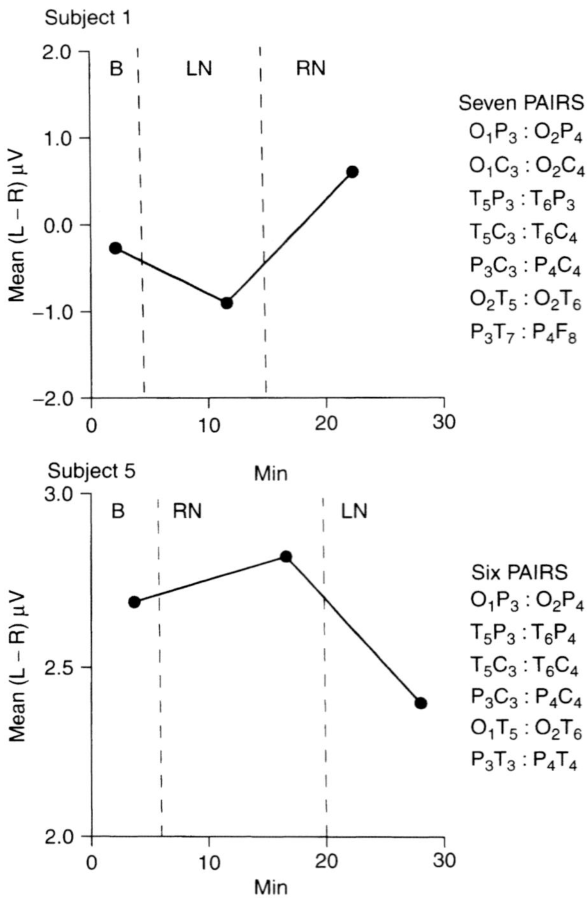


FIG. 36. Effect of UFNB on EEG asymmetry. Subjects 1 and 5: Use of the Bic-Mini-CEARS computer system. With subject 1 the mean difference between the left- and right-hemisphere EEG amplitudes were measured from seven pairs of EEG recordings and is plotted during UFNB. Each sample is 2 min of EEG. The subject was originally breathing predominantly through the right nostril so L-UFNB was first employed followed by R-UFNB. With subject 5 the mean difference between the left- and right-hemisphere EEG amplitudes were measured with six pairs of EEG recordings and is plotted during UFNB. B, baseline; RN, right nostril breathing; LN, left nostril breathing. Each sample is from 2 min of EEG. The subject was originally breathing through the left nostril so R-UFNB was first employed followed by L-UFNB. Reprinted from *Human Neurobiology*, 6, 1987, 165–171, Selective hemispheric stimulation by unilateral forced nostril breathing, Werntz, D. A., Bickford, R. G., Shannahoff-Khalsa, D. S., Figure 5. With kind permission of Springer Science and Business Media.

activation in respect to the active nostril. Preliminary results are presented in Fig. 37 for 148-channel MEG activity with the gamma band power averaged/channel over the respective recording periods using an adjusted energy scale for comparing the three plots of the experiment. The same subject was employed in both experiments. In the three panels on the right side of the figure, the middle portion shows data for 31 min of using a UFNB technique discovered by yogis (Shannahoff-Khalsa, 1991b, 1997, 2006; Shannahoff-Khalsa *et al.*, 1999) for treating obsessive compulsive disorder, called the "OCD breath" (OCDB). This is compared with a 10-min period of preexercise rest (top plot) and a 10-min period of postexercise rest (bottom plot). The same rest-exercise-rest sequence is presented on the left side of the figure, using the right nostril (not claimed to have effects on OCD) instead of the left, again using the same one BPM pattern that consists of the strict implementation of 15-sec inspiration, 15-sec breath retention, 15-sec expiration, and 15-sec breath held out for 31 consecutive minutes. Compared to rest phase I, the left nostril breathing pattern clearly activates greater right frontal hemispheric activity. The reverse is observed for the right nostril pattern. In addition, both breath patterns produce a greater bilateral and diffused hemispheric activation in the rest phase II. However, in rest phase II there is substantially greater bilateral activation after using the right nostril breathing pattern. This is consistent with the yogic view that right nostril breathing is more "stimulating" compared to the left (Shannahoff-Khalsa, 2006). This work is a preliminary result from a collaboration of D.S.K. with a group at the University of Catania, Sicily, and details of the analyses are published in Baglio *et al.* (2002). Some of these color plots were previously published (Shannahoff-Khalsa, 2006).

Figures 38–43 also show MEG power during the three periods of the same experiment, but with the left nostril breathing exercise experiment on the top of the figure and the right nostril breathing exercise experiment on the bottom of the figure, respectively, as a linear time series of the power with arrows drawn to specific channels on the head map. Here the color plot of the power is presented in a linear time series of channels with channel 1 on the left side of

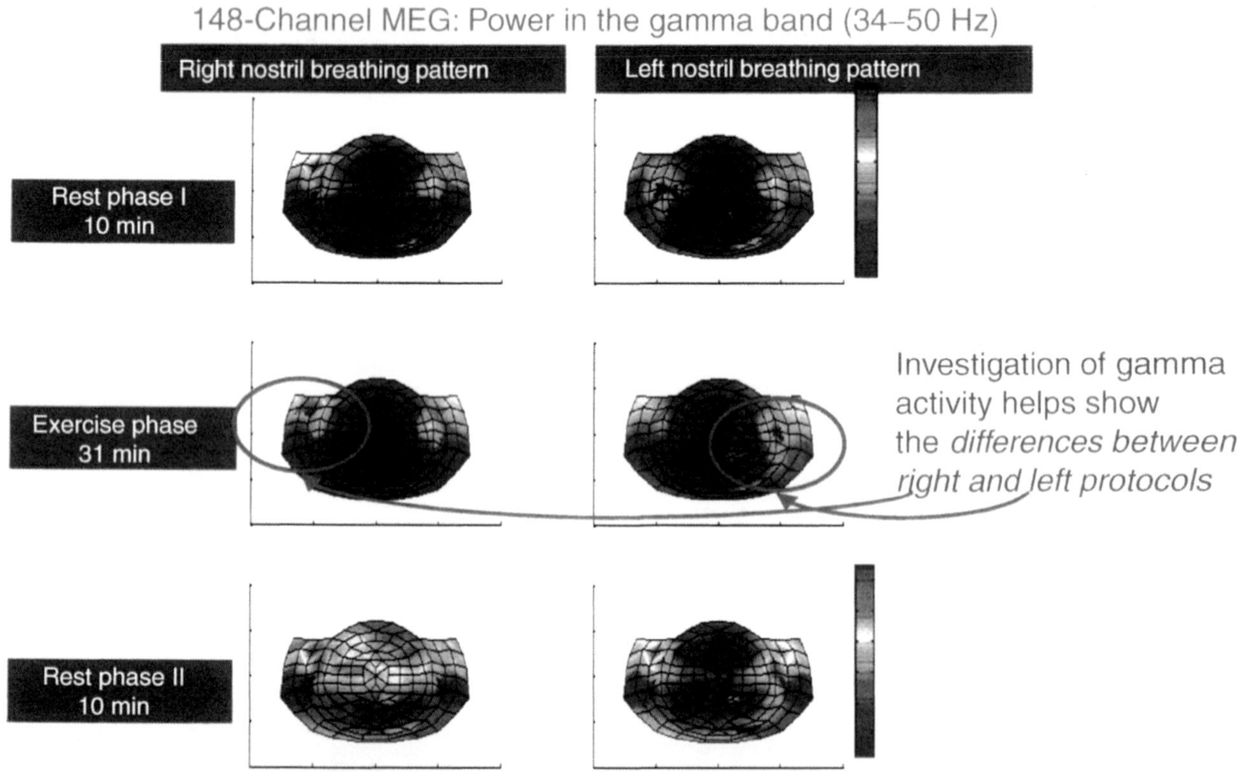


FIG. 37. Gamma band (34–50 Hz) activity in whole-head representations of MEG power. Comparatively increased power is induced during the exercise period in the frontal and prefrontal areas of the contralateral hemisphere. Reprinted from Kundalini Yoga Meditation: Techniques Specific for Psychiatric Disorders, Couples Therapy, and Personal Growth by David Shannahoff-Khalsa; Copyright © 2006. Used by permission of W. W. Norton & Company, Inc. (See Color Insert.)

the figure and channel 148 on the far most right side of the color plot. In the color portion of the plot the preexercise 10-min rest phase of the experiment is shown as the topmost portion of the data with the exercise periods in the middle and the last 10 min of the post-exercise phase of the experiment at the lowest portion of the color plot. Therefore, from top down, the data are presented, respectively, for power for 10 min (rest phase I) + 31 min (exercise period) + 10 min (rest phase II). Power is calculated for each 1-min segment of the data with red color used to mark the highest power and violet as the lowest power using the scale ROYGBIV.

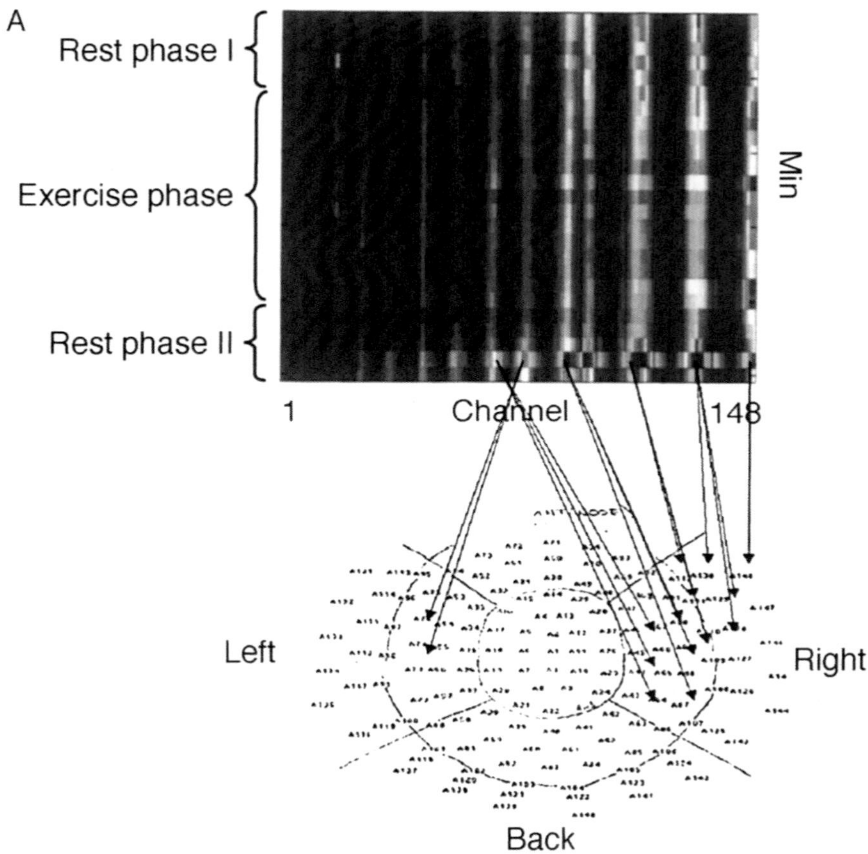


Fig. 38. (*Continued*)

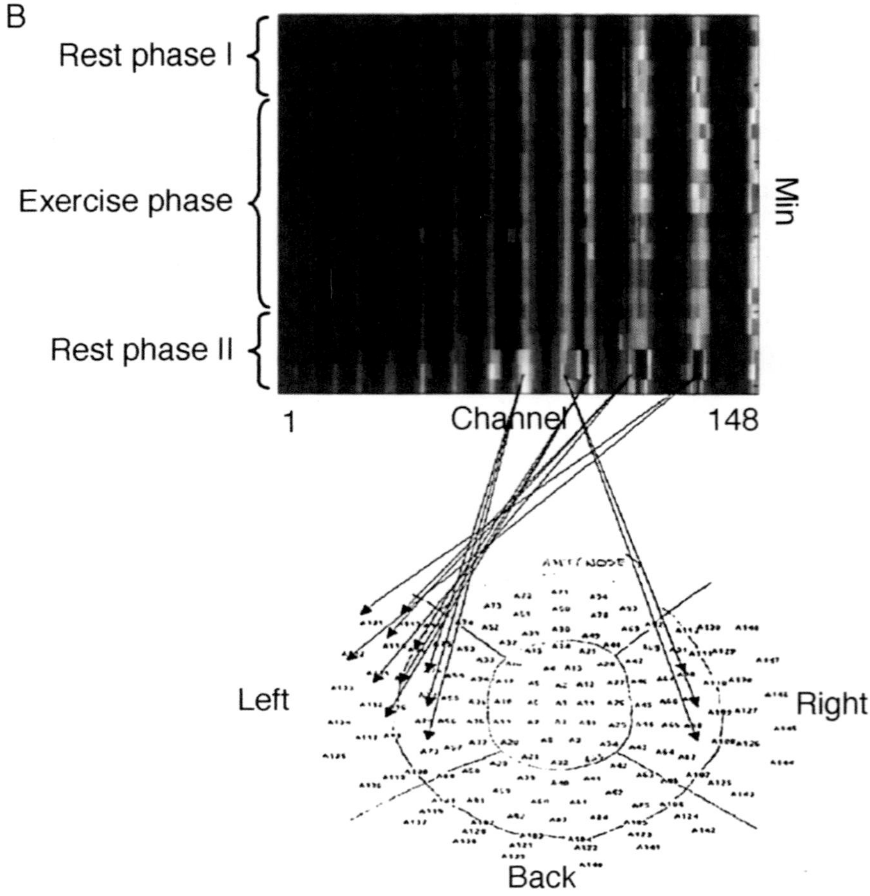


FIG. 38. Total energy or the broadband response (0.1–54 Hz) in channel-space representations of MEG power. Channels within 20% of maximum power in postexercise rest period are mapped with arrows to their spatial locations in the lower part of the figure. Note here that the left nostril breathing pattern is presented on the top (A) of the figure and the right nostril breathing pattern is presented here on the bottom (B) of the figure. Both (A) and (B) demonstrate the contralateral activation patterns for either the left or right nostril breathing patterns, respectively. Adapted from Kundalini Yoga Meditation: Techniques Specific for Psychiatric Disorders, Couples Therapy, and Personal Growth by David Shannahoff-Khalsa; Copyright © 2006. Used by permission of W. W. Norton & Company, Inc. (See Color Insert.)

In Figs. 38–43, the channels with 20% of the maximum power in the postexercise rest period are mapped with arrows drawn to their spatial locations in the lower part of the figure. In Figs. 38–43, the arrows show that the contralateral hemisphere is primarily activated for either the left or right nostril breathing exercise patterns. Figure 38 shows the contralateral activation pattern for total energy, Figs. 39–43 show the same relative effect for the delta frequency band (0.1–4.0 Hz), the theta band (4.0–8.0 Hz), alpha band (8.0–12.0 Hz), beta band (12.0–20.0 Hz), and gamma bands (30.0–54.0 Hz), respectively. There is a contralateral activation pattern for all frequency bands. However, the alpha band shows much greater activation in the occipital regions and this is due to the visualization of a screen indicating the timing for the four 15-sec

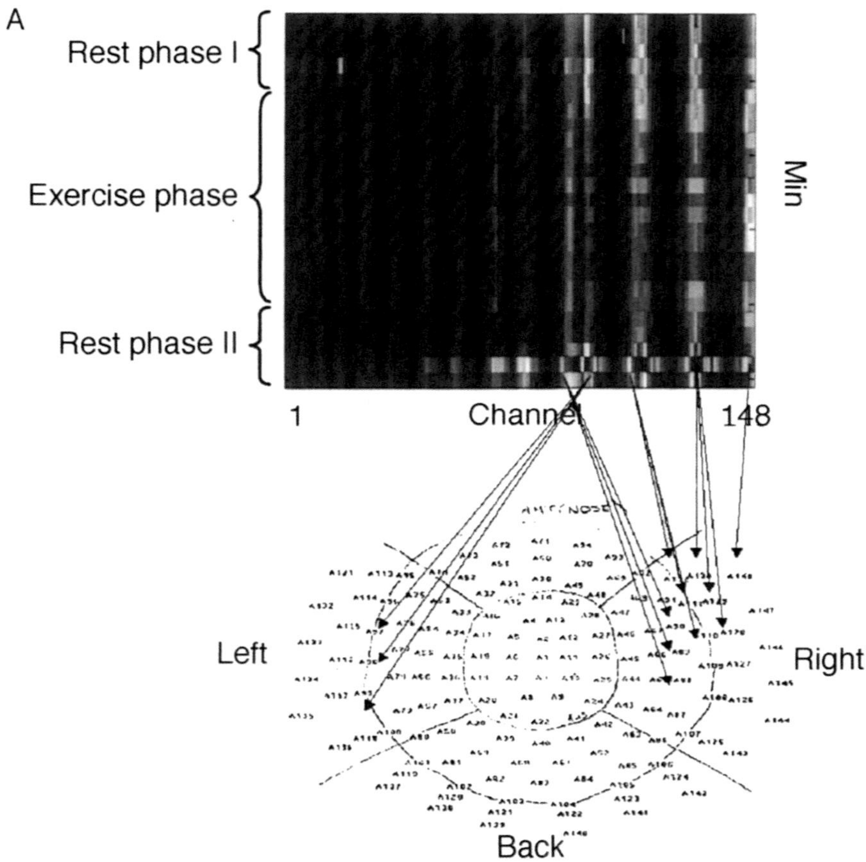


Fig. 39. (*Continued*)

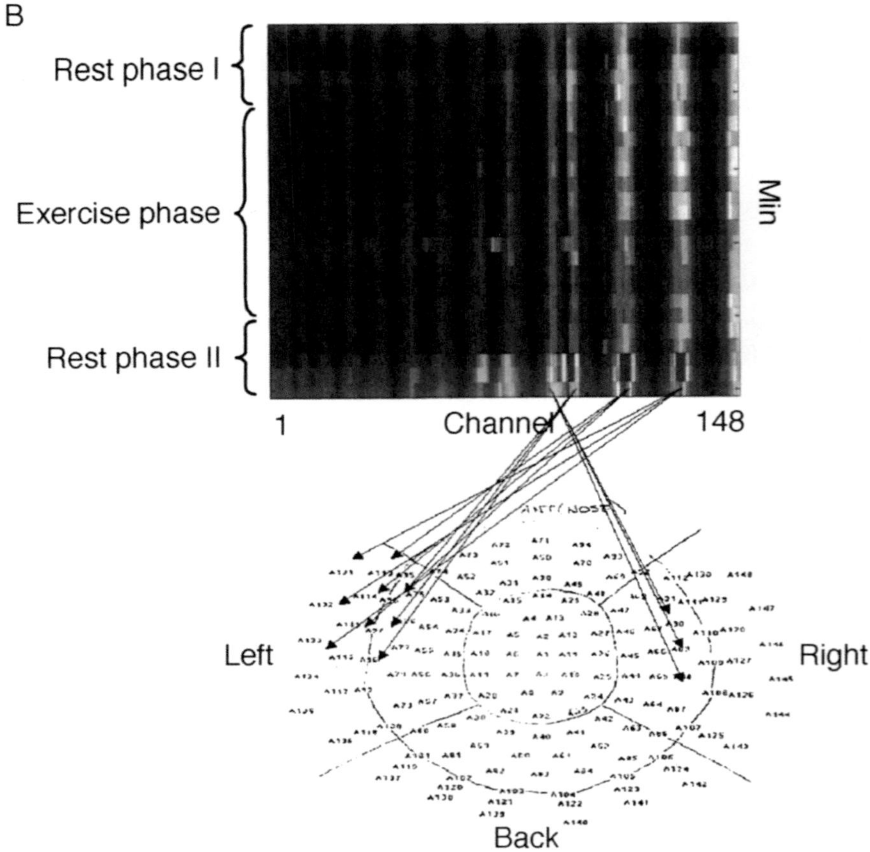


FIG. 39. The left nostril breathing pattern is presented on the top (A) of the figure and the right nostril breathing pattern is presented here on the bottom (B) of the figure for delta band (0.1–4.0 Hz) activity. Channels within 20% of maximum power in postexercise rest period are mapped with arrows to their spatial head map locations in the lower part of the figure. Note the contralateral activation patterns for either the left or right nostril breathing patterns for the delta frequency band. Adapted from Kundalini Yoga Meditation: Techniques Specific for Psychiatric Disorders, Couples Therapy, and Personal Growth by David Shannahoff-Khalsa; Copyright © 2006. Used by permission of W. W. Norton & Company, Inc. (See Color Insert.)

respective breathing phases of the experiment. The majority of the increased activation, that is, channels with the greatest 20% of the power during the phase II portion of the experiment, shows primarily an activation pattern in the frontal and prefrontal brain regions in the hemispheres contralateral to the active nostril.

Using an earlier version of MEG instrumentation that employed 74 channels of MEG (as galvanometers as opposed to the magnetometers in the 148-channel instrument) that are arranged in two separate 14-cm disks, with 37 channels per hemisphere, the same subject was studied performing the "OCDB" pattern, that is, only using the left nostril technique with the four 15-sec phases of the breath cycle repeated for 31 consecutive minutes. However, here the subject was laying on his right side, as the two 37-channel disks are arranged where one disk descends from the ceiling above the subject's left side of the head and the other was positioned below on the subject's right side of the head. Again, the 31-min exercise was performed with the eyes open and at the perfected rate of one

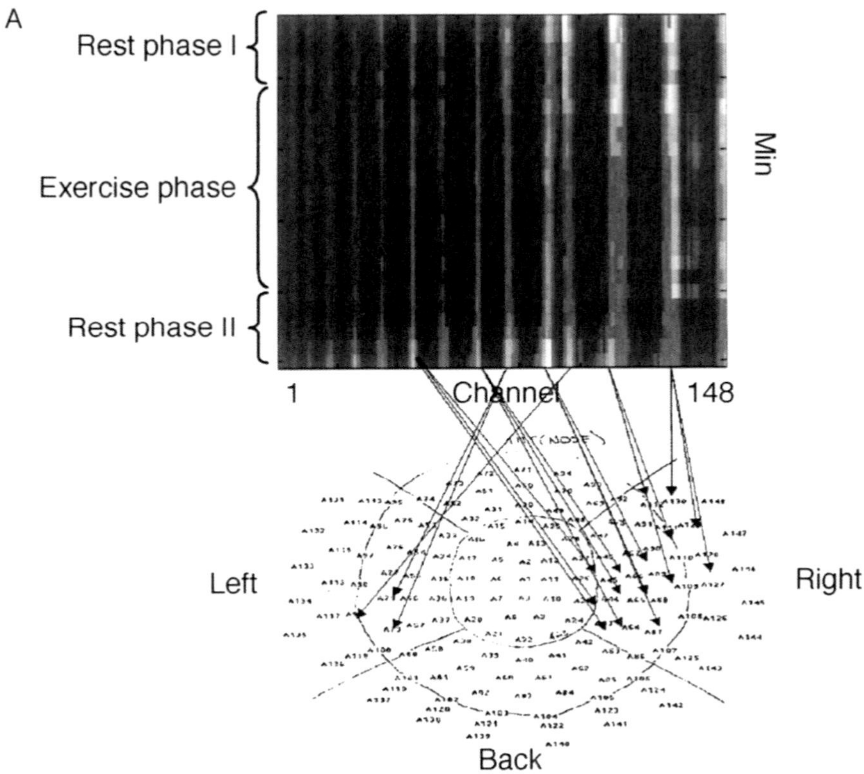


Fig. 40. (*Continued*)

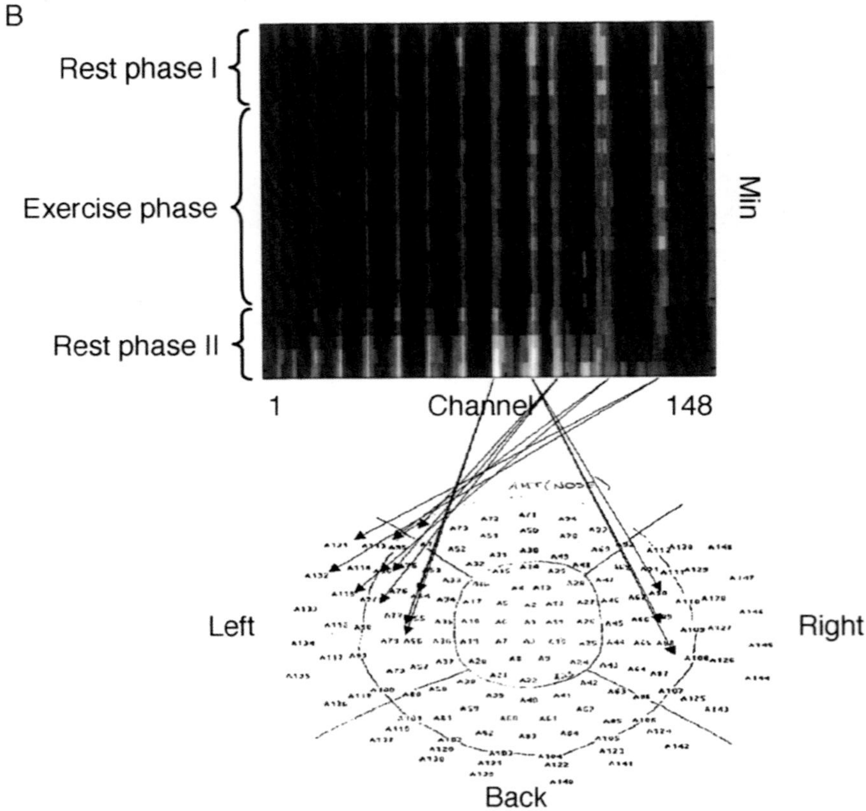


FIG. 40. The left nostril breathing pattern is presented on the top (A) of the figure and the right nostril breathing pattern is presented here on the bottom (B) of the figure for the theta band (4.0–8.0 Hz) activity. Channels within 20% of maximum power in postexercise rest period are mapped with arrows to their spatial head map locations in the lower part of the figure. Note the contralateral activation patterns for either the left or right nostril breathing patterns for the theta frequency band. (See Color Insert.)

BPM for 31 consecutive minutes with a 10-min preexercise recording period and another 10-min recording of the postexercise rest period. Figure 44 shows four color plots. The left side of the figure shows the data for the left hemisphere with the 10-min preexercise rest period plotted at the top of the figure and the 10-min postexercise rest period plotted on the bottom half of the figure. The right side of the figure has the respective data plotted for the right hemisphere. In this figure the vertical color columns starting from the left of each figure are of channels progressing across the figure to the rightmost column for channel 37. The data are presented as mean power (0.1–50 Hz) for each 15-sec epoch pictured with a square of the respective color for each of the 15-sec epochs and time one starts at the top of the figure. However, here the data are plotted with the highest power represented by violet, and the color red is used to represent the lowest power, or as "VIBGYOR" (higher to lower power). This is the reverse compared to the plots for Figs. 37–43. Each plot in Fig. 44 has 40 rows of data, since there are 10 min for each period and four 15-sec epochs per minute. Note

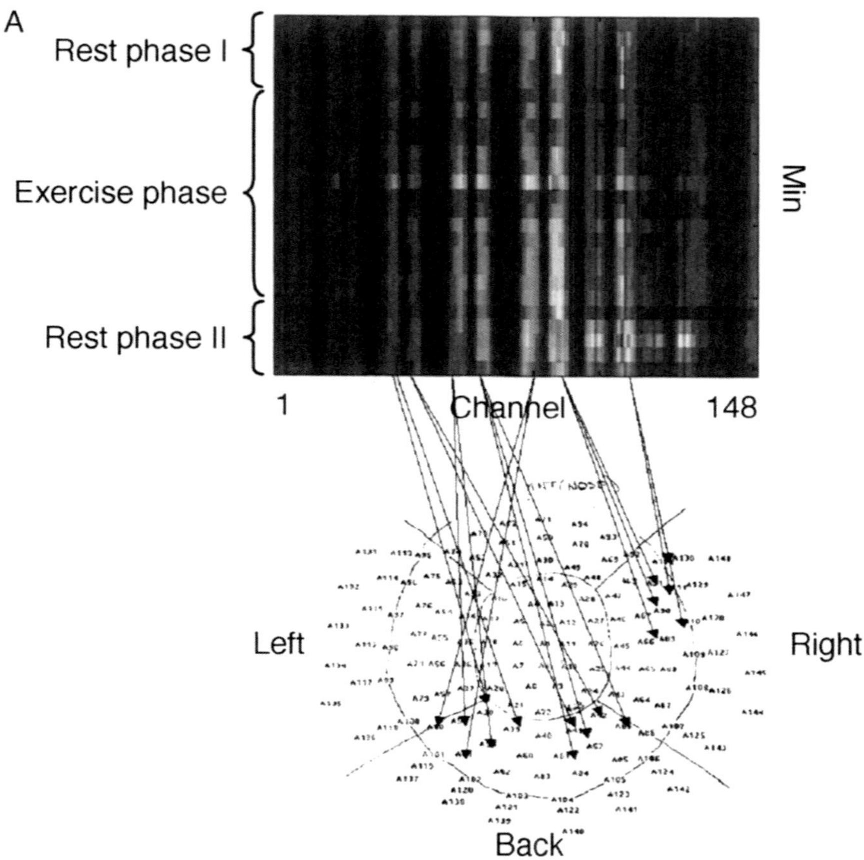


Fig. 41. (*Continued*)

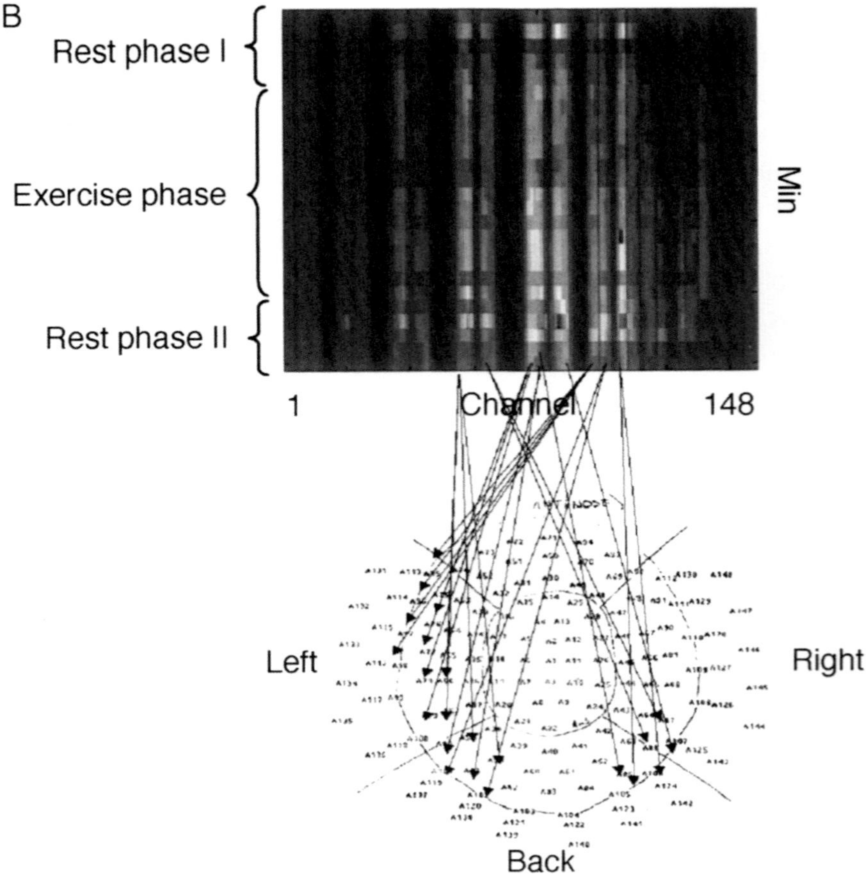


FIG. 41. The left nostril breathing pattern is presented on the top (A) of the figure and the right nostril breathing pattern is presented here on the bottom (B) of the figure for the alpha band (8.0–12.0 Hz) activity. Channels within 20% of maximum power in postexercise rest period are mapped with arrows to their spatial head map locations in the lower part of the figure. Note the contralateral activation patterns for either the left or right nostril breathing patterns for the alpha frequency band. (See Color Insert.)

the left and right hemispheres are fairly similar for the same rows of data for the rest periods, and the same rows usually show the same relative patterns of power activation for greater or lesser energy. Figure 45 is a presentation of the 31 min for the left nostril breathing portion of the experiment, again with the left hemisphere on the left side of the figure and the right hemisphere on the right side of the figure. And again, the top of the figure represents the start of the exercise period descending on the page to the end of the 31-min exercise period, with each row representing a 15-sec epoch of MEG power. However, here it is qualitatively visually apparent that the right hemisphere shows the greater power across the channels. This again demonstrates a pattern of contralateral hemispheric activation for the active nostril. Figure 46 shows the 31-min exercise periods for the left hemisphere (left side of page) and right hemisphere (right side of page). However, here there are four separate pictures on each side, and from the top down, they profile the four phases individually, as collections of the respective 15-sec phases in rows. The top

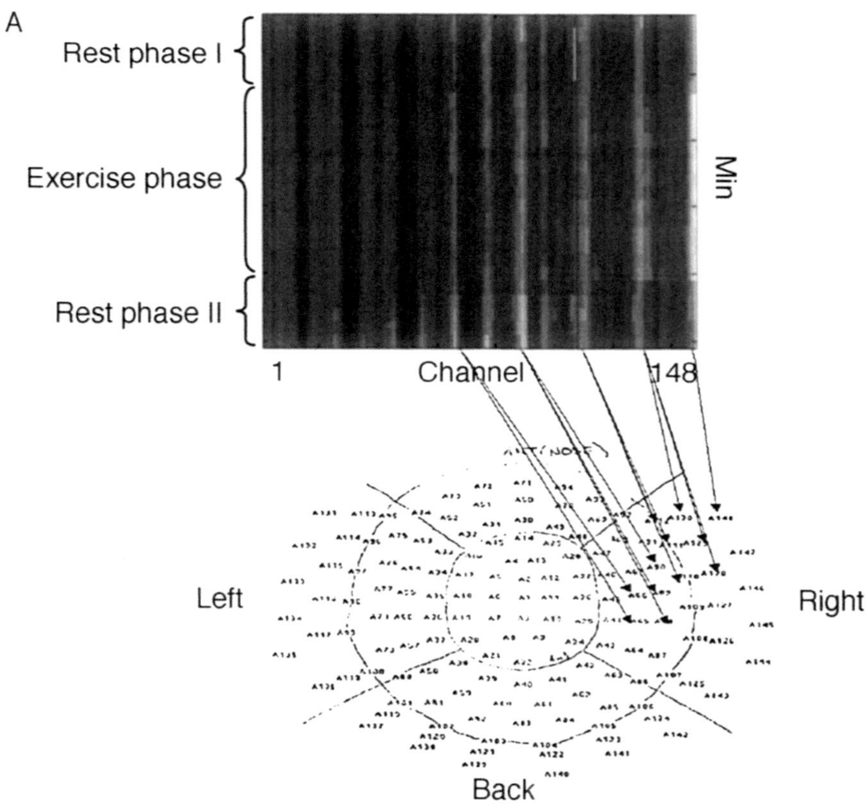


FIG. 42. (*Continued*)

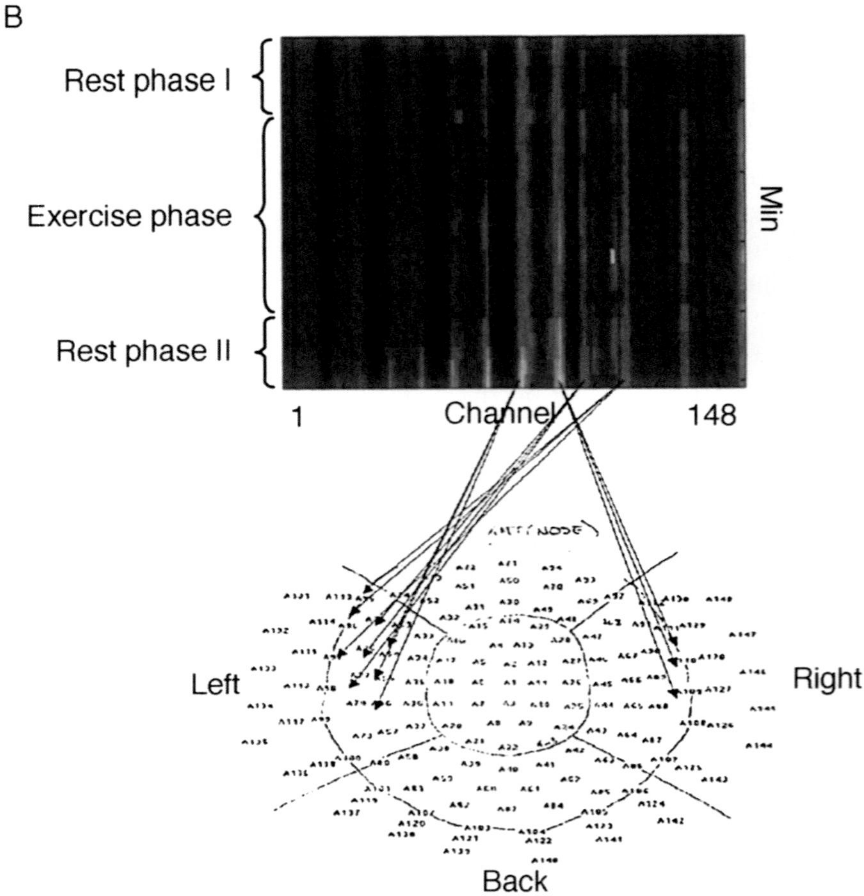


FIG. 42. The left nostril breathing pattern is presented on the top of the figure and the right nostril breathing pattern is presented here on the bottom of the figure for beta band (12.0–20.0 Hz) activity. Channels within 20% of maximum power in postexercise rest period are mapped with arrows to their spatial head map locations in the lower part of the figure. Note the contralateral activation patterns for either the left or right nostril breathing patterns for the beta frequency band. Adapted from Kundalini Yoga Meditation: Techniques Specific for Psychiatric Disorders, Couples Therapy, and Personal Growth by David Shannahoff-Khalsa; Copyright © 2006. Used by permission of W. W. Norton & Company, Inc. (See Color Insert.)

pictures are the 31 individual 15-sec inspiration phases, the second picture down is the 31 individual 15-sec breath retention phases, the third down is the 31 individual 15-sec expiration phases, and the bottom pictures are the 31 individual 15-sec breath hold out phases.

The topmost row for each of the four figures on each side is the first minute of the exercise phase, and the second row would be the second minute, and the last or bottom row is the last minute of the 31-min exercise period for the respective phase. Again, the profiles on the right side (right hemisphere) show greater MEG power compared to the left-hemisphere profiles. However, it appears that the inspiration phases for the left hemisphere exhibit the greatest overall power, and apparently much of the power effect comes from the stimulation of the inspiration phase.

Figure 47 shows the MEG data used in the experiment for the same subject plotted in Figs. 44, 45, and 46. However, here the data are averaged for every 15-sec epoch for mean power across all

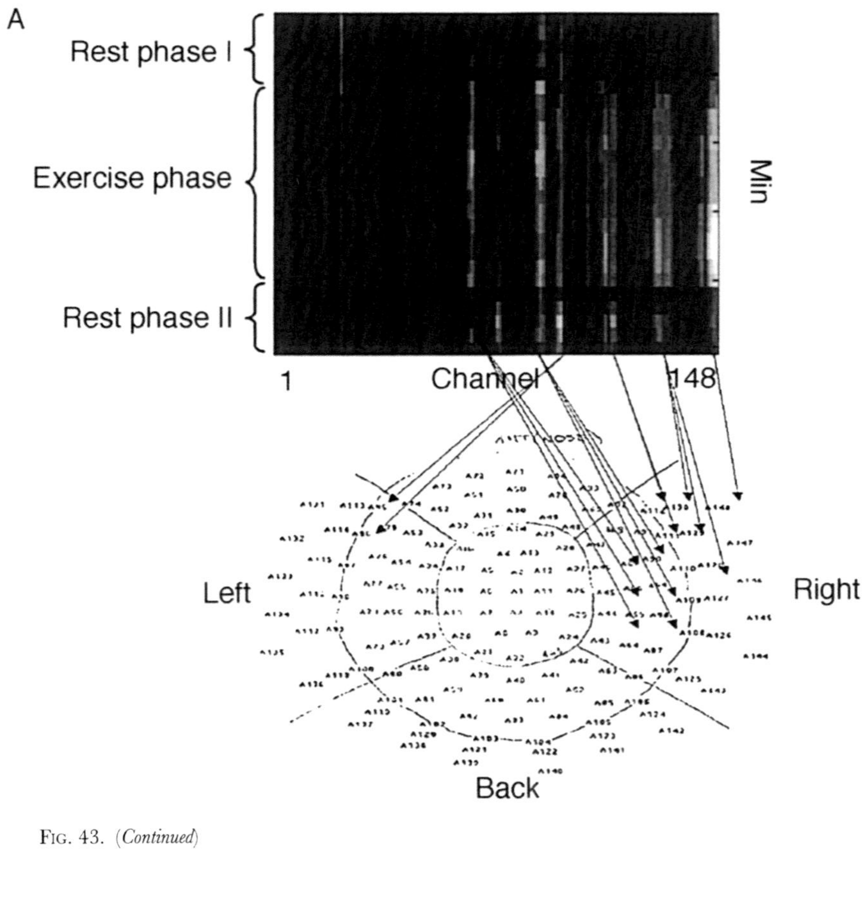


FIG. 43. (*Continued*)

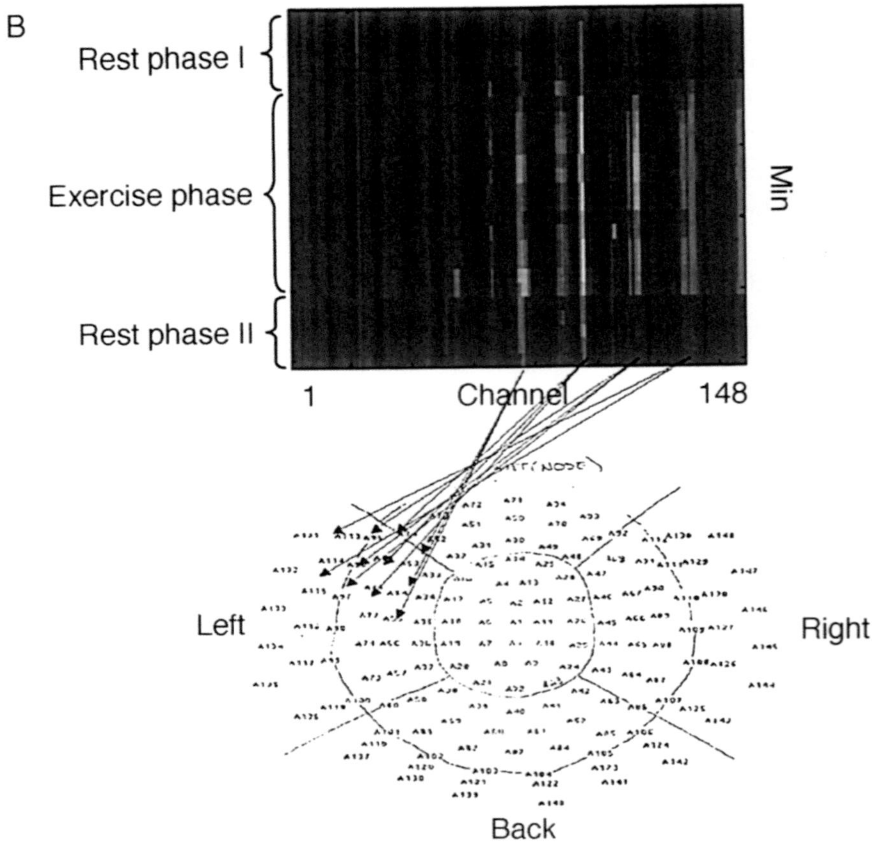


FIG. 43. The left nostril breathing pattern is presented on the top (A) of the figure and the right nostril breathing pattern is presented here on the bottom (B) of the figure for gamma band (30.0–54.0 Hz) activity. Channels within 20% of maximum power in postexercise rest period are mapped with arrows to their spatial head map locations in the lower part of the figure. Note the contralateral activation patterns for either the left or right nostril breathing patterns for the gamma frequency band. Adapted from Kundalini Yoga Meditation: Techniques Specific for Psychiatric Disorders, Couples Therapy, and Personal Growth by David Shannahoff-Khalsa; Copyright © 2006. Used by permission of W. W. Norton & Company, Inc. (See Color Insert.)

channels for each hemisphere, respectively. The sampling rate was 251 Hz. Therefore, each 15-sec epoch includes the mean value of 3765 measures for each of the 37 channels, and the plot presents the mean value for the 37 channels. The top figure is the data set for the left hemisphere, and the bottom figure is the data plotted for the right

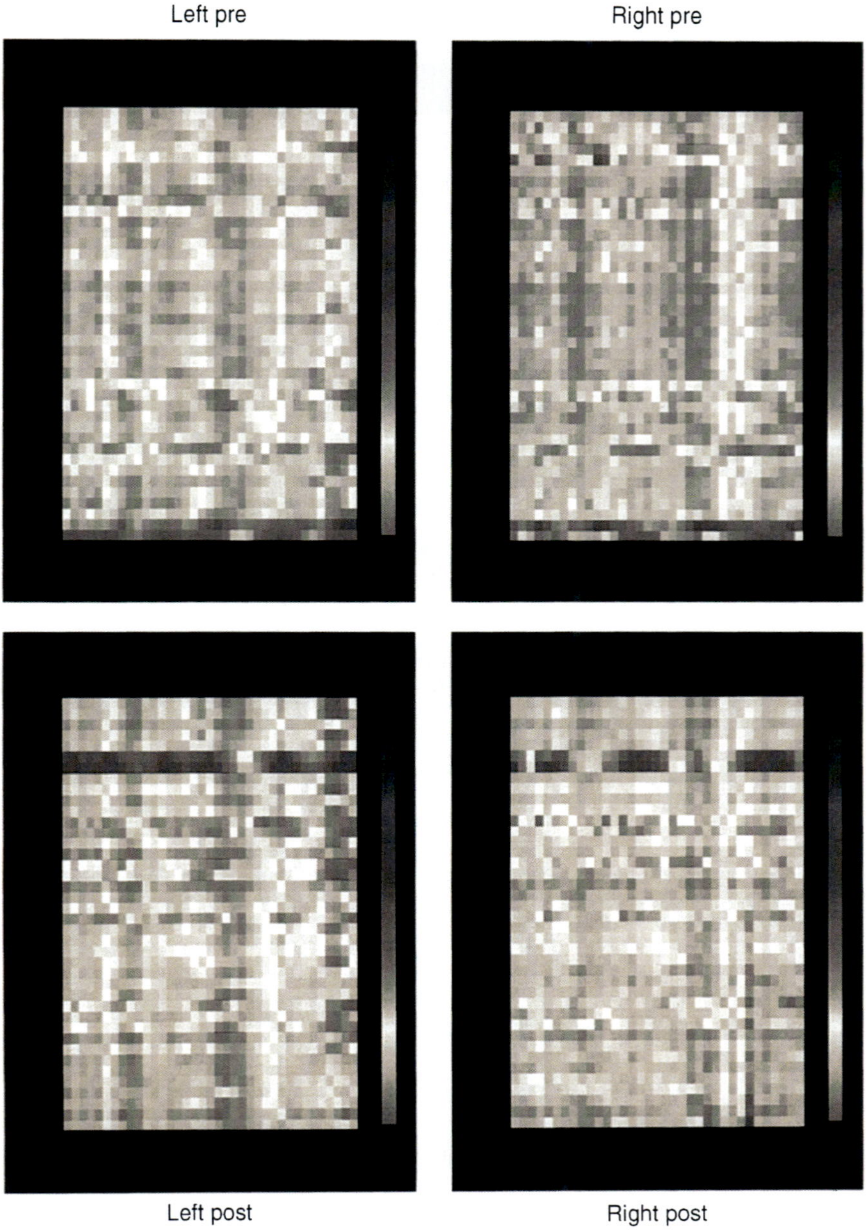


FIG. 44. Plots of 74 channels of MEG, with 37 channels per hemisphere. The data are from a subject performing the "OCDB." The subject was laying on his right side, as a 37-channel disk was arranged to record from each hemisphere with the eyes open and at the perfected rate of one BPM for

hemisphere. Both the top and bottom figures each have three separate zones. Points 0–600 present the mean profile for the 10 min of the preexercise rest phase, data points 600–2460 profile the 31 min of the OCDB exercise period, and points 2460–3060 profile the final 10 min of the postexercise rest period. While the single gross representation of data for the two rest phases appear to be nearly identical, it is clear that the two plots of the exercise period are substantially different. The power in the right hemisphere is dramatically increased across the recording period compared to the left hemisphere, and the structure also shows a substantial difference. This indicates a selective activation of the right hemisphere using the OCDB, which again supports the pattern of contralateral hemispheric activation using the active nostril.

Two studies suggest that EEG activity generated by nasal (versus oral) breathing is produced by a neural mechanism in the superior nasal meatus (Kristof *et al.*, 1981; Servit *et al.*, 1981). This activating effect could also be produced by air insufflation into the upper nasal cavity without inflating the lung. Local anesthesia of the nasal mucosal membrane suppressed the cortical effects of airflow stimulation. They also showed how deep breathing through one side of the nose could activate abnormalities in epileptic patients with unilateral focal or lateralized paroxysmal abnormalities in the fronto- or occipitotemporal region. "The abnormalities of this type were significantly more activated from the ipsilateral nasal cavity" (Servit *et al.*, 1981). However, these paroxysmal abnormalities were

31 consecutive minutes with a 10-min preexercise recording period and another 10-min recording with a postexercise rest period. The figure shows four plots. The left side of the figure shows the data for the left hemisphere with a plot of the 10-min preexercise rest period plotted at the top and the 10-min postexercise rest period plotted on the bottom left half. The right side of the figure has the respective data plotted for the right hemisphere. In this figure, the color columns going from the left of each figure are channel 1 with the rightmost column of channel 37. The data are presented as power for each 15-sec epoch of the data pictured with a square for the color. Here the data are plotted with the highest power represented by violet, and the color red is used to represent the lowest power, or as "VIBGYOR" (higher power to lower power) which is the reverse compared to the plots for Figs. 37–43. Each plot in this figure has 40 rows of data, since there are 10 min and four 15-sec epochs plotted per minute. Note the left and right hemispheres are fairly similar for the same rows of data for each rest period. The same rows usually show the same patterns of activation for greater energy. (See Color Insert.)

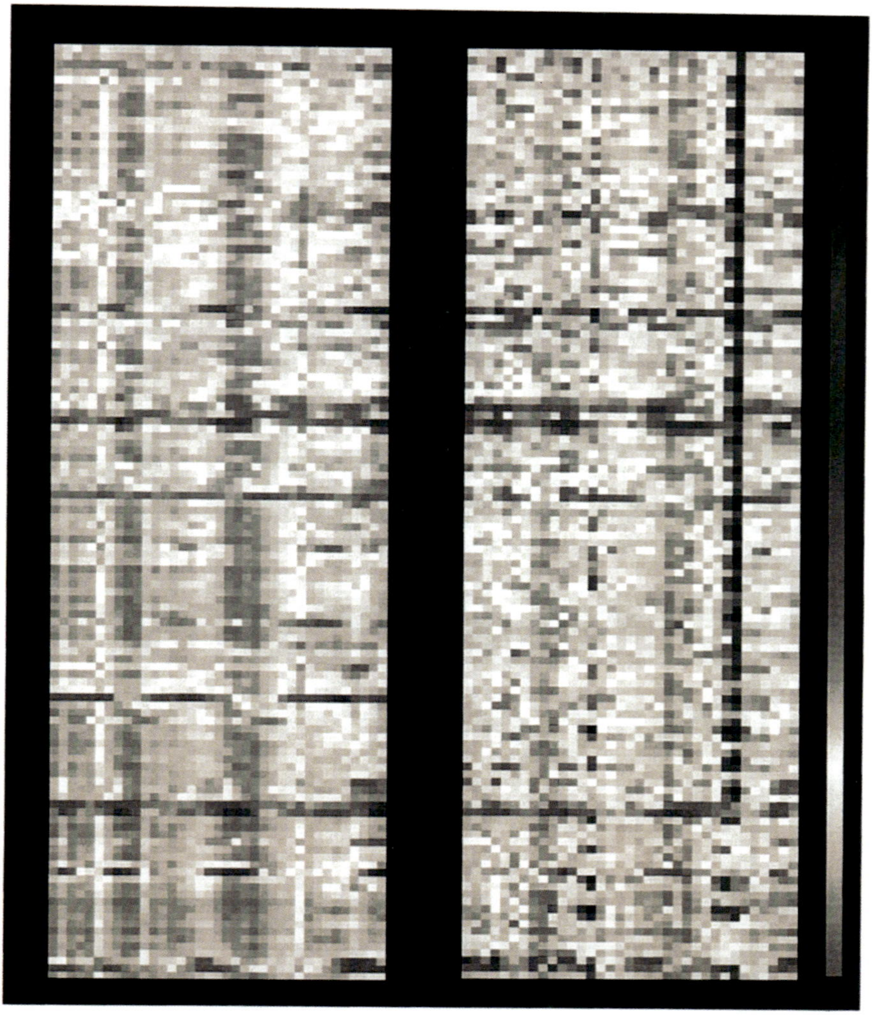

FIG. 45. Presentation of 31 min for the left nostril breathing portion of the experiment, again with the left hemisphere on the left side and the right hemisphere on the right side of the figure. And again, the top of the figure represents the start of the exercise period descending on the page to the end of the 31-min exercise period with each row representing a 15-sec epoch of the power. Here it is qualitatively apparent that the right hemisphere shows the greater power across the channels, which again demonstrates a pattern of contralateral activation for the active nostril. (See Color Insert.)

also generated with contralateral breathing to the foci in 60% of the patients. These abnormalities are not equivalent to the sustained contralateral increases in EEG produced in the study by Werntz

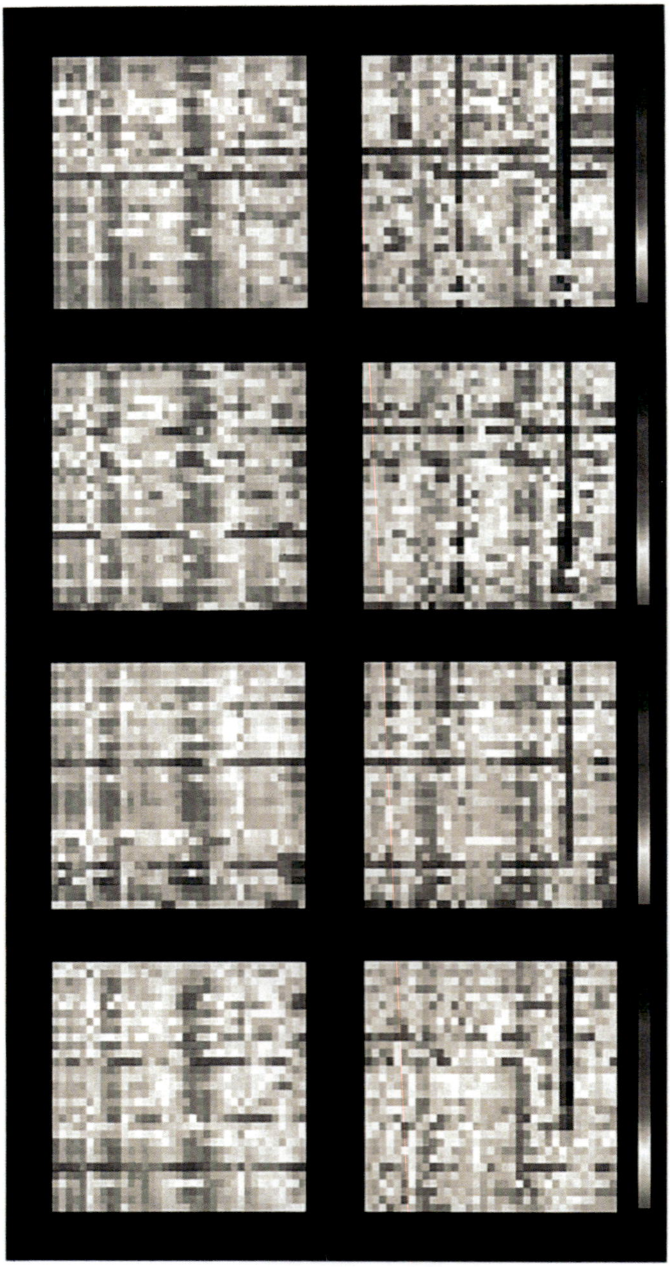

FIG. 46. This shows the 31-min exercise periods for the left hemisphere (left side of page) and right hemisphere (right side of page). The top pictures are the 31 15-sec inspiration phases, the second down are the 31 15-sec breath retention phases, the third down are the 31 15-sec expiration phases, and the

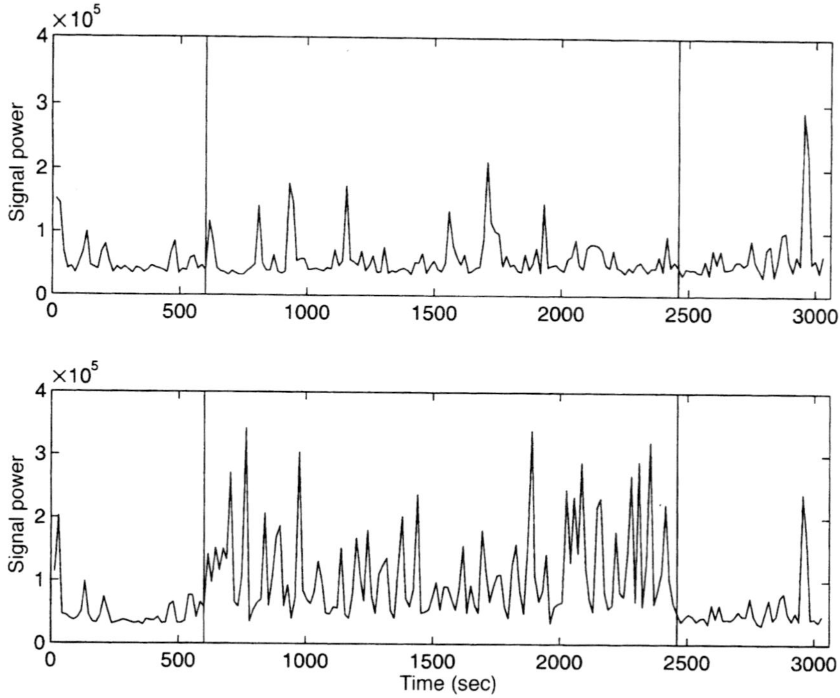


FIG. 47. This shows MEG data for the OCDB and the 10-min pre- and 10-min postexercise rest phases. The data sampled at 251 Hz (bandwidth 0.1–50.0 Hz) are averaged for every 15-sec epoch for the mean power across all channels for each hemisphere. Each data point in the figure is the mean value of 3765 measures for each and the mean of all 37 channels is plotted. The top figure is the data set for the left hemisphere, and the bottom figure is the data set plotted for the right hemisphere. Points 0–600 present the mean profile for all channels for 10 min of the preexercise rest phase, data points 600–2460 profile 31 min of the OCDB exercise period, and points 2460–3060 profile the final 10 min of the postexercise rest period. During the exercise period the power in the right hemisphere is dramatically increased across the recording period compared to the left hemisphere, and the structure also shows a substantial difference.

*et al.* (1987), as this paroxysmal activity manifests as intermittent spikes in only a small fraction of the record with epileptic patients. However, it is an example of how lateralized EEG activity can be affected by unilateral nasal airflow. The contralateral increase in

---

bottom pictures are the 31 15-sec breath hold out phases. The topmost row for each figure is the first minute of the exercise phase, and the second row would be the second minute, and the last or bottom row is the last minute of the 31-min exercise period for the respective phase. (See Color Insert.)

relatively greater EEG power (Werntz *et al.*, 1987) as a marker of greater or lesser mental activity was controversial. The yogic postulate states that UFNB activates the contralateral hemisphere and thus increases cognitive performance in the contralateral hemisphere. One study (Klein *et al.*, 1986) showed under resting conditions that right nasal dominance is coupled to relatively greater verbal performance (left brain activity), and left nasal dominance was coupled to relatively greater spatial skills (right brain activity). Two later studies (Jella and Shannahoff-Khalsa, 1993; Shannahoff-Khalsa *et al.*, 1991) using 30 min of UFNB, also with naive subjects, showed that right-UFNB (R-UFNB) increased left-hemispheric cognitive performance and that left-UFNB (L-UFNB) increased right-hemispheric performance. Three other groups also studied the effects of UFNB on cognitive performance or mood (Block *et al.*, 1989; Sanders *et al.*, 1994; Schiff and Rump, 1995).

In 1989, one study of UFNB on cognitive performance showed a mixed pattern of hemispheric activation with males appearing to have an ipsilateral increase in performance, but "unilateral breathing influences female performance contralaterally, but only on the spatial task" (Block *et al.*, 1989). These results were obtained after only 5 min of UFNB. In contrast to the results of past studies they state "These differences within and between sexes may exist because unilateral nostril breathing differently activates the two hemispheres and thereby facilitates performance, or because attempts of the brain to control the NC unilaterally interfere with performance." However, in 1994, an attempt to replicate the study by Block *et al.* (1989) exactly as conducted found no nostril-to-condition related performance for either males or females with a 5-min exercise period using identical psychological tasks (Sanders *et al.*, 1994). The study by Klein *et al.* found similar nostril dominance and hemisphere (contralateral) relations for both sexes during rest (Klein *et al.*, 1986). It is not likely that the ANS circuitry differs between sexes. In addition, another study found that UFNB through the dominant nostril also led to greater cognitive performance in the contralateral hemisphere (Schiff and Rump, 1995). However, this study did not investigate the UFNB effects in the nondominant congested nostril. In sum, it may be concluded that the results of these studies are in part dependent on the true lateralized nature of the cognitive tests employed, the breathing times and efforts, and keeping the nostril blocked during the final testing period to help maximize the effects.

An EEG study (Velikonja *et al.*, 1993) also failed to find a nostril-hemisphere effect. However, that study only captured four 1-min samples of EEG by having subjects lie in the lateral recumbent position while occluding the contralateral nostril. They only analyzed high alpha (10–12 Hz) and low beta (12–18 Hz) EEG frequency bands. This study also differs from that of Werntz *et al.* (1987) in that it did not analyze a continuous measure of EEG activity over all the entire recording period. One minute data samples, compared to a continuous recording of relative left/right power, can easily lead to mis-sampling due to the Mayer wave (0.1–0.008 Hz) activity that produces substantial intermittent increases in power. Longer, continuous, and filtered recordings are less affected by this normal autonomic high-frequency event when relative hemispheric powers are compared.

In 1991, another study (Stancak *et al.*, 1991) compared UFNB to bilateral breathing and reported that the peak power of beta 2 activity in the frontal leads was lower during UFNB than in bilateral breathing. They also reported that they found a homolateral relationship between nostril activity and EEG theta activity, but attributed this result to "increased upper airway resistance and to lateralized modulation of the subcortical generators of EEG theta rhythm during unilateral nostril breathing."

In 1997, a study on memory attempted to detect the hemisphere-specific effects of UFNB; however, the testing was done on a day after 10 successive days of the intervention (Naveen *et al.*, 1997). They compared R-UFNB, L-UFNB, alternate nostril breathing (inhaling through the left nostril and exhaling through the right nostril followed by inhaling through the right nostril and exhaling through the left nostril, with a continuation of this alternating sequence), breath awareness, and a control group with no breathing practices. All four breathing groups showed only increases in spatial skills where an "average increase in spatial memory scores for the trained groups was 84%." Again, hemisphere-related cognitive testing was not done during a breathing exercise, but only one day later after 10 days of practice.

It appears that nasal airflow may stimulate sympathetic dominance on the homolateral (ipsilateral) body-brain half. A mechanistic principle supporting the effects of UFNB is that this technique produces ipsilateral cortical vasoconstriction (via increased sympathetic tone) and thus reduced blood flow, and therefore reduced cortical activity in the ipsilateral brain hemisphere. It has been suggested that increased parasympathetic activation occurs simultaneously in the contralateral hemisphere to compensate for this sympathetic activation, which then helps to maintain adequate cerebral perfusion in total brain (Shannahoff-Khalsa, 2001).

Two clinical trials have employed the use of a specific L-UFNB pattern for the treatment of OCD with substantial and significant clinical reductions in obsessions and compulsions when measured with the Yale-Brown Obsessive Compulsive Scale, along with significant reductions in other psychological symptoms measured with other scales, and either a reduction or elimination of medication (Shannahoff-Khalsa and Beckett, 1996; Shannahoff-Khalsa *et al.*, 1999).

When considering the peripheral effects of UFNB, the earliest western scientific study to demonstrate a normal half-sided reaction in autonomic function was that of the relationship of the nose and lung (Drettner, 1970; Samzelius-Lejdstrom, 1939; Sercer, 1930; Stoksted, 1960). There is a unilateral nasal-pulmonary reflex mechanism which is clearly elicited when there is a forced inhalation through one nostril that has been shown to produce a significant increase in inflation in the homolateral lung. The lung is one organ where sympathetic influences lead to vasodilatation rather than vasoconstriction, thus leading to greater blood flow in the homolateral lung and therefore greater inflation and expansion. Samzelius-Lejdstrom studied 182 individuals and showed that the movements of one thoracal half were much more inflated compared to the contralateral lung in 94% of subjects. She also reported that in cases of tuberculosis where there is primarily a lateralized deficit, there is a simultaneous pathological phenomenon of the homolateral nasal and thoracal halves. One group studied rabbits under experimental conditions and showed that if coal dust was inhaled through one nasal opening, it was deposited in much larger quantities in the homolateral lung (Wotzilka and Schramek, 1930).

Backon and colleagues (Backon, 1988; Backon and Kullok, 1989; Backon *et al.*, 1989) have demonstrated the effects of UFNB on several autonomic dependent phenomena. Backon showed how R-UFNB significantly increased blood glucose levels and how L-UFNB lowered it (Backon, 1988), and that R-UFNB reduced involuntary eye blink rates and that L-UFNB increased eye blink rates (Backon and Kullok, 1989). They also showed how R-UFNB leads to an average and significant decrease of 23% in intraocular pressure and that L-UFNB increases it by an average but not significant value of 4.5% (Backon *et al.*, 1989). Others have also found that R-UFNB reduced intraocular pressure, but L-UFNB failed to increase it significantly (Chen *et al.*, 2004; Mohan *et al.*, 2001). We conducted three experiments using impedance cardiography to monitor the beat-to-beat effects of UFNB on the heart (Shannahoff-Khalsa and Kennedy, 1993). Two experiments employed a respiratory rate of 6 BPM and one experiment employed a rapid rate (2–3 breaths/sec) with shallow abdominal-based respiratory efforts, using a yogic technique called "breath of fire" or "kapalabhati." These studies all showed that R-UFNB increased HR compared to L-UFNB which lowered HR. We also showed that stroke volume and end diastolic volume are higher with L-UFNB at 6 BPM. These stimulation effects parallel those described above with the stellate ganglion in dogs, where stimulation of the right stellate ganglion leads to a greater increase in HR compared to stimulation of the left stellate ganglion (Levy and Martin, 1979; Levy *et al.*, 1966). Another study showed that L-UFNB significantly reduced HR in the subjects that were initially right nostril dominant, but failed in those who were initially left nostril dominant, and also failed to show any effects of

R-UFNB in subjects who were either left or right nostril dominant initially (Mohan and Wei, 2002). In yet another study, it was found that R-UFNB increased and L-UFNB decreased systolic and diastolic blood pressure, but only in women with no differential effects found in men (Dane *et al.*, 2002).

In addition, R-UFNB, L-UFNB, and alternate nostril breathing have been compared for their possible effects on metabolism as measured by oxygen consumption (Telles *et al.*, 1994). They found that with the effects of having "27 respiratory cycles, repeated 4 times a day for one month," that R-UFNB produced a 37% increase in baseline oxygen consumption, and that L-UFNB produced a 24% increase, and alternate nostril breathing increased baseline values by 18%. They also found that the L-UFNB group showed an increase in volar galvanic skin resistance, interpreted as a reduction in the sympathetic activity supplying the sweat glands. In another study they found that a one time 45-min practice of R-UFNB increased oxygen consumption by 17%, increased systolic blood pressure by 9.4 mm Hg, and decreased digital pulse volume by 45.7% (Telles *et al.*, 1996). That study did not include left UFNB.

These UFNB results, and the relevant understanding of the ANS innervation of the heart, help explain the findings of an open clinical trial using alternate nostril breathing as an effective therapy for treating angina pectoris (Friedell, 1948). Friedell reported an interesting clinical result. He found that "diaphragmatic breathing with attention to both phases of respiration and the intervening pauses" coupled with "alternately closing one nostril while inhaling slowly through the other" had profound effects on patients with angina pectoris. The 11 patients in this study all experienced relief from symptoms using this breathing practice and were able to eventually curtail the use of nitroglycerin. It is likely that the effect of the alternate nostril breathing technique can directly affect the lateralized sympathetic and vagal input to the heart, thereby inducing a balance in ANS activity. This breath pattern may help to reset the electrical patterns affecting the heart muscle.

In 1957, Riga published observations on unilateral chronic nasal obstruction which he thought might predispose people to a variety of disorders. Patients presented with a range of symptoms which he classified as:

> local disorders; nasal respiratory insufficiency, hypertrophic rhinitis of the obstructed nostril and allergic disorders, and neighboring disorders; spontaneous painful sensitivity in the periphery, sinusitis, catarrh of the Eustachian tube, hypacousia and otorrhea, bronchorrhea all on the obstructed side, and distant disorders; intellectual asthenia with frequent amnesia, headaches, hyperthyroidism, cardiopulmonary asthenia with tachycardia and asthmatic disorder with sometimes hypertrophy of the left cavity of the heart and pulmonary emphysema, hepatic and gall bladder, gastritis, enterocolitis, sexual disorders, dysmenorrhea, and decrease of virility (Riga, 1957).

Eighty-nine percent of the cases with right nasal obstruction were found to be afflicted to some degree with this widespread and apparently unrelated array, but only 26% of the cases with left nasal obstruction were afflicted. This suggests that a right-sided obstruction may more seriously affect health. It is possible that chronic unilateral obstruction may alter both the peripheral ANS activity and the balance of the cerebral rhythm. Deviated septums are common and may impair health in unexpected ways by off-setting the CNS–ANS rhythm.

One fascinating study of a 31-year-old woman, unaware of the phenomena of cerebral rhythms and nasal cycles showed the capacity to apparently exert a self-control of psychophysiological states (Gott *et al.*, 1984). She was self-trained, without fully understanding her achievement, and was able to voluntarily select and hold either of two qualitatively different state of consciousness that when studied in the laboratory gave evidence of differential dominance of the left or right hemisphere. "Asymmetries of EEG alpha and task performance scores indicated a state dependent shift in functional lateralization." The woman reported "that her state switch had been involuntary from early childhood. At age 16 she learned to select her state at will, thereby improving her school work and personal behavior." "Evoked response studies showed directional changes in the rate of interhemispheric transmission correlated with state-related hemisphere dominance. These findings demonstrated the capability for voluntary endogenous control of cerebral dominance under natural conditions" (Gott *et al.*, 1984). This finding is similar to the case reports of Ischlondsky. However the MPD patients apparently adapted a form of this mechanism for lateralized switching that was not consciously controlled (Ischlondsky, 1955). An advanced yogi can consciously select which hemisphere he wants to use within the span of one breath. He can switch back and forth fully activating one side of his brain with each breath cycle. The autonomic phenomenon becomes a consciously regulated activity. This level of development reflects a very advanced stage in the discipline of "self-regulation." Also, in normal individuals, where there is a transition state with the right and left hemispheres exhibiting equal balance, this state is supposedly very short-lived, lasting for no more than 1 or 2 min (Shannahoff-Khalsa, 1991a). However, the advanced yogi can consciously choose to operate from this state for prolonged periods. Perhaps this is the most advanced stage of lateralized development.

### B. Stimulation of the Autonomic Reflex Point on the Fifth Intercostal Space

In ancient times, yogis had also learned that lateral recumbency induces ipsilateral nasal congestion and contralateral decongestion, and that by applying pressure to the fifth intercostal space at the axilla, it is possible to affect changes in the nasal cycle and concommitant mental states. Novice practioners were taught to lean on the "yoga danda," a crutch-like device for altering the nasal cycle and cerebral rhythm. This noninvasive mechanism was used by the less adept to shift mind–body states. Who has not noticed the lateral recumbent effects on nasal congestion when suffering with the effects of the common cold, where the nostril on the recumbent "down" side is the one that quickly becomes or remains congested. No doubt everyone assumes this congestion reflex is the result of gravity, where mucous drains in the sinuses to the lower sinus and nostril. Perhaps the first western reports of such postural effects on the nasal cycle were in the original papers on the nasal cycle (Heetderks, 1927; Kayser, 1889, 1895), and then later in classic papers on sweat reflexes and body surface pressures where ipsilateral nasal airflow resistance is produced by application of pressure to the chest wall (Konno, 1969; Takagi and Sakurai, 1950), and with postural effects of pressure in the shoulder region and tested specifically in the axilla (Rao and Potdar, 1970).

While yogis had learned to mimic the lateral recumbent effects when remaining upright, while either standing or sitting, this ability to induce changes while vertical was not reported until the work of Rao and Potdar in 1970. They had studied ancient yogic texts and became aware of the use of the wooden crutch called the "yoga danda." They were aware that it was used "for correcting the right or left nasal airflow" (Rao and Potdar, 1970). They state "The crutchlike device used for producing deep pressure in the axilla was a T-shaped adjustable wooden prop. It was placed under either armpit so that the subject rested the weight of his shoulder on it." They observed how the pressure in the axilla could induce changes that lead to decongestion in the contralateral nostril. In one set of experiments:

> while the subjects maintained the lateral horizontal posture of the body, the tissue around the shoulder and arm were freed of the squeezing effect. To accomplish this, the subjects were placed in the lateral posture on two tables separated in such a manner that body weight was borne on their temporal region, lateral abdomen, and lateral part of thigh and leg. The lower neck region, shoulder, and hand were free of any weight or pressure. No increase in flow resistance through the down side of the nose was found after 10 min in this position (Rao and Potdar, 1970).

They believed that the effect is likely autonomic and solely the result of pressure on the surface near the shoulder in the axillary region. They discussed the possible neural pathways involved.

Later, two leading otolaryngologists, well trained with modern methods of measuring nasal airflow, performed a series of complex experiments to study the effects of lateral recumbancy on nasal airflow in great detail (Cole and Haight, 1984, 1986; Haight and Cole, 1984, 1986). In a set of experiments they compared 45 sec versus 12 min of lateral recumbency; the effect on nasal resistance of progressively lengthening the periods of lateral recumbency; short periods of lateral recumbency immediately after the reciprocating phase of the nasal cycle; the magnitude of nasal resistance changes after rotation of hips or of whole body; determined if pressure, warmth, or touch are effective in inducing ipsilateral nasal congestion and contralateral decongestion; and whether these effects could be blocked by injection of a local anesthetic or by topical nasal decongestants (Haight and Cole, 1986). They found that in the 45-sec versus 12-min study, that "the resistive changes reversed within approximately 60 sec of the termination of lateral recumbency, but after 12 min they persisted for 15 min or more." They conclude here that "there are two nasal responses to lateral recumbency, a 'transient' and a 'sustained,' and that the difference is due to temporal summation" (Haight and Cole, 1986). Also, when observing effects of progressive lengthening, they found "that with progressively longer periods of lateral recumbency the nasal response increased in magnitude, endured for longer, and a sustained phase reversal was produced." Also, when checking short periods of lateral recumbency immediately after the reciprocating phase of the nasal cycle, they found that ipsilateral nasal congestion is usually adopted, but also that the nasal cycle continues after long lateral recumbent periods, often after 2 h. They also found that both the transient changes and the sustained reversals are prevented by local anesthetic blockade of the cervical sympathetic ganglion. They conclude that the efferent pathway for both responses is via the sympathetic fibers to the erectile tissue of the nasal mucosa. And that the receptors are located deep in the subcutaneous tissue but superficial to thoracic viscera. In addition, they did not find that warmth alone could elicit the changes in nasal patency and that pressures to the head, arms, or legs were not effective, nor to the abdomen or lower dorsum. They concluded that the pressure-sensitive zones are located in the ventral, dorsal, and lateral aspects of the pelvic and pectoral girdles and thoracic wall. They also state that "This topographical distribution is strikingly similar to that which induces contralateral sweating in response to localized pressure: the 'hemi-hydrotic reflex.' Therefore there is a possibility that these responses share a common afferent pathway" (Haight and Cole, 1986). They also mention that deviated septums and unilateral fixed nasal obstruction in some patients may well have pathological significance in sleep.

### C. Vagal Nerve Stimulation

The dynamic view of ANS–CNS interactions may help us to better understand the therapeutic potential of VNS and its potential risks. While the vagus nerve is usually thought of mostly as an efferent fiber system, the vagus is actually a mixed nerve and about 80% of the fibers are actually afferent sensory fibers carrying information to the brain from the head, neck, thorax, and abdomen (Foley and DuBois, 1937). This afferent fiber system is what makes VNS a potentially useful therapeutic tool. The influences of the left and right vagus nerves are not identical and VNS studies have empirically led to the selective use of the left cervical (mid-inferior region) branch for prolonged and intermittent stimulation to help avoid cardiac instabilities (Henry, 2002).

VNS has been shown to be an important therapeutic tool for the treatment of pharmacoresistant epilepsy and it has shown to yield an average decline in seizure frequency of 25–30% when patients ($N = 313$) are treated with a high stimulation rate (30 Hz, 30 sec on/5 min off; 500 μsec pulse width) compared to a low stimulation rate (1 Hz, 30 sec on/90–180 min off; 130 μsec pulse width) which yields only a 6–15% reduction in seizure frequency (Ben-Menachem *et al.*, 1995; Handforth *et al.*, 1998; Morris and Mueller, 1999). VNS is well tolerated, however, it is not a substitute for anti-epileptic medication (Hatton *et al.*, 2006). Long-term VNS therapy for epileptic patients resulted in a 35% reduction in seizure frequency at 1 year, 44.3% at 2 years, and 44.1% at 3 years. The proportion of patients-with sustained seizure frequency reductions of 50% or greater was 23% at 3 months, 36.8% at 1 year, 43.2% at 2 years, and 42.7% at 3 years. Thus, it appears that the acute 3-month response increases up to the second year of treatment, after which response rates tend to plateau (DeGiorgio *et al.*, 2000; Morris and Mueller, 1999; Salinsky *et al.*, 1996). Also, the postive response during acute treatment suggests that this can be maintained for longer periods (Salinsky *et al.*, 1996). It is claimed that long-term treatment was well tolerated, with continuation rates of 96.7% at 1 year, 84.7% at 2 years, and 72.1% at 3 years (Morris and Mueller, 1999). VNS is also claimed to be effective in children aged 3–18 years with median reductions in seizure frequency at 3, 6, 12, and 18 months of 23%, 31%, 34%, and 42%, respectively (Cyberonics, 2004).

VNS has also been studied with treatment-resistant depression patients. To date, two trials have been published. The first was an uncontrolled pilot study ($N = 60$) looking at the acute effects in 10 weeks ($N = 60$) (Rush *et al.*, 2000; Sackeim *et al.*, 2001), and the second was a larger, double-masked, sham-controlled, 10-week trial ($N = 235$) (Rush *et al.*, 2005). Fifty-nine of the 60 patients in the pilot completed the study, and 18 (30.5%) were considered responders [a $\geq$50% reduction in baseline Hamilton Depression Scale (HAMD)-28 total scores], and 9 (15.3%) remitted (HAMD-28 total score $\leq$10). Improvement was gradual, with a mean of 48.1 days until the response was significant. None of the patients withdrew due to adverse events. The larger study compared VNS with sham treatment with either unipolar depression patients or bipolar patients in the depressed phase. There were 112 patients in the treatment group (high/stronger stimulation rates) and 110 in the sham group (low/weaker stimulation rates) (Rush *et al.*, 2005). The device was activated (single-blinded) after a 2-week postimplantation recovery period and stimulation parameters were adjusted during the first 3 weeks postactivation and fixed for the remaining 8 weeks of the trial. While the device was well tolerated, there was no short-term demonstration of efficacy in the response rates ($\geq$50% reduction in baseline HAMD-28), with the active group showing 15.2% and the sham group a 10.0% improvement. However, when long-term rates of efficacy were calculated with the 59 patients who completed the short-term pilot study (Rush *et al.*, 2000; Sackeim *et al.*, 2001), and met response criteria as early responders (3 months) or as late responders (1 year) and followed for 2 years (Nahas *et al.*, 2005), the 3-month response rates of 30.5% increased to 44.1% at 1 year and were 42.4% at 2 years (Nahas *et al.*, 2005). Also, when maintenance of response was considered, 55.6% of early responders and 78.6% of late responders continued as responders at the 2 year mark (Sackeim *et al.*, 2004). When rates of remission were considered in a subset of 30 patients (remission is defined as ≤10 on the HAMD-28), there was a significant increase from 17% at 3 months (5 of 30 patients) to 29% at 1 year (8 of 28 patients) (Marangell *et al.*, 2002). Similar sustained results in the larger study (Rush *et al.*, 2005) were observed with the follow-up of 205 patients where the treatment group showed a response rate for remission of 27.2% and the sham group showed 15.8%. One might conclude that VNS therapy holds some promise for treatment refractory depression. However, the mechanisms of effect are not completely understood.

Since VNS causes brain effects in regions also believed to regulate anxiety, and there were major reductions in anxiety in the first depression study, a multisite open trial in treatment-resistant anxiety-disorder patients was launched involving 30 anxiety-disorder patients with a primary diagnosis of either OCD, posttraumatic stress disorder (PTSD), or panic disorder (George *et al.*, 2003). No results are reported to date for this trial, however, others have also discussed the potential utility of VNS for OCD (Husted and Shapira, 2004; Pallanti *et al.*, 2004). And VNS has also been suggested as a therapy for treating obesity, pain, Alzheimer's disease, and other neuropsychiatric disorders (George *et al.*, 2003).

However, VNS requires general anesthesia that may also include other surgical procedures after initial placement. Therefore, recent attention has been directed toward potential perioperative complications postimplantation, and other anesthetic considerations during initial placement, and anesthetic management issues for patients with a preexisting VNS device (Hatton *et al.*, 2006).

The stimulation parameters of VNS (high/stronger stimulation rates vs low/weaker stimulation rates) are important factors and they are discussed in depth in the efficacious treatment of epilepsy and depression (Cyberonics, 2004; George *et al.*, 2003; Henry, 2002; Nemeroff *et al.*, 2006). The concepts of pulsatility and structured stimulation patterns are also important parameters with some of the more advanced UFNB techniques. An example of the possible complexity of UFNB patterns that requires altered rates of pulsatile stimulation are detailed in the following description of what is probably the most highly structured, but not the most difficult to perform UFNB technique. This technique is claimed to be effective for inducing a "comprehensive, comparative, and intuitive mind" (Shannahoff-Khalsa, 1991b).

*Description*: This technique has four sections with the first three sections each including three additional parts. First the right nostril is blocked and the breathing pattern is only through the left nostril and includes a series of broken breaths (or steps where the breath is inspired sequentially in relatively equal parts) but only during the inspiration phase with this technique. To help clarify this procedure, for example using the "4-part breath" (see below), the first inspiration involves taking in approximately ¼ of a full lung volume, followed by the second ¼ volume, and then the third ¼ volume, and finally the fourth ¼ volume. However, when this is actually practiced, it is not a requirement that the lungs are filled to maximum capacity, but to near full capacity which is less stressful.

*Section 1* (total time is 9 min): (Part A) Inhale through the left nostril in four parts and out the left nostril in one part, and continue this pattern for 3 min. (Part B) Inhale through the left nostril in eight parts and exhale out of the left nostril in one part for 3 min. (Part C) Inhale through the left nostril in 16 parts and exhale out of the left nostril in one part for 3 min.

*Section 2* (total time is 9 min): Immediately repeat the entire procedure, for parts A, B, and C of Section 1, but start by breathing only through the right nostril while blocking the left nostril during all three parts, respectively.

*Section 3* (total time is 9 min): Relaxing both hands in the lap, complete the breathing pattern of parts A, B, and C used in Sections 1 and 2, again each for 3 min but without blocking either nostril.

*Section 4* (total time is 4 min): Keep the hands relaxed in the lap. Curl the tongue in a "U" shape and extend it out of the mouth, inhale in four parts through the curled tongue, then close the mouth and exhale in one part through the nose, and continue the four parts in through the curled tongue and one part out through the nose for 4 min. The total time for this technique (Sections 1–4) is 31 min.

Supposedly, the effects of the 4-part, 8-part, and 16-part breath patterns all have differential influences on the cortex, and the use of the two nostrils independently in series (L-UFNB proceeding R-UFNB), later followed by the section without blocking either nostril all together have a balancing effect on the cortex and peripheral ANS. And the pattern through the mouth supposedly has beneficially effects on the thyroid and parathyroid glands. One might conclude that if such highly unique patterns are supposedly effective in UFNB techniques, unique patterns may also be found to be beneficial with VNS, and perhaps may differ in benefit with a range of disorders.

In addition to the effects of SUAA using UFNB on the brain, heart, and the other organs and systems innervated by the ANS, and in the treatment of OCD (Shannahoff-Khalsa and Beckett, 1996; Shannahoff-Khalsa *et al.*, 1999), the modern method of VNS has shown a marked benefit in the treatment of pharmacoresistant epilepsy (Group, 1999), major depression (George *et al.*, 2000; Rush *et al.*, 2000), and may show potential with OCD and other anxiety disorders (Husted and Shapira, 2004). "It is concluded that although the precise mechanism of action of VNS is still unknown, the search for the mechanism has the potential to lend new insight into the neuropathology of depression" (Groves and Brown, 2005). One might conclude that the effects of VNS may also be mediated by similar mechanisms to those of UFNB—a generalized differential activation of one-half of the ANS. In fact, yogis refer to the vagus nerve as the "mind nerve" (Yogi Bhajan, personal communication), and this may suggest that VNS has a relatively simple unilateral influence that may be useful for many disorders, both psychological and physiological. Yogis clearly claim that the various UFNB patterns all have differential and beneficial health benefits, and especially with the psychiatric disorders.

In sum, one might conclude that SUAA is a simple and useful method that can be used to exploit the unique, independent, and lateralized autonomic innervation to the organs, tissues, and brain. It appears that UFNB works through mechanical receptors in the nasal mucosa that lead to the hypothalamus, and this center then employs the SNS directly through the ipsilateral pathways to peripheral and central sites of influence. It may also be the case that a passive compensatory activation through PNS also influences the respective organs, brain, and periphery. Henry comments:

> Anatomical pathways provide the left cervical vagus afferent and efferent fibers with access to (a) parasympathetic control of the heart and multiple other visceral organs, (b) pharyngeal muscles of vocalization, (c) a limited somatosensory representation of the head and neck, and (d) a widespread array of autonomic, reticular, and limbic structures of the brainstem and both hemispheres. Therapeutic VNS appears to have remarkably little effect on the vagal parasympathetic visceroeffectors. The common reversible adverse effects of VNS mainly involve vocalization and somatic sensation. Experimental and human studies most strongly support altered activities of the reticular activating system, the central autonomic network, the limbic system, and the diffuse noradrenergic projection system as modalities of seizure antagonism (Henry, 2002).

However, it may also be important to explore any potential effects that VNS has on the natural endogenous ultradian rhythms, both those expressed in the periphery and those of the CNS. It is likely that such effects exist and that they may play a central role in the regulation of a range of disorders where imbalances occur. The ANS–CNS rhythm manifests as an internal pendulum of lateral activities, and it may be a shift in this rhythmic-like activity that helps play a useful therapeutic role (Shannahoff-Khalsa, 1991a,b). It is known that UFNB can indeed affect the balance of various ANS–CNS functions and yogis had viewed this pendulum as a balance of "yin and yang" like activities that are central to health, which we can now view within the extended concept of the BRAC hypothesis.

## VI. Reflections, Conclusions, and Future Directions

The development of the lateralized ultradian rhythms of the nervous system is a major evolutionary step in the nervous system and in our physiological development. The first western reference to this phenomenon apparently comes from the work of Kayser, a German physician, at the turn of the nineteenth century with his observation on the nasal cycle and his description of how this cyclical activity reflects the "alternation of vasomotor tone throughout the periphery on the two sides of the body" (Kayser, 1889, 1895). While the nasal cycle has been studied at some length by many researchers in prominent institutions around the world, those efforts have been primarily directed toward a better understanding of nasal physiology in the hopes of finding better solutions for respiratory diseases. However, the true significance of the nasal cycle has been mostly ignored after Kayser's publication. One exception to this "compartmentalized" study of the nose was the work of another German researcher on the "half-sided rhythms of the vegetative nervous system" (Beickert, 1951). Observations were made at 30-min intervals and Beickert found how lateralized differences in secretions of the nose and eye varied in phase with the nasal cycle. He also observed how a stellate ganglion block could lead to autonomic-related lateral changes in the nose, pupils, vessels of the arms and middle ear, perspiration, and nasal secretions. Beickert also discovered in normal healthy subjects who were subjected to "pharmaceuticals which irritate the vegetative nervous system," that the left side is more capable of swelling and deswelling than the right side. But in atrophies (ozaena-pathologies) the more extensive swell-width has been surprisingly observed, always on the right side and not as in normal cases on the left side (Beickert, 1951). This may be another clue to better understanding autonomic physiology in healthy and disease states. This apparent bias in disease-related lateralization is reminiscent of Riga's discovery in patients with chronic unilateral nasal occlusion, where patients with right occlusion seem to suffer more from an array of local and distantly related symptoms than patients with chronic left nasal occlusion (Riga, 1957).

Beickert also commented that "for the supply area of the external and internal carotid arteries, as well as for the brain vessels, side contrasting innervations resulting from one-sided stimulation of the vegetative nervous system have not been found." However, he also comments "In the head and neck area, this side rhythm will probably be found, and all experimental and therapeutical investigations will bring unexplicable and contradicting results if the described peculiarities of the vegetative innervation in the head are neglected, and when the measurements are taken during different phases of the cycles" (Beickert, 1951). Beickert also referenced similar observations (Springorum and Centenera, 1938) on the differential activities in the two kidneys as expected correlates, and thus presented us with a rather wide scope of the lateralized autonomic rhythm. We can conclude that for the most part rather interesting and striking observations on the nose and peripheral organ systems left little imprint on the research strategies of neurophysiologists and those with interests in psychophysiological states.

The later work by researchers on sleep with the REM and NREM cycles and the proposal of the BRAC hypothesis also apparently missed the insights of the early German physiologists. I must clarify here that our study on the nasal cycle and its postulated relationship to the ultradian rhythm of alternating cerebral hemispheric activity was motivated by yogic teachings that claimed that the nasal cycle was a marker for the cerebral rhythm, lateralized rhythms of ANS activity, and for psychophysiological states. Our study on the nasal cycle coupling to the cerebral rhythm using EEG was initiated in 1976 as a thesis dissertation by Deborah A. Werntz at my suggestion, and was conducted also in collaboration with Reginald G. Bickford and Floyd E. Bloom (Werntz *et al.*, 1980, 1983). When this work was conceived, we were unaware of the early sleep study results in humans by Goldstein and colleagues who used EEG to show an alternation of cerebral dominance during sleep and a hemispheric coupling to sleep stages (Goldstein *et al.*, 1970, 1972), or the early work by others on "unihemispheric" sleep in whale and dolphins (see Section II.B.1). Shortly after we started our study, I remember hearing a story about a researcher who was informed by someone else with a background in yoga that the nasal cycle was related to the REM–NREM sleep cycle. That researcher then carefully studied the nasal cycle in two medical school students, but only during waking hours and found a 3–4 h cycle. He concluded that since the REM–NREM cycle is a "90-min rhythm," it could not be related to the nasal cycle. This same kind of error has lead to much confusion in the physiological and psychophysiological studies in the ultradian domain. The fact that there is so much wobble and nonstationarity with the ultradians has led to much confusion because these rhythms have been studied with various species, ages, bodily systems, laboratory conditions, health and disease states, during waking or sleep, and with different sampling rates. Another major problem has been the virtual lack of multivariate physiological studies where systems could be studied simultaneously during both waking and sleep. Also, many researchers assume that unless two parameters are either perfectly in phase, or 180° out of phase, the two phenomena are entirely independent. The possibility of a lag period must also be considered, and when the swings in amplitudes are not identical, this too does not discount the possible coupling of two different systems. The use of spectral time series analysis is important here to help establish the possibility of a single or mutually coupled oscillators. Because we had the yogic insight on the lateralized rhythms of the ANS and CNS, and how the nasal cycle is a marker for states, and we also conducted multivariate studies, we were able to present a new view for psychophysiological states and what now appears to be a more general ANS–CNS rhythm. Clearly, the yogic insight that comes from the nasal cycle now sheds new light on how we can better and more inclusively define psychophysiological states with the critical regulatory correlate of the lateralized neural rhythms, and the nasal cycle as the key marker here for potentially defining states, that is, either a left or a right nostril-dominant mode. These rhythms and their translational aspects are important and exciting keys toward understanding physiology, performance studies, treating psychiatric disorders, and perhaps a wide range of other disorders. There is an obvious irony to the nasal cycle. This rhythm is very subtle, yet it plays a very dominant role in our lives. It regulates our moods, emotions, drives, energetic states, levels of mental and physical performance efficiencies, and our behavior. If the importance of the nasal cycle is indicative of the importance of other yogic discoveries, we would be well served if we pay more attention to what we can harvest from these ancient teachings. Apparently old discoveries, some of which have been ignored, like those by Kayser and Beickert, are more important than expected. Perhaps others perceived them as only bizarre anomalies only related to that external structure of the nose? This book also describes other striking findings that have apparently been overlooked that tell us the same story of differential lateral activation. The finding on the harlequin color change in newborns is clearly a remarkable observation (Neligan and Strang, 1952), as is the study on the lateralized autonomic shifts with complementary personalities in patients with MPD (Ischlondsky, 1955).

These observations suggest the possibility that disease can be lateralized in the periphery as a result of an imbalance where one side may somehow be more stressed than the other, or that one side may be inherently weaker or more susceptible to specific forms of stress and disease. Some personality profiles or states of psychopathology may reflect overactivation and abuse of one hemisphere and this is mentioned in Section IV. But is there clinical evidence toward a lateralized bias in autonomic malfunction otherwise? Eccles and Eccles (1981) in referring to lateralized autonomic tone state that "under stress or with marked hypothalamic instability this balance may be disrupted and result in the marked autonomic asymmetry seen in migraine or Meniere's syndrome." Such a disruption in autonomic balance may explain the asymmetrical autonomic response observed in migraine with unilateral flushing, nasal congestion, and visual distortion. Cluster headaches are characterized as recurrent, unilateral attacks of severe pain that almost always occur on the same side of the head with lacrimation, nasal congestion, conjunctival infection, ptosis, miosis, and rhinorrhea also occurring on the same side (Kittrelle *et al.*, 1985). Another curious and suggestive finding from the perspective of an ergotrophic-related state is the autonomic instability of asthmatics during sleep. Asthmatics seem to suffer more bronchoconstriction during REM sleep (Shapiro *et al.*, 1986). Normal bronchodilation occurs via increased sympathetic tone which enhances respiration, contrary to the vasoconstrictive effects of sympathetic fibers in most tissues. During REM sleep, therefore, a weakened or "stressed" autonomic fiber system may not "hold its own." However, even though this is not a lateralized effect of autonomic stress in the lungs, the principle of autonomic stress and lability and specific rhythmic phases holds, as REM is considered the active phase of the BRAC. Dexter and Weitzman (1970) found that REM sleep stages are also temporally related to nocturnal migraines and cluster headaches. In their study, sidedness was noted in only four of the seven subjects. All four experienced right-sided pain, ptosis, lacrimation, rhinorrhea, and sometimes sweating over the right side of the face and forehead. One patient showed an alternating hemicranial headache. No report as to side was given for the other two patients. Right-sided peripheral pain with these other symptoms also suggest the sympathetic fibers had been "weakened or strained" and hence releasing vessels causing acute dilatation. Symptoms of such headaches (and asthma) are often treated with sympathomimetics to gain relief. Baust (1974) states that even though heart rate is highest during REM sleep, sympathetic tone is at its lowest, at least in the cat. This suggests that during REM sleep there is a propensity for failed sympathetic tone which primarily manifests on the right side at least in this small group of subjects. This is equivalent to a lateralized stress of sympathetic function.

In bilaterally structured organs presenting with pathologies, there are commonly unilateral effects, such as with pneumonia, kidney disease, hyper- and hypothyroid conditions, inflammation of the ovary or testicle, tumors, or skin rashes. The unilateral stress of autonomic function deserves attention in these cases. There may be constellations of psychosomatic disorders that are more strongly coupled to right or left autonomic stress and dysfunction.

In a study of 980 female patients with unilateral breast cancer, results show a left/right ratio of 1.26:1 (Senie *et al.*, 1980). The data suggest that there are differences in the sensitivity of left and right mammary glands to hormonal stimulation resulting in an inequality of tissue at risk to develop carcinoma. Also when asynchronous bilateral carcinoma was documented, the disease first occurred more often in the left breast. As this study indicates a differential sensitivity to hormonal influence, it is also possible that an autonomic correlate plays a role. In another study of breast cancer, adenocarcinoma had a ratio of (L/R) 1.778:1 (McManus, 1977). Lateralization was also studied in 601 cases of carcinoma of the nasal cavity and paranasal sinuses where squamous, anaplastic carcinomata, and adenocarcinoma had a pronounced left-sided predominance in the ethmoid and to a much lesser extent in the nose (Robin and Shortridge, 1979).

The significant differences in breast or nasal carcinoma are at best suggestive that a lateralized influence of autonomic stress plays a role. However, in a study of 151 cases of herpes zoster, with 92 cases on the right and 59 on the left side of the body, stress is very likely to be an important influence (Wilson, 1986).

When we first started the work on the nasal cycle and cerebral rhythm, we were equally aware of the yogic claim of UFNB, which we also pursued in the laboratory. Again, who would have expected that altering the pattern of nasal airflow might have such importance and significance? The awareness in the west of the breath as a tool for altering mind–body states, or psychophysiological states, has been missing. However, in yoga, the role of the breath is elementary as a therapeutic tool. In the west, we rarely pay any attention to the breath.

What can we conclude about the discoveries in this book and the ultradian literature at large? First, it is easy to conclude that we must conduct many more multivariate studies during both waking and sleep that also include the transition periods between waking and sleep to also study the continuity here of the ANS–CNS rhythm between these two psychophysiological states. These studies will most likely give us the most useful information if they are conducted in humans, both in healthy and diseased states, and of course while including the nasal cycle as a central marker. We need to study the ANS via the nasal cycle with at least 4-Hz sampling; the CNS using EEG, MEG, or other noninvasive high-frequency sampling methods; the cardiovascular system using beat-to-beat noninvasive sampling with impedance cardiography and noninvasive instruments that can also give us beat-to-beat measures of the blood pressures; intravenous blood sampling (or salivary testing) to study neuroendocrine hormones, INS, glucose, neurotransmitters; and last but not least, parameters of the immune system. These systems are all very accessible and they may give us additional unique insights to how the major systems of the body are coregulated and integrated under healthy, stressed, and diseased conditions. While the ultradian rhythms of the gastrointestinal system were briefly reviewed earlier (see Section II.C), it is worth noting that urinary volumes and osmolarity exhibit with ultradians in the hourly domain and that they also correlate with dreaming (Mandell *et al.*, 1966). In addition, the ultradian rhythms of plasma renin activity (PRA) and aldosterone are also tightly coupled to the REM–NREM sleep cycle and are sleep-stage dependent (Brandenberger *et al.*, 1998):

> NREM sleep is invariably linked to increasing PRA levels, and declining levels are observed when sleep becomes slighter. Spontaneous and provoked awakenings blunt the rise in PRA normally associated with NREM sleep. Thus, PRA curves exactly reflect the pattern of sleep stage distribution. When the sleep cycles are regular, PRA levels oscillate at a regular period. For incomplete sleep cycles, PRA curves reflect all irregularities in sleep structure. It appears that this association cannot be broken. In normal man, modifying the renal renin content only modulates the amplitude of the nocturnal oscillations without disturbing their relation to sleep stages. This relation persists in some pathological cases, such as narcolepsy and moderate hypertension (Brandenberger, 1991).

These authors state "It is suggested that a central generator synchronizes endocrine, renal, autonomic and sleep processes" (Brandenberger *et al.*, 1998).

The chronobiology of system-to-system interrelationships is likely to be an important and productive frontier that has yet to be explored in any great depth. We have only begun to scratch the surface in this area. One of the most recent observations on the nasal cycle (Dane and Balci, 2007), where greater left nostril dominance during waking has been observed with autistic patients is a hint to what we may find that may help lead to novel therapies where little progress has been made to date in treatment. Autism spectrum disorders are now said to affect 1 in every 150 children up to age eight in the United States (Rice *et al.*, 2007).

The use of UFNB as a tool to treat OCD is another remarkable discovery that has its origins in yogic studies (Shannahoff-Khalsa, 1997, 2003, 2006, 2007; Shannahoff-Khalsa and Beckett,

1996; Shannahoff-Khalsa *et al.*, 1999). We employed a technique that yogis had claimed was "disorder-specific" for the treatment of OCD, and it was included in a multipart protocol that I designed to help improve the possibility of a clinical success for patients with a very difficult-to-treat psychiatric disorder that is also perhaps known to be the least susceptible to placebo treatment effects. So not only had yogis discovered that the breath is a link between the mind and body, but that it can also be a very useful tool for treating psychiatric disorders, improving health, and mental wellness in general. There is now significant information published (Shannahoff-Khalsa, 1991b, 2003, 2004, 2005, 2006, 2007) on the use of these techniques as tools for treating OCD and other psychiatric disorders. There are different multipart protocols published for treating the following disorders: (1) acute stress disorder, (2) OCD, (3) major depressive disorder, (4) bipolar disorders, (5) chronic fatigue syndrome, (6) treating the addictive impulse control and eating disorders, (7) attention deficit hyperactivity and comorbid disorders, (8) and PTSD (Shannahoff-Khalsa, 2006). There are also 60 different Kundalini yoga meditation techniques published in the same text that all deserve much greater attention as potential therapeutic tools for treating disease and perhaps even more importantly for use as preventative measures for maintaining health (Shannahoff-Khalsa, 2006). The idea that yogis had discovered "disorder-specific" techniques is likely to lead to much skepticism and criticism. This same "knee-jerk" reaction was the case for many when the original idea was posed for monitoring the nasal cycle as a marker for an undiscovered cerebral rhythm in humans during the waking state (Werntz *et al.*, 1983).

## A. Seven Examples of Highly Structured Yogic Breathing Techniques

The following are examples of ancient yogic breathing techniques that may prove useful in both preventing illness and treating specific conditions. All of these highly structured respiratory control techniques were published previously in a peer-reviewed scientific book (Shannahoff-Khalsa, 1991b).

1. *Technique for Treating Insanity and Alleviating Emotional Stress and Anxiety*

*Description*: Sit erect and maintain a straight spine. Relax the arms and the hands in the lap. Focus the eyes on the tip of the nose (the end which you cannot see). Open the mouth as wide as possible, slightly stressing the temporal-mandibular joint, touch the tongue tip to the upper palate where it is hard and smooth. Breathe through the nose only, while making the breath long, slow, and deep. Let the mental focus be on the sound of the breath, listen to the sound of the inhale and exhale. Maintain this for at least 3–5 min with a maximum of 8 min at first trial. With practice it can be built up to 31 min maximum.

2. *Technique for Fatigue and Listlessness*

*Description*: Sit erect with a straight spine. Place the palms together at the center of the chest, touching the sternum lightly, with the fingers pointing up and away at 60°. The eyelids are lightly closed with the visual focus where the nose meets the eyebrows. As you inhale break the breath into four equal parts, hold the breath for 1–2 sec and then exhale by breaking the breath again into four equal parts, and then hold the breath out for 1–2 sec before inhaling again. If desired, instead of counting 1, 2, 3, 4 to gauge the rhythm, try using the sounds Sa, Ta, Na, Ma in their place. Mentally vibrate these four sounds on the inhale and again on the exhale, it increases the benefits. Their innate effect on the psyche is to help guide and correct the consciousness. On each part of the inhale or exhale pull the naval point in slightly. One full cycle or breath takes about 7–8 sec. Continue this pattern for 3–5 min. Then inhale deeply and press the palms together with maximum force for 10 sec. Relax for 15–30 sec. Then repeat this entire procedure two more times. When finished, if necessary, immediately lie flat on the back with eyes closed and relax the entire body for 2 min. Pregnant women or individuals with high blood pressure can do this exercise, but must refrain from pressing the palms together at the end.

3. *Technique for Obsessive-Compulsive Disorders*

*Description*: Sit erect with a straight spine in a comfortable position, either with the legs crossed while sitting on the floor or in a straight back chair with both feet flat on the floor. Close the eyes. Use the right thumb tip to block the end of the right nostril, other fingers point up straight, allow the arm to relax (elbow should not be sticking up and out to the side creating unnecessary tension). Inhale very slowly, long, and deep through the left nostril, hold in long, exhale out slowly and completely through the same nostril only (left nostril), hold out long. The mental focus should be on the sound of the breath. Continue this pattern with a maximum time of 31 min for each sitting. Initially, begin with a comfortable rate and time, but where the effort presents a fair challenge. Holding the breath in or out long varies from person to person. Ideal time per complete breath cycle is one minute where each section of the cycle lasts for 15 sec. When first beginning to practice this technique, 5 sec for each of the four phases of the breath cycle is a good accomplishment which then leads to a respiration rate of three breaths per minute. This technique has been subjected to clinical trial as part of a multipart protocol and has shown a 71% mean group improvement in OCD symptoms using the Yale-Brown Obsessive Compulsive Scale (Shannahoff-Khalsa *et al.*, 1999, 2006).

4. *Technique for Expanding and Integrating the Mind*

*Description*: Sit erect with a straight spine and close the eyes and bring the mental focus to the area where the root of the nose meets the eyebrows (the third eye point). Relax the hands in the lap. Begin breathing through a curled tongue that is extended out of the mouth. The sides of the tongue are curled up and the tongue then makes a "U" shape. Break the inhale into eight equal parts for the inspiration. Then bring the tongue into the mouth, close it, and exhale in eight equal parts through the nose. Do not pause after completing the full inhale or exhale. Continue the cycle—eight parts in through the curled tongue and eight parts out the nose, taking about 10 sec for one complete round. If desired, try using the sounds Sa, Ta, Na, Ma (two times on inhale and two times on the exhale) instead of counting 1, 2, 3, 4, 5, 6, 7, 8 for each part of the breath. Mentally pair the sound of the breath with each of the different syllables in the proper sequence or just mentally listen to the sound of the breath itself. If you cannot curl the sides of the tongue up in this fashion take the inspiration only through the nose in eight parts, keeping the mouth closed, and exhale out of the nose in eight equal parts. Curling the tongue is a genetically determined ability. If you can curl the tongue in this way it will also help stimulate the thyroid and parathyroid glands. Start with 3–5 min, build the time up to 10–15 min, and then up to 31 min maximum. Upon completing this technique, take at least three long, slow, and deep breaths through the nose and then relax.

5. *Technique for Stimulating the Immune System*

*Description*: Before doing this technique it is best to practice technique number (4). It should be attempted just after the end section of (4) after the last three long, deep breaths are taken. On the last exhale, attempt to hold the breath out fairly completely, but relaxed, for a minimum of 1 min. Again sit with a straight spine and keep the eyes closed. The time held out is the secret here, the longer the better. With practice 3 min can be reached. The minimum time to achieve the desired effect is 1 min before the nervous system recognizes this signal. Since this is done by volition, no panic is experienced. The practitioner realizes he/she can quit at any time if desired. But only part of the brain recognizes this fact. Another part of the brain triggers an "emergency reset button" in the hypothalamus to engage all healing systems, which includes the immune system. In ancient times, yogis taught this technique for treating malignant but not benign tumors. It was said to be a direct means for stimulating the immune system. This procedure can easily be practiced three times per day. This technique is not for pregnant women, beyond 4 months.

6. *Technique for a Comprehensive, Comparative, and Intuitive Mind*

*Description*: This is an advanced exercise and requires substantial effort. Practice of this exercise is more rigorous and is best attempted after having developed the endurance to complete exercise (4) for 15 min. Its format is complex and the times should be followed exactly and supervised by another to properly indicate time periods, until experience is gained. It has four sections with the first three sections broken into three additional parts. The sitting posture and eye position is similar to exercise (4). Begin by using the thumb of the right hand to block the right nostril, making sure to lower the elbow to reduce strain on the arm for this time period. The breathing pattern is a series of broken breaths, the rate is about one part per second with the four-part breath and then less thereafter.

- Section 1 (total time is 9 min).

Part A: Inhale through the left nostril in four parts and exhale out through the left nostril in one part, continue this pattern for 3 min. Part B: Inhale through the left nostril in eight parts and exhale out through the left nostril in one part, continue this pattern for 3 min. Part C: Inhale through the left nostril in 16 parts and exhale out through the left nostril in one part, continue this pattern for 3 min.

- Section 2 (total time is 9 min).

Repeat the entire procedure, parts A, B, and C of Section 1 completely but start by breathing through the right nostril instead and use the left thumb to block the left nostril for this entire period.

- Section 3 (total time is 9 min).

Relaxing both hands in the lap complete the breathing pattern of the three parts given in A, B, and C, without blocking either nostril. The initial phase of the nasal cycle is not a concern in this exercise or in the previous ones. One side of the nose may be more difficult to breathe through.

• Section 4 (total time is 4 min).

Relax the hands in the lap. Curl the tongue (as in yogic exercise number 4) and extend it from the mouth, inhale in four parts close the mouth and exhale in one part out the nose, four parts in through the curled tongue and one part out the nose continue for 4 min. The total time for Sections 1–4 is 31 min.

When finished completely relax on the back for 10–30 min.

### 7. *Technique for Regenerating the CNS*

*Description*: Sit erect as in the previous exercises. Keep the eyes half open and focus on the tip of the nose (the end you cannot see). The eye muscles may become sore in the beginning of practice, but this will disappear with time. The hand position is as follows: males grasp the left thumb with the right hand closing the fingers of the right hand over the left thumb (which is now enclosed) and fingers also encompass right thumb; females reverse the hand posture clasping the right thumb inside, etc. Inhale and break the breath into 16 equal parts, then exhale and break the breath into 16 equal parts. Breathe only through the nose. Do not hold the breath once having completed the inhale or exhale. Continue breathing in this way. Each complete breath takes about 20 sec. If desired, instead of counting 1–16, mentally vibrate the sounds of Sa, Ta, Na, Ma, four cycles on the inhale and four cycles on the exhale. Begin with a few minutes and build up slowly to 31 min maximum time and no longer. Once having completed the technique, take several long and deep breaths, then relax. Stop if you feel like you are becoming light-headed. This exercise was reported to help regenerate the CNS for those who have been damaged by drugs and alcohol. It is also said that if it is practiced for 31 min/day for 120 days, a person's intuition will begin to remarkably improve.

Yogis had also discovered a technique which children and others can use to learn to help consciously regulate the phase of the nasal cycle. The practitioner sits erect with a straight spine and the hands are interlocked and placed directly against the abdominal region at the diaphragm or solar plexus level with the elbows near the ribs. The fingers of both hands are alternating where the right thumb is on the top followed by the left thumb, and then the right index finger, and the left index finger, etc., until the left little finger is on the bottom. This orientation of the fingers is to be employed even if the individual naturally interlocks the fingers with the opposite orientation, that is, with the left thumb dominating and the right little finger on the bottom. A tight pressure is maintained on both hands during the interlock, that is, the hands are held tightly together with some tension in the fingers. However, all other muscles in the body are relaxed. The eyes are closed and the individual concentrates on the flow of the breath at the tip of the nose. First, the natural phase of the nasal cycle is observed for several minutes. Then the practitioner attempts to consciously breathe through the congested nostril for several minutes. Once he is successful in changing dominance, he should then reverse the dominance again for several minutes. Eventually, the practitioner can learn to quickly alter the phase of dominance, and eventually the hand posture is no longer required. Yogi Bhajan suggested that this technique can be taught to children and to have them learn to master it by the age of three, so that they always have greater control over their emotional states and mental activities (Bhajan, 1980).

The ancients had clearly gained insights toward the mind and body and to the nature of our consciousness that deserves our serious attention. We may gain significantly from pursuing these techniques in the treatment of psychiatric disorders and for their inherent structure for what we can learn about the mind, the brain, and how to better treat diseases in general, and how to better promote health. Today we are learning that the concepts of the ancients, for example that of the nasal cycle and UFNB, have substantial value. Although the world of yogic medicine has a language that is different than that of modern science, it does not mean that these terms cannot be translated to help advance our understanding of the human nervous system and our ability to augment and facilitate its functions in order to better improve our lives. While it is true that we need a contemporary view of ancient concepts, it is now more obvious than ever that the experimentalists of the past have more to offer than we had ever imagined. Today, from a medical and scientific point of view, our future holds the possibility for developing a more stress-resistant and disease-resistant individual.

## References


Achermann, P., Finelli, L. A., and Borbely, A. A. (2001). Unihemispheric enhancement of delta power in human frontal sleep EEG by prolonged wakefulness. *Brain Res.* **913**(2), 220–223.

Adrian, E., and Matthews, B. (1934a). Berger rhythm: Potential changes from occipital lobes in man. *Brain* **57,** 355–385.

Adrian, E. D., and Matthews, B. H. (1934b). The interpretation of potential waves in the cortex. *J. Physiol.* **81**(4), 440–471.

Ahern, G. L., and Schwartz, G. E. (1979). Differential lateralization for positive versus negative emotion. *Neuropsychologia* **17**(6), 693–698.

Alexiev, A. D., and Roth, B. (1978). Some peculiar changes in the pattern of respiration connected with REM sleep. A preliminary report. *Electroencephalogr. Clin. Neurophysiol.* **44**(1), 108–111.

Armitage, R. (1986). Ultradian rhythms in EEG and performance: An assessment of individual differences in the basic rest activity cycle. PhD. Department of Psychol. Carleton University, Ottawa, Ontario.

Armitage, R., Bell, I., Campbell, K., and Stelmack, R. (1990). Asymmetrical auditory probe evoked potentials during REM and NREM sleep. *Sleep* **13**(1), 69–78.

Armitage, R., Emslie, G. J., Hoffmann, R. F., Weinberg, W. A., Kowatch, R. A., Rintelmann, J., and Rush, A. J. (2000). Ultradian rhythms and temporal coherence in sleep EEG in depressed children and adolescents. *Biol. Psychiatry* **47**(4), 338–350.

Armitage, R., Hoffmann, R., Loewy, D., and Moffitt, A. (1989). Variations in period-analysed EEG asymmetry in REM and NREM sleep. *Psychophysiology* **26**(3), 329–336.

Armitage, R., Hoffmann, R. F., and Rush, A. J. (1999). Biological rhythm disturbance in depression: Temporal coherence of ultradian sleep EEG rhythms. *Psychol. Med.* **29**(6), 1435–1448.

Aschoff, J., and Gerkema, M. (1985). "On the Diversity and Uniformity of Ultradian Rhythms." Springer-Verlag, Berlin.

Aserinsky, E., and Kleitman, N. (1953). Regularly occurring periods of eye motility, and concomitant phenomena, during sleep. *Science* **118**(3062), 273–274.

Aserinsky, E., and Kleitman, N. (1955a). A motility cycle in sleeping infants as manifested by ocular and gross bodily activity. *J. Appl. Physiol.* **8**(1), 11–18.

Aserinsky, E., and Kleitman, N. (1955b). Two types of ocular motility occurring in sleep. *J. Appl. Physiol.* **8**(1), 1–10.

Ashley, C. C., and Lea, T. J. (1978). A method for studying the cyclic changes in nasal resistance in the anaesthetized pig. *J. Physiol.* **282,** 1p–2p.

Backon, J. (1988). Changes in blood glucose levels induced by differential forced unilateral nostril breathing, a technique which affects both brain hemisphericity and autonomic activity. *Med. Science Res.* **16,** 1197–1199.

Backon, J., and Kullok, S. (1989). Effect of forced unilateral nostril breathing on blink rates: Relevance to hemispheric lateralization of dopamine. *Int. J. Neurosci.* **46**(1–2), 53–59.

Backon, J., Matamoros, N., and Ticho, U. (1989). Changes in intraocular pressure induced by differential forced unilateral nostril breathing, a technique that affects both brain hemisphericity and autonomic activity. A pilot study. *Graefes Arch. Clin. Exp. Ophthalmol.* **227**(6), 575–577.

Baglio, S., Bucolo, M., Fortuna, L., Frasca, M., La Rosa, M., and Shannahoff-Khalsa, D. (2002). MEG signals spatial power distribution and gamma band activity in yoga breathing exercises. *In* "Conference Proceedings of the IEEE Eng Medicine and Biology Society," Houston, October 23–26, 2002.

Bailey, D., Harry, D., Johnson, R. E., and Kupprat, I. (1973). Oscillations in oxygen consumption of man at rest. *J. Appl. Physiol.* **34**(4), 467–470.

Bakalkin, G., Tsibezov, V. V., Sjutkin, E. A., Veselova, S. P., Novikov, I. D., and Krivosheev, O. G. (1984). Lateralization of LH-RH in rat hypothalamus. *Brain Res.* **296**(2), 361–364.

Bamford, O. S., and Eccles, R. (1982). The central reciprocal control of nasal vasomotor oscillations. *Pflugers Arch.* **394,** 139–143.

Banquet, J. (1983a). Interhemispheric asymmetry during sleep. *In* "Sleep 1982 6th European Congress Sleep Research" (W. Koella, Ed.), pp. 178–181. Karger, Basel.

Banquet, J. P. (1983b). Inter- and intrahemispheric relationships of the EEG activity during sleep in man. *Electroencephalogr. Clin. Neurophysiol.* **55**(1), 51–59.

Barcaro, U., Denoth, F., Murri, L., Navona, C., and Stefanini, A. (1986). Changes in the interhemispheric correlation during sleep in normal subjects. *Electroencephalogr. Clin. Neurophysiol.* **63**(2), 112–118.

Baust, W. (1974). Autonomic function during sleep. 2nd Europ. Congr. Sleep Res. Sleep 1974 Rome. pp. 24–33. Karger, Basel.

Baust, W., and Bohnert, B. (1969). The regulation of heart rate during sleep. *Exp. Brain Res.* **7**(2), 169–180.

Baust, W., and Rohrwasser, W. (1969). Gastric motility and pH during natural human sleep. *Pflugers Arch.* **305**(3), 229–240.

Bear, D. M. (1983). Hemispheric specialization and the neurology of emotion. *Arch. Neurol.* **40**(4), 195–202.
Beattie, J. (1932). Hypothalamic mechanisms. *Can. Med. Assoc. J.* **26,** 400–405.
Beattie, J., and Kerr, A. (1936). The effects of diencephalic stimulation on urinary bladder tonus. *Brain* **59,** 302–314.
Beattie, J., and Sheehan, D. (1934). The effects of hypothalamic stimulation on gastric motility. *J. Physiol.* **81**(2), 218–227.
Beattie, J., Duel, A. B., and Ballance, C. (1932). The effects of stimulation of the hypothalamic pupillo-dilator centre after successful anastomoses between the cervical sympathetic and certain motor nerves. *J. Anat.* **66**(Pt. 3), 283–299.
Beickert, P. (1951). Halbseitenrhythmus der vegetativen innervation. *Arch. Ohr. Nos. Kehl. Hdk.* **157,** 404–411.
Ben-Menachem, E., Hamberger, A., Hedner, T., Hammond, E. J., Uthman, B. M., Slater, J., Treig, T., Stefan, H., Ramsay, R. E., Wernicke, J. F., and Wilder, B. J. (1995). Effects of vagus nerve stimulation on amino acids and other metabolites in the CSF of patients with partial seizures. *Epilepsy Res.* **20**(3), 221–227.
Bench, C. J., Frackowiak, R. S., and Dolan, R. J. (1995). Changes in regional cerebral blood flow on recovery from depression. *Psychol. Med.* **25**(2), 247–261.
Benton, L. A., and Yates, F. E. (1990). Ultradian adrenocortical and circulatory oscillations in conscious dogs. *Am. J. Physiol.* **258**(3 Pt. 2), R578–R590.
Bhajan, Y. (1980). "Survival Kit: Meditations and Exercises for Stress and Pressure of the Times." Kundalini Research Institute, Espanola, NM.
Blinowska, K., and Marsh, D. J. (1985). Ultra- and circadian fluctuations in arterial pressure and electromyogram in conscious dogs. *Am. J. Physiol.* **249** (6 Pt. 2), R720–R725.
Block, R. A., Arnott, D. P., Quigley, B., and Lynch, W. C. (1989). Unilateral nostril breathing influences lateralized cognitive performance. *Brain Cogn.* **9**(2), 181–190.
Bohus, B., Benua, R. F., Fokkema, D. S., Koolhaas, J. M., Nyakas, C., van Oortmerssen, G. A., Prins, A. J. A., de Ruiter, A. J. H., Scheurink, A. J. W., and Steffens, A. B. (1987). Neuroendocrine states and behavioral and physiological stress responses. *In* "Progress in Brain Research" (E. de Kloet, V. Wiegant, and D. de Wied, Eds.), Vol. 72, pp. 57–70. Elsevier, Amsterdam.
Bojsen-Moller, F., and Fahrenkrug, J. (1971). Nasal swell-bodies and cyclic changes in the air passage of the rat and rabbit nose. *J. Anat.* **110,** 25–37.
Borod, J. C., Kent, J., Koff, E., Martin, C., and Alpert, M. (1988). Facial asymmetry while posing positive and negative emotions: Support for the right hemisphere hypothesis. *Neuropsychologia* **26**(5), 759–764.
Bossom, J., Natelson, B. H., Levin, B. E., and Stokes, P. E. (1983). Ultradian rhythms in cognitive functions and their relationship to visceral processes. *Physiol. Behav.* **31**(1), 119–123.

Bouayad-Amine, D., Cupissol, D., Nougier-Soule, J., Bres, J., Gestin-Boyer, C., René, C., Assens, C., and Serrou, B. (1993). Ultradian variations of interleukin-1 beta concentration (IL-1 beta), interferon gamma (IFN-gamma) and soluble IL-2 receptors (RIL-2) in healthy volunteers humans. *C. R. Seances Soc. Biol. Fil.* **187,** 542–553.

Boyar, R., Finkelstein, J., Roffwarg, H., Kapen, S., Weitzman, E., and Hellman, L. (1972a). Synchronization of augmented luteinizing hormone secretion with sleep during puberty. *N. Engl. J. Med.* **287**(12), 582–586.

Boyar, R., Perlow, M., Hellman, L., Kapen, S., and Weitzman, E. (1972b). Twenty-four hour pattern of luteinizing hormone secretion in normal men with sleep stage recording. *J. Clin. Endocrinol. Metab.* **35**(1), 73–81.

Brandenberger, G. (1991). Renin and its relations to the internal structure of sleep. *Presse Med.* **20**(36), 1778–1782.

Brandenberger, G., Charloux, A., Gronfier, C., and Otzenberger, H. (1998). Ultradian rhythms in hydromineral hormones. *Horm. Res.* **49**(3–4), 131–135.

Breasted, J. (1930). "The Edwin Smith Surgical Papyrus," Volumes 2. The University of Chicago Press, Chicago.

Broten, T. P., and Zehr, J. E. (1989). Autonomic modulation of ultradian blood pressure and heart rate oscillations in dogs. *Am. J. Physiol.* **256**(5 Pt. 2), R1127–R1137.

Broughton, R. (1975). Biorhythmic variations in consciousness and psychological functions. *Can. Psychol. Rev.* **16,** 217–239.

Buchsbaum, M. S., Gillin, J. C., Wu, J., Hazlett, E., Sicotte, N., Dupont, R. M., and Bunney, W. E. (1989). Regional cerebral glucose metabolic rate in human sleep assessed by positron emission tomography. *Life Sci.* **45**(15), 1349–1356.

Bulloch, K. (1985). Neuroanatomy of lymphoid tissue: A review. *In* "Neural Modulation of Immunity" (R. Guillemin, M. Cohen, and T. Melnechuk, Eds.), pp. 111–141. Raven Press, New York.

Cannon, W. (1929). "Bodily Changes in Pain, Hunger, Fear and Rage." Appleton, New York.

Cannon, W. (1932). "The Wisdom of the Body." Norton, New York.

Chapple, W. (1977). Role of asymmetry in the functioning of invertebrate nervous systems. *In* "Lateralization in the Nervous System" (S. Harnad, R. W. Doty, L. Goldstein, J. Jaynes, and G. Krauthamer, Eds.), pp. 3–22. Academic Press, New York.

Chen, J. C., Brown, B., and Schmid, K. L. (2004). Effect of unilateral forced nostril breathing on tonic accommodation and intraocular pressure. *Clin. Auton. Res.* **14**(6), 396–400.

Chou, H. F., McGivern, R., Berman, N., and Ipp, E. (1991). Oscillations of circulating plasma insulin concentrations in the rat. *Life Sci.* **48**(15), 1463–1469.

Cole, P., and Haight, J. S. (1984). Posture and nasal patency. *Am. Rev. Respir. Dis.* **129**(3), 351–354.

Cole, P., and Haight, J. S. (1986). Posture and the nasal cycle. *Ann. Otol. Rhinol. Laryngol.* **95**(3 Pt. 1), 233–237.

Cowdry, R. W., Gardner, D. L., O'Leary, K. M., Leibenluft, E., and Rubinow, D. R. (1991). Mood variability: A study of four groups. *Am. J. Psychiatry* **148**(11), 1505–1511.

Critchley, H. D., Taggart, P., Sutton, P. M., Holdright, D. R., Batchvarov, V., Hnatkova, K., Malik, M., and Dolan, R. J. (2005). Mental stress and sudden cardiac death: Asymmetric midbrain activity as a linking mechanism. *Brain* **128**(Pt. 1), 75–85.

Cyberonics (2004). Physician's Manual VNS Therapy™ Pulse Model 102 Generator and VNS Therapy™ Pulse Duo Model 102R Generator, Cyberonics.

Dane, S., and Balci, N. (2007). Handedness, eyedness and nasal cycle in children with autism. *Int. J. Dev. Neurosci.* **25**(4), 223–226.

Dane, S., Caliskan, E., Karasen, M., and Oztasan, N. (2002). Effects of unilateral nostril breathing on blood pressure and heart rate in right-handed healthy subjects. *Int. J. Neurosci.* **112**(1), 97–102.

Debener, S., Beauducel, A., Nessler, D., Brocke, B., Heilemann, H., and Kayser, J. (2000). Is resting anterior EEG alpha asymmetry a trait marker for depression? Findings for healthy adults and clinically depressed patients. *Neuropsychobiology* **41**(1), 31–37.

DeGiorgio, C. M., Schachter, S. C., Handforth, A., Salinsky, M., Thompson, J., Uthman, B., Reed, R., Collins, S., Tecoma, E., Morris, G. L., Vaughn, B., Naritoku, D. K., *et al.* (2000). Prospective long-term study of vagus nerve stimulation for the treatment of refractory seizures. *Epilepsia* **41**(9), 1195–1200.

Dement, W., and Kleitman, N. (1957a). Cyclic variations in EEG during sleep and their relation to eye movements, body motility, and dreaming. *Electroencephalogr. Clin. Neurophysiol. Suppl.* **9**(4), 673–690.

Dement, W., and Kleitman, N. (1957b). The relation of eye movements during sleep to dream activity: An objective method for the study of dreaming. *J. Exp. Psychol.* **53**(5), 339–346.

Dexter, J. D., and Weitzman, E. D. (1970). The relationship of nocturnal headaches to sleep stage patterns. *Neurology* **20**(5), 513–518.

Dietl, H., Prast, H., and Philippu, A. (1993). Pulsatile release of catecholamines in the hypothalamus of conscious rats. *Naunyn Schmiedebergs Arch. Pharmacol.* **347**(1), 28–33.

Dolce, G., and Waldeier, H. (1974). Spectral and multivariate analysis of EEG changes during mental activity in man. *Electroencephalogr. Clin. Neurophysiol.* **36**(6), 577–584.

Drettner, B. (1970). Pathophysiological relationship between the upper and lower airways. *Ann. Otol. Rhinol. Laryngol.* **79**(3), 499–505.

Eccles, R. (2000). Nasal airflow in health and disease. *Acta Otolaryngol.* **120**(5), 580–595.

Eccles, R., and Eccles, K. S. (1981). Asymmetry in the autonomic nervous system with reference to the nasal cycle, migraine, anisocoria and Meniere's syndrome. *Rhinology* **19**(3), 121–125.

Eccles, R., and Lee, R. L. (1981). The influence of the hypothalamus on the sympathetic innervation of the nasal vasculature of the cat. *Acta Otolaryngol.* **91,** 127–134.

Eriksson, E., Eden, S., Modigh, K., and Haggendal, J. (1980). Ultradian rhythm in rat hypothalamic dopamine levels. *J. Neural Transm.* **48**(4), 305–310.

Escalante-Mead, P. R., Minshew, N. J., and Sweeney, J. A. (2003). Abnormal brain lateralization in high-functioning autism. *J. Autism Dev. Disord.* **33**(5), 539–543.

Ferres, M. (1958). The effect of pressure on sweating. *J. Physiol.* **143,** 39P–40P.

Flor-Henry, P. (1969a). Psychosis and temporal lobe epilepsy. A controlled investigation. *Epilepsia* **10**(3), 363–395.

Flor-Henry, P. (1969b). Schizophrenic-like reactions and affective psychoses associated with temporal lobe epilepsy: Etiological factors. *Am. J. Psychiatry* **126**(3), 400–404.

Flor-Henry, P. (1986). Epilepsy and schizophrenia. *In* "Handbook of Studies on Schizophrenia, Part 1" (G. Burrows, T. Norman, and G. Rubenstein, Eds.), pp. 201–214. Oxford, Elsevier Science Publishers, Amsterdam, New York.

Flor-Henry, P. (1987). Cerebral dynamics, laterality and psychopathology: A commentary. *In* "Cerebral Dynamics, Laterality, and Psychopathology" (R. Takahashi, P. Flor-Henry, J. Gruzelier, and S. Niwa, Eds.), pp. 1–21. Elsevier Science Publishers, Amsterdam.

Flor-Henry, P., Lind, J. C., and Koles, Z. J. (2004). A source-imaging (low-resolution electromagnetic tomography) study of the EEGs from unmedicated males with depression. *Psychiatry Res.* **130**(2), 191–207.

Foley, J., and DuBois, F. (1937). Quantitative studies of the vagus nerve in the cat. I. The ration of sensory and motor studies. *J. Comp. Neurol.* **67,** 49–67.

Folkard, S. (1979). Time of day and level of processing. *Mem. Cogn.* **7,** 247–252.

Friedell, A. (1948). Automatic attentive breathing in angina pectoris. *Minn. Med.* **31,** 875–881.

Friedman, S., and Fisher, C. (1967). On the presence of a rhythmic, diurnal, oral instinctual drive cycle in man. A preliminary report. *J. Am. Psychoanal. Assoc.* **15**(2), 317–343.

Frye, R., and Doty, R. (1992). The influence of ultradian autonomic rhythms, as indexed by the nasal cycle, on unilateral lfactory thresholds. *In* "Chemical

Signals in Vertebrates" (R. Doty and D. Muller-Schwarze, Eds.), pp. 595–598. Plenum Press, New York.

Furnival, C. M., Linden, R. J., and Snow, H. M. (1973). Chronotropic and inotropic effects on the dog heart of stimulating the efferent cardiac sympathetic nerves. *J. Physiol.* **230**(1), 137–153.

Gallego, A. J., Cavallari, F. E., Valera, F. C., Demarco, R. C., and Anselmo-Lima, W. T. (2006). Study of nasal cycles in children by acoustic rhinometry. *Am. J. Rhinol.* **20**(6), 560–562.

Gazzaniga, M. S. (1995). Consciousness and the cerebral hemispheres. *In* "The Cognitive Neurosciences" (M. S. Gazzaniga, Ed.), pp. 1391–1400. MIT Press, Cambridge.

Gazzaniga, M. S., Bogen, J. E., and Sperry, R. W. (1962). Some functional effects of sectioning the cerebral commissures in man. *Proc. Natl. Acad. Sci. USA* **48,** 1765–1769.

Gellhorn, E. (1967). "Principles of Autonomic-Somatic Integration." University of Minnesota Press, Minneapolis.

George, M. S., Rush, A. J., Sackeim, H. A., and Marangell, L. B. (2003). Vagus nerve stimulation (VNS): Utility in neuropsychiatric disorders. *Int. J. Neuropsychopharmacol.* **6**(1), 73–83.

George, M. S., Sackeim, H. A., Marangell, L. B., Husain, M. M., Nahas, Z., Lisanby, S. H., Ballenger, J. C., and Rush, A. J. (2000). Vagus nerve stimulation. A potential therapy for resistant depression? *Psychiatr. Clin. North Am.* **23**(4), 757–783.

Gerendai, I. (1980). Unilateral complete isolation of the medial basal hypothalamus interferes with the compensatory ovarian growth following unilateral ovariectomy. *Neurendocrinol. Lett.* **2,** 39–43.

Gerendai, I. (1984). Lateralization of neuroendocrine control. *In* "Cerebral Dominance: The Biological Foundations" (N. Geschwind and M. Galaburda, Eds.), pp. 167–178. Harvard University Press, Cambridge, Mass.

Gerendai, I. (1986). "Laterality in the Neuroendocrine System." Wenner-Glen Center International Symposium on The, Dual Brain.

Gerendai, I., and Halasz, B. (1997). Neuroendocrine asymmetry. *Front. Neuroendocrinol.* **18**(3), 354–381.

Gertner, R., Podoshin, L., and Fradis, M. (1984). A simple method of measuring the nasal airway in clinical work. *J. Laryngol. Otol.* **98**(4), 351–355.

Globus, G. G., Drury, R. L., Phoebus, E. C., and Boyd, R. (1971). Ultradian rhythms in human performance. *Percept. Mot. Skills* **33**(3), 1171–1174.

Goldstein, L., Burdick, J. A., and Lazslo, M. (1970). A quantitative analysis of the EEG during sleep in normal subjects. *Acta Physiol. Acad. Sci. Hung.* **37**(3), 291–300.

Goldstein, L., Stoltzfus, N. W., and Gardocki, J. F. (1972). Changes in interhemispheric amplitude relationships in the EEG during sleep. *Physiol. Behav.* **8**(5), 811–815.

Gomez, B., Alborch, E., Diesuez, G., and Lluch, S. (1976). Presence of alpha- and beta-adrenergic tone in the walls of cerebral vessels. *In* "The Cerebral Vessel Wall" (J. Cervos-Navarro, J. Betz, F. Matakas, and R. Wullenbweber, Eds.), pp. 139–142. Raven Press, New York.

Goodner, C. J., Walike, B. C., Koerker, D. J., Ensinck, J. W., Brown, A. C., Chideckel, E. W., Palmer, J., and Kalnasy, L. (1977). Insulin, glucagon, and glucose exhibit synchronous, sustained oscillations in fasting monkeys. *Science* **195**(4274), 177–179.

Gordon, H. W., and Stoffer, D. S. (1989). Ultradian rhythms of right and left hemisphere function. *Int. J. Neurosci.* **47**(1–2), 57–65.

Gordon, H. W., Corbin, E. D., and Lee, P. A. (1986). Changes in specialized cognitive function following changes in hormone levels. *Cortex* **22**(3), 399–415.

Gordon, H. W., Frooman, B., and Lavie, P. (1982). Shift in cognitive asymmetries between wakings from REM and NREM sleep. *Neuropsychologia* **20**(1), 99–103.

Gott, P. S., Hughes, E. C., and Whipple, K. (1984). Voluntary control of two lateralized conscious states: Validation by electrical and behavioral studies. *Neuropsychologia* **22**(1), 65–72.

Gottesmann, C., and Gottesman, I. (2007). The neurobiological characteristics of rapid eye movement (REM) sleep are candidate endophenotypes of depression, schizophrenia, mental retardation and dementia. *Prog. Neurobiol.* **81**(4), 237–250.

Grabow, J. D., Aronson, A. E., Greene, K. L., and Offord, K. P. (1979). A comparison of EEG activity in the left and right cerebral hemispheres by power-spectrum analysis during language and non-language tasks. *Electroencephalogr. Clin. Neurophysiol.* **47**(4), 460–472.

Granat, M., Lavie, P., Adar, D., and Sharf, M. (1979). Short-term cycles in human fetal activity. *Am. J. Obs. Gynecol.* **134,** 696–701.

Green, W. J., and Stajduhar, P. P. (1966). The effect of ECT on the sleep-dream cycle in a psychotic depression. *J. Nerv. Ment. Dis.* **143**(2), 123–134.

Gresham, S. C., Agnew, H. W., Jr., and Williams, R. L. (1965). The sleep of depressed patients. An EEG and eye movement study. *Arch. Gen. Psychiatry* **13**(6), 503–507.

Group, V. N. S. S. (1999). A randomized controlled trial of chronic vagus nerve stimulation for treatment of medically intractable seizures. *Neurology* **45,** 224–230.

Groves, D. A., and Brown, V. J. (2005). Vagal nerve stimulation: A review of its applications and potential mechanisms that mediate its clinical effects. *Neurosci. Biobehav. Rev.* **29**(3), 493–500.

Gruzelier, J. (1983). A critical assessment and integration of lateral asymmetries in schizophrenia. *In* "Hemisyndromes: Psychobiology, Neurology, and Psychiatry" (M. Myslobodsky, Ed.), pp. 265–326. Academic Press, New York.

Gruzelier, J. (1987). Commentary on neuropsychological and information processing deficits in psychosis and neuro-psychological syndrome relationships to schizophrenia. *In* "Cerebral Dynamics Laterality, and Psychopathology" (R. Takahashi, P. Flor-Henry, J. Gruzelier, and S. Niwa, Eds.), pp. 23–52. Oxford, Elsevier Science Publishers, Amsterdam, New York.

Gruzelier, J., and Venables, P. (1974). Bimodality and lateral asymmetry of skin conductance orienting activity in schizophrenics: Replication and evidence of lateral asymmetry in patients with depression and disorders of personality. *Biol. Psychiatry* **8**(1), 55–73.

Hagstadius, S. (1989). "Brain Function and Dysfunction." PhD. Departments of Psychiatry and Geropsychiatrics. University of Lund, Lund, Sweden.

Hagstadius, S., and Risberg, J. (1989). Regional cerebral blood flow characteristics and variations with age in resting normal subjects. *Brain Cogn.* **10**(1), 28–43.

Haight, J. J., and Cole, P. (1984). Reciprocating nasal airflow resistances. *Acta Otolaryngol.* **97**(1–2), 93–98.

Haight, J. S., and Cole, P. (1986). Unilateral nasal resistance and asymmetrical body pressure. *J. Otolaryngol. Suppl.* **16,** 1–31.

Halaris, A., Ed. (1987). "Chronobiology and Psychiatric Disorders." Elsevier, New York, Amsterdam, London.

Halasz, B., and Szentagothai, J. (1959). Histological demonstration of a nervous signal transmission from the adrenal cortex to the hypothalamus. *Z. Zellforsch. Mikrosk. Anat.* **50,** 297–306.

Halberg, F. (1964). Organism as circadian systems: Temporal analysis of their physiologic and pathologic responses, including injury and death. *In* "Symposium, Medical Aspects of Stress in the Military Climate," pp. 1–36. Walter Reed, Army Institute of Research, Washington, DC.

Halbreich, U. (1987). The circadian rhythm of cortisol and MHPG in depressive and normals. *In* "Chronobiology and Psychiatric Disorders" (A. Halaris, Ed.), pp. 49–67. Elsevier, New York, Amsterdam, London.

Hall, D. P., Jr., Sing, H. C., and Romanoski, A. J. (1991). Identification and characterization of greater mood variance in depression. *Am. J. Psychiatry* **148**(10), 1341–1345.

Hall, N. R., and Goldstein, A. L. (1983). The thymus-brain connection: Interactions between thymosin and the neuroendocrine system. *Lymphokine Res.* **2**(1), 1–6.

Hamlin, R. L., and Smith, C. R. (1968). Effects of vagal stimulation on S-A and A-V nodes. *Am. J. Physiol.* **215**(3), 560–568.

Handforth, A., DeGiorgio, C. M., Schachter, S. C., Uthman, B. M., Naritoku, D. K., Tecoma, E. S., Henry, T. R., Collins, S. D., Vaughn, B. V., Gilmartin, R. C., Labar, D. R., Morris, G. L., III, *et al.* (1998). Vagus nerve stimulation therapy for partial-onset seizures: A randomized active-control trial. *Neurology* **51**(1), 48–55.

Hansen, B. S., Manning, P. A., and Achtman, M. (1982). Promoter-distal region of the tra operon of F-like sex factor R100 in *Escherichia coli* K-12. *J. Bacteriol.* **150**(1), 89–99.

Hartmann, E., Verdone, P., and Snyder, F. (1966). Longitudinal studies of sleep and dreaming patterns in psychiatric patients. *J. Nerv. Ment. Dis.* **142**(2), 117–126.

Hasegawa, M., and Kern, E. B. (1978). Variations resistance in man: A rhinomanometric study of cycle in 50 human subjects. *Rhinology* **16,** 20–29.

Hatta, T. (1984). Lateral eye movement and hemisphere asymmetry: Effects of question type, task type, emotion type, and individual differences. *Cortex* **20**(4), 543–556.

Hatton, K. W., McLarney, J. T., Pittman, T., and Fahy, B. G. (2006). Vagal nerve stimulation: Overview and implications for anesthesiologists. *Anesth. Analg.* **103**(5), 1241–1249.

Heetderks, D. R. (1927). Observations on the reaction of the nasal mucous membranes. *Am. J. Med. Sci.* **174,** 231–244.

Hellbrugge, T. (1974). The development of circadian and ultradian rhythms of premature and full-term infants. *In* "Chronobiology" (L. E. Scheving, F. Halberg, and J. E. Pauly, Eds.), pp. 339–341. Igaku Shoin, Tokyo.

Henriques, J. B., and Davidson, R. J. (1997). Brain electrical asymmetries during cognitive task performance in depressed and nondepressed subjects. *Biol. Psychiatry* **42**(11), 1039–1050.

Henry, T. R. (2002). Therapeutic mechanisms of vagus nerve stimulation. *Neurology* **59**(6 Suppl. 4), S3–S14.

Hess, W. (1947). "Vegetative Functionen und Zwischenhirn." Benno Schwabe, Basel.

Hess, W. (1948). "Die Funktionelle Organization Des Vegetativen Nervensystems." Benno Schwabe, Basel.

Hess, W. R. (1949). Das Zwischenhirn, Basel, Schwabe.

Hess, W. R. (1954). "Diencephalon, Autonomic and Extrapyridimal Functions." Grune and Stratton, New York.

Hiatt, J. F., and Kripke, D. F. (1975). Ultradian rhythms in walking gastric activity. *Psychosom. Med.* **37**(4), 320–325.

Hondeghem, L. M., Mouton, E., Stassen, T., and De Geest, H. (1975). Additive effects of acetylcholine released by vagal nerve stimulation on atrial rate. *J. Appl. Physiol.* **38**(1), 108–113.

Honma, K., and Honma, S. (1985). Ultradian rhythms in locomotor activity, deep body temperature and plasma corticosterone level in rats: Two different origins? *In* "Ultradian Rhythms in Physiology and Behavior" (H. Schulz and P. Lavie, Eds.), pp. 77–94. Springer-Verlag, Berlin, Heidelberg.

Horne, J. A., and Whitehead, M. (1976). Ultradian and other rhythms in human respiration rate. *Experientia* **32**(9), 1165–1167.

Husted, D., and Shapira, N. (2004). A review of the treatment for refractory obsessive-compulsive disorder: From medicine to deep brain stimulation. *CNS Spectr.* **9**(11), 833–847.

Ischlondsky, N. (1955). The inhibitory process in the cerebrophysiological laboratory and in the clinic. *J. Nerv. Ment. Dis.* **121,** 5–18.

Iskra-Golec, I., and Smith, L. (2006). Ultradian and asymmetric rhythms of hemispheric processing speed. *Chronobiol. Int.* **23**(6), 1229–1239.

Jackson, J. (1884). Evolution and dissolution of the nervous system (Croonian Lectures). Reprinted in 1958: *In* "Selected Writings of John Hughlings Jackson" (J. Taylor, Ed.), Basic Books, New York.

Jaspan, J. B., Lever, E., Polonsky, K. S., and Van Cauter, E. (1986). *In vivo* pulsatility of pancreatic islet peptides. *Am. J. Physiol.* **251**(2 Pt. 1), E215–E226.

Jella, S. A., and Shannahoff-Khalsa, D. S. (1993). The effects of unilateral forced nostril breathing on cognitive performance. *Int. J. Neurosci.* **73**(1–2), 61–68.

Jouvet, M. (1973). Essai sur le re've. *Arch. Ital. Biol.* **III,** 564–576.

Kalen, P., Rosegren, E., Lindvall, O., and Bjorklund, A. (1989). Hippocampal noradrenaline and serotonin release over 24 hours as measured by the dialysis technique in freely moving rats: Correlation to behavioural activity state, effect of handling and tail-pinch. *Eur. J. Neurosci.* **1**(3), 181–188.

Kalin, N. H., Shelton, S. E., Barksdale, C. M., and Brownfield, M. S. (1987). A diurnal rhythm in cerebrospinal fluid corticotrophin-releasing hormone different from the rhythm of pituitary-adrenal activity. *Brain Res.* **426**(2), 385–391.

Karacan, I., Hursch, C. J., Williams, R. L., and Thornby, J. I. (1972). Some characteristics of nocturnal penile tumescence in young adults. *Arch. Gen. Psychiatry* **26**(4), 351–356.

Karplus, J., and Kreidl, A. (1909). Gehirn und sympathicus. I. Zwischenhirnbasis und halssympatheticus. *Pfluger Arch. Gesamte Physiol.* **129,** 138–144.

Karplus, J., and Kreidl, A. (1910). Gehirn und sympathicus. II. Ein sympathicuszentrum im zwischenhirn. *Pfluger Arch. Gesamte Physiol.* **135,** 401–416.

Karplus, J., and Kreidl, A. (1912). Gehirn und sympathicus. III. Sympathicusleitung im gehirn und halsmark. *Pfluger Arch. Gesamte Physiol.* **143,** 107–127.

Karplus, J., and Kreidl, A. (1914). Uber totallexstirpationen einer und beider grosshirnhemispharen an affen (Macacus rhesus). *Arch. Anat. Phsyiol. (Physiol Abt)* 5–212.

Kawase, T. (1952). Further studies on pressure sweat reflex. *Jap. J. Physiol.* **3,** 1–9.

Kayser, R. (1889). Uber den Weg der Athmungsluft durch die Nase. *Z. Ohrerlheilh.* **20,** 96–106.

Kayser, R. (1895). Die exacta messung der luftdurchgangigkeit der nase. *Arch. Laryngol. Rhinol.* **3,** 101–120.

Kennedy, B., Ziegler, M. G., and Shannahoff-Khalsa, D. S. (1986). Alternating lateralization of plasma catecholamines and nasal patency in humans. *Life Sci.* **38**(13), 1203–1214.

Kern, W., Offenheuser, S., Born, J., and Fehm, H. L. (1996). Entrainment of ultradian oscillations in the secretion of insulin and glucagon to the nonrapid eye movement/rapid eye movement sleep rhythm in humans. *J. Clin. Endocrinol. Metab.* **81**(4), 1541–1547.

Keuning, J. (1968). On the nasal cycle. *J. Intern. Rhinol.* **6,** 99–136.

Kimura, F., Praputpittaya, C., Mitsugi, N., Hashimoto, R., and Suzuki, R. (1985). Relationship between ultradian rhythms of the sleep-wakefulness cycle and growth hormone and corticosterone secretion in rats. *In* "Ultradan Rhythms in Physiology and Behavior" (H. Schulz and P. Lavie, Eds.), pp. 61–76. Springer-Verlag, Berlin.

Kittrelle, J. P., Grouse, D. S., and Seybold, M. E. (1985). Cluster headache. Local anesthetic abortive agents. *Arch. Neurol.* **42**(5), 496–498.

Klein, R., and Armitage, R. (1979). Rhythms in human performance: 1 1/2-hour oscillations in cognitive style. *Science* **204**(4399), 1326–1328.

Klein, R., Pilon, D., Prosser, S., and Shannahoff-Khalsa, D. (1986). Nasal airflow asymmetries and human performance. *Biol. Psychol.* **23**(2), 127–137.

Kleitman, N. (1961). "The Nature of Dreaming." Churchill, London.

Kleitman, N. (1963). "Sleep and Wakefulness." The University of Chicago Press, Chicago, London.

Kleitman, N. (1967a). "Phylogenetic, Ontogenetic and Environmental Determinants in the Evolution of Sleep-Wakefulness Cycles." The Williams and Wilkins Co., Baltimore.

Kleitman, N. (1967b). Phylogenetic, ontogenetic and environmental determinants in the evolution of sleep-wakefulness cycles. *Res. Publ. Assoc. Res. Nerv. Ment. Dis.* **45,** 30–38.

Kleitman, N. (1967c). The basic rest—activity cycle and physiological correlates of dreaming. *Exp. Neurol.* **4**(Suppl.), 2–4.

Kleitman, N. (1967d). Basic rest activity cycle in relationship to sleep and wakefulness. *In* "Sleep: Physiology and Pathology" (A. Kales, Ed.), Lippincott, Philadelphia.

Kleitman, N. (1982). Basic rest-activity cycle—22 years later. *Sleep* **5**(4), 311–317.

Knobil, E. (1987). A hypothalamic pulse generator governs mammalian reproduction. *News Physiol. Sci.* **2,** 42–43.

Knott, V. J., and Lapierre, Y. D. (1987). Computerized EEG correlates of depression and antidepressant treatment. *Prog. Neuropsychopharmacol. Biol. Psychiatry* **11**(2–3), 213–221.

Kobayashi, T., Tsuji, Y., and Endo, S. (1985). Sleep cycles as a basic unit of sleep. *In* "Ultradian Rhythms in Physiology and Behavior" (H. Schulz and P. Lavie, Eds.), pp. 260–269. Plenum, New York.

Koenigsberg, H. W., Teicher, M. H., Mitropoulou, V., Navalta, C., New, A. S., Trestman, R., and Siever, L. J. (2004). 24-h Monitoring of plasma norepinephrine, MHPG, cortisol, growth hormone and prolactin in depression. *J. Psychiatr. Res.* **38**(5), 503–511.

Koles, Z. J., Lind, J. C., and Flor-Henry, P. (2004). A source-imaging (low-resolution electromagnetic tomography) study of the EEGs from unmedicated men with schizophrenia. *Psychiatry Res.* **130**(2), 171–190.

Konno, A. (1969). Air flow and resistance in the nasal cavity. 2. Bilateral rhinometry using a pneumotachometer. Its principles and clinical application. *Nippon Jibiinkoka Gakkai Kaiho* **72**(1), 49–65.

Korenberg, M. J. (1988). Identifying nonlinear difference equation and functional expansion representations: The fast orthogonal algorithm. *Ann. Biomed. Eng.* **16**(1), 123–142.

Korenberg, M. J. (1989). A robust orthogonal algorithm for system identification and time-series analysis. *Biol. Cybern.* **60**(4), 267–276.

Korenberg, M. J., and Paarmann, L. D. (1989a). Applications of fast orthogonal search: Time-series analysis and resolution of signals in noise. *Ann. Biomed. Eng.* **17**(3), 219–231.

Korenberg, M. J., and Paarmann, L. D. (1989b). An orthogonal ARMA identifier with automatic order estimation for biological modeling. *Ann. Biomed. Eng.* **17**(6), 571–592.

Kripke, D. (1982). Ultradian rhythms in behavior and physiology. *In* "Rhythmic Aspects of Behavior" (F. Brown and R. Graeber, Eds.), pp. 313–343. Lawrence Erlbaum Associates, Hillsdale, New Jersey.

Kripke, D. F. (1974). Ultradian rhythms in sleep and wakefulness. *In* "Advances in Sleep Research" (E. Weitzman, Ed.), Vol. 1, pp. 305–325. Spectrum, New York.

Kripke, D. F., Lavie, P., Parker, D., Huey, L., and Deftos, L. J. (1978). Plasma parathyroid hormone and calcium are related to sleep stage cycles. *J. Clin. Endocrinol. Metab.* **47**(5), 1021–1027.

Kristof, M., Servit, Z., and Manas, K. (1981). Activating effect of nasal air flow on epileptic electrographic abnormalities in the human EEG. Evidence for the reflect origin of the phenomenon. *Physiol. Bohemoslov.* **30**(1), 73–77.

Kronfol, Z., Hamsher, K. D., Digre, K., and Waziri, R. (1978). Depression and hemispheric functions: Changes associated with unilateral ECT. *Br. J. Psychiatry* **132,** 560–567.

Kuno, Y. (1934). "The Physiology of Human Perspiration." J and A Churchill, London.

Lang, D. A., Matthews, D. R., Burnett, M., and Turner, R. C. (1981). Brief, irregular oscillations of basal plasma insulin and glucose concentrations in diabetic man. *Diabetes* **30**(5), 435–439.

Larsson, L. (1980). New aspects on the neural, paracrine and endocrine regulation of islet function. *In* "Frontiers in Hormone Research" (U. Tj and B. Van Wimersma Griedanus, Eds.), Vol. 7, pp. 14–29. Karger, Basel.

Lavie, P. (1976). Ultradian rhythms in the perception of two apparent motions. *Chronobiologia* **3**(3), 214–218.

Lavie, P. (1979). Ultradian rhythms in alertness—a pupillometric study. *Biol. Psychol.* **9**(1), 49–62.

Lavie, P. (1989). Ultradian rhythms in arousal—the problem of masking. *Chronobiol. Int.* **6**(1), 21–28.

Lavie, P., and Kripke, D. F. (1981). Ultradian circa 11/2 hour rhythms: A multi-oscillatory system. *Life Sci.* **29**(24), 2445–2450.

Lavie, P., Kripke, D. F., Hiatt, J. F., and Harrison, J. (1978). Brief report: Gastric rhythms during sleep. *Behav. Biol.* **23**(4), 526–530.

Lavie, P., Levy, C., and Coolidge, F. (1975). Ultradian rhythms in the perception of the spiral aftereffect. *Physiol. Psychol.* **3,** 144–146.

Lavie, P., Matanya, Y., and Yehuda, S. (1984). Cognitive asymmetries after wakings from REM and NONREM sleep in right-handed females. *Int. J. Neurosci.* **23**(2), 111–115.

Lavie, P., and Sutter, D. (1975). Differential responding to the beta movement after waking from REM and nonREM sleep. *Am. J. Psychol.* **88**(4), 595–603.

Lavie, P., and Tzischinsky, O. (1984). Cognitive asymmetries after waking from REM and NONREM sleep: Effects of delayed testing and handedness. *Int. J. Neurosci.* **23**(4), 311–315.

Leconte, P., and Lambert, C. (1988). Chronopsychologie, style cognitif et differenciation interhemispherique. *Psychologie et Education* **4,** 195–197.

Leon-Carrion, J., and Vela-Bueno, A. (1991). Cannabis and cerebral hemispheres: A chrononeuropsychological study. *Int. J. Neurosci.* **57**(3–4), 251–257.

Levin, B. E., Goldstein, A., and Natelson, B. H. (1978). Ultradian rhythm of plasma noradrenaline in rhesus monkeys. *Nature* **272**(5649), 164–166.

Levin, B. E., Rappaport, M., and Natelson, B. H. (1979). Ultradian variations of plasma noradrenaline in humans. *Life Sci.* **25**(7), 621–627.

Levin, E., Kirsner, J., Palmer, W., and Butler, C. (1948). The variability and periodicity of the nocturnal gastric secretion in normal individuals. *Gastroenterology* **10,** 939–951.

Levin, E., Kirsner, J. B., and Palmer, W. L. (1950). The continuous twelve-hour nocturnal gastric secretion in normal individuals and in patients with duodenal ulcer after a 24-hour fast. *Gastroenterology* **15**(3), 454–457.

Levy, M., and Martin, P. (1979). "Neural Control of the Heart." American Physiological Society, Bethesda, MD.

Levy, M. N., Ng, M. L., and Zieske, H. (1966). Functional distribution of the peripheral cardiac sympathetic pathways. *Circ. Res.* **19**(3), 650–661.

Livnat, A., Zehr, J. E., and Broten, T. P. (1984). Ultradian oscillations in blood pressure and heart rate in free-running dogs. *Am. J. Physiol.* **246**(5 Pt. 2), R817–R824.

Loganovsky, K. N., Volovik, S. V., Manton, K. G., Bazyka, D. A., and Flor-Henry, P. (2005). Whether ionizing radiation is a risk factor for schizophrenia spectrum disorders? *World J. Biol. Psychiatry* **6**(4), 212–230.

Lyamin, O. I., Mukhametov, L. M., Siegel, J. M., Nazarenko, E. A., Polyakova, I. G., and Shpak, O. V. (2002). Unihemispheric slow wave sleep and the state of the eyes in a white whale. *Behav. Brain Res.* **129**(1–2), 125–129.

Macris, N. T., Schiavi, R. C., Camerino, M. S., and Stein, M. (1970). Effect of hypothalamic lesions on immune processes in the guinea pig. *Am. J. Physiol.* **219**(5), 1205–1209.

Magee, D. F., and Naruse, S. (1983). Neural control of periodic secretion of the pancreas and the stomach in fasting dogs. *J. Physiol.* **344,** 153–160.

Mandell, A. J., Chaffey, B., Brill, P., Mandell, M. P., Rodnick, J., Rubin, R. T., and Sheff, R. (1966). Dreaming sleep in man: Changes in urine volume and osmolality. *Science* **151**(717), 1558–1560.

Manseau, C., and Broughton, R. (1983). Ultradian variations in human daytime EEGs: A preliminary report. *In* "Sleep 1982 European Congress Sleep Research" (W. P. Koella, Ed.), pp. 196–198. Karger, Basel.

Marangell, L. B., Rush, A. J., George, M. S., Sackeim, H. A., Johnson, C. R., Husain, M. M., Nahas, Z., and Lisanby, S. H. (2002). Vagus nerve stimulation (VNS) for major depressive episodes: One year outcomes. *Biol. Psychiatry* **51**(4), 280–287.

Marx, J. L. (1982). Autoimmunity in left-handers. Left-handedness may be associated with an increased risk of autoimmune disease. Is testosterone the link between the two? *Science* **217**(4555), 141–142.

Maxim, P. E., Bowden, D. M., and Sackett, G. P. (1976). Ultradian rhythms of solitary and social behavior in rhesus monkeys. *Physiol. Behav.* **17**(2), 337–344.

Mayer, S. (1876). Studien zur physiologie des herzens und der blutgefasse: V. Über spontane blut druckschwankungen. *Saech Akad Wiss Sitz Liepsig Math Naturw* **74,** 281–307.

McIntyre, M., Pritchard, P. B., III, and Lombroso, C. T. (1976). Left and right temporal lobe epileptics: A controlled investigation of some psychological differences. *Epilepsia* **17**(4), 377–386.

McManus, I. C. (1977). Predominance of left-sided breast tumours. *Lancet* **2** (8032), 297–298.

Meier-Koll, A. (1989a). Ultradian rhythms in cerebral laterality tested by a verbal dichotic listening paradigm. *Int. J. Neurosci.* **47**(1–2), 115–124.

Meier-Koll, A. (1989b). Ultradian laterality cycle in stereotyped behavior of a severely mentally retarded patient. *Int. J. Neurosci.* **47**(1–2), 103–113.

Meier-Koll, A., and Pohl, P. (1979). Chronobiological aspects of stereotyped motor behaviour in mentally retarded children. *Int. J. Chronobiol.* **6**(3), 191–209.

Mershon, J. L., Sehlhorst, C. S., Rebar, R. W., and Liu, J. H. (1992). Evidence of a corticotropin-releasing hormone pulse generator in the macaque hypothalamus. *Endocrinology* **130**(5), 2991–2996.

Merskey, H., and Watson, G. D. (1979). The lateralisation of pain. *Pain* **7**(3), 271–280.

Mizunuma, H., DePalatis, L. R., and McCann, S. M. (1983). Effect of unilateral orchidectomy on plasma FSH concentration: Evidence for a direct neural connection between testes and CNS. *Neuroendocrinology* **37**(4), 291–296.

Mohan, S., and Wei, L. (2002). Modulation of pulse rate by unilateral nostril breathing. *J. Indian Psychol.* **20**(1), 32–37.

Mohan, S. M., Reddy, S. C., and Wei, L. Y. (2001). Modulation of intraocular pressure by unilateral and forced unilateral nostril breathing in young healthy human subjects. *Int. Ophthalmol.* **24**(6), 305–311.

Monakhov, K., and Perris, C. (1980). Neurophysiological correlates of depressive symptomatology. *Neuropsychobiology* **6**(5), 268–279.

Morris, G. L., III, and Mueller, W. M. (1999). Long-term treatment with vagus nerve stimulation in patients with refractory epilepsy. The Vagus Nerve Stimulation Study Group E01–E05. *Neurology* **53**(8), 1731–1735.

Mukhametov, L. M., Lyamin, O. I., and Polyakova, I. G. (1985). Interhemispheric asynchrony of the sleep EEG in northern fur seals. *Experientia* **41**(8), 1034–1035.

Mukhametov, L. M., Supin, A. Y., and Polyakova, I. G. (1977). Interhemispheric asymmetry of the electroencephalographic sleep patterns in dolphins. *Brain Res.* **134**(3), 581–584.

Myslobodsky, M. S., and Horesh, N. (1978). Bilateral electrodermal activity in depressive patients. *Biol. Psychol.* **6**(2), 111–120.

Nahas, Z., Marangell, L. B., Husain, M. M., Rush, A. J., Sackeim, H. A., Lisanby, S. H., Martinez, J. M., and George, M. S. (2005). Two-year outcome of vagus nerve stimulation (VNS) for treatment of major depressive episodes. *J. Clin. Psychiatry* **66**(9), 1097–1104.

Nance, D. M., Bhargava, M., and Myatt, G. A. (1984). Further evidence for hypothalamic asymmetry in endocrine control of the ovary. *Brain Res. Bull.* **13**(5), 651–655.

Natelson, B. H. (1985). Neurocardiology. An interdisciplinary area for the 80s. *Arch. Neurol.* **42**(2), 178–184.

Naveen, K. V., Nagarathna, R., Nagendra, H. R., and Telles, S. (1997). Yoga breathing through a particular nostril increases spatial memory scores without lateralized effects. *Psychol. Rep.* **81**(2), 555–561.

Neligan, G. A., and Strang, L. B. (1952). A harlequin color change in the newborn. *Lancet* **2**(21), 1005–1007.

Nelson, J., Phillips, R., and Goldstein, L. (1977). Interhemispheric EEG laterality relationships following psychoactive agents and during operant performance in rabbits. *In* "Lateralization in the Nervous System" (S. Harnad, R. Doty, L. Goldstein, J. Jaynes, and G. Krauthamer, Eds.), pp. 451–470. Academic Press, New York.

Nemeroff, C. B., Mayberg, H. S., Krahl, S. E., McNamara, J., Frazer, A., Henry, T. R., George, M. S., Charney, D. S., and Brannan, S. K. (2006). VNS therapy in treatment-resistant depression: Clinical evidence and putative neurobiological mechanisms. *Neuropsychopharmacology* **31**(7), 1345–1355.

Netter, F. H. (1972). "The Ciba Collection of Medical Illustrations." Ciba, Summit, New Jersey.

Neveu, P. J., Taghzouti, K., Dantzer, R., Simon, H., and Le Moal, M. (1986). Modulation of mitogen-induced lymphoproliferation by cerebral neocortex. *Life Sci.* **38**(21), 1907–1913.

Nicholls, M. E., Ellis, B. E., Clement, J. G., and Yoshino, M. (2004). Detecting hemifacial asymmetries in emotional expression with three-dimensional computerized image analysis. *Proc. Biol. Sci.* **271** (1540), 663–668.

Nystrom, C., Matousek, M., and Hallstrom, T. (1986). Relationships between EEG and clinical characteristics in major depressive disorder. *Acta Psychiatr. Scand.* **73**(4), 390–394.

Ohki, M., Ogoshi, T., Yuasa, T., Kawano, K., and Kawano, M. (2005). Extended observation of the nasal cycle using a portable rhinoflowmeter. *J. Otolaryngol.* **34**(5), 346–349.

Orr, W. C., and Hoffman, H. J. (1974). A 90-min cardiac biorhythm: Methodology and data analysis using modified periodograms and complex demodulation. *IEEE Trans. Biomed. Eng.* **21**(2), 130–143.

Orr, W. C., Hoffman, H. J., and Hegge, F. W. (1974). Ultradian rhythms in extended performance. *Aerosp. Med.* **45**(9), 995–1000.

Ortega, S., and Cabrera, M. (1990). Ultradian rhythms in the EEG and task performance. *Chronobiologia* **17,** 183–194.

Oswald, I., Merrington, J., and Lewis, H. (1970). Cyclical "on demand" oral intake by adults. *Nature* **225**(5236), 959–960.

Otto, M. W., Dougher, M. J., and Yeo, R. A. (1989). Depression, pain, and hemispheric activation. *J. Nerv. Ment. Dis.* **177**(4), 210–218.

Pallanti, S., Hollander, E., and Goodman, W. K. (2004). A qualitative analysis of nonresponse: Management of treatment-refractory obsessive-compulsive disorder. *J. Clin. Psychiatry* **65**(Suppl. 14), 6–10.

Parker, D., and Rossman, L. (1973). "Physiology of Human Growth Hormone Release in Sleep." Fourth International Congress of Endocrinology, Excerpta Medica, Amsterdam.

Parker, D. C., Rossman, L. G., and Vanderlaan, E. F. (1974). Relation of sleep-entrained human prolactin release to REM-nonREM cycles. *J. Clin. Endocrinol. Metab.* **38**(4), 646–651.

Pawel, M. A., Sassin, J. F., and Weitzman, E. D. (1972). The temporal relation between HGH release and sleep stage changes at nocturnal sleep onset in man. *Life Sci. I.* **11**(12), 587–593.

Penaz, J. (1978). Mayer waves: History and methodology. *Automedica* **2,** 135–141.

Piepenbrock, N., Valatx, J. L., Malquarti, V., and Jouvet, M. (1985). Effects of hypothalamic paraventricular lesions on sleep in rats. *Neurosci. Lett.* **62**(2), 151–156.

Pivik, R. T., Busby, K. A., Gill, E., Hunter, P., and Nevins, R. (1996). Heart rate variations during sleep in preadolescents. *Sleep* **19**(2), 117–135.

Pollock, V. E., and Schneider, L. S. (1990). Quantitative, waking EEG research on depression. *Biol. Psychiatry* **27**(7), 757–780.

Polonsky, K. S., Given, B. D., and Van Cauter, E. (1988). Twenty-four-hour profiles and pulsatile patterns of insulin secretion in normal and obese subjects. *J. Clin. Invest.* **81**(2), 442–448.

Polosa, C. (1984). Rhythms in the activity of the autonomic nervous system: Their role in the generation of systemic arterial pressure waves. *In* "Mechanisms of Blood Pressure Waves" (K. Miyakawa, H. Koepchen, and C. Polosa, Eds.), pp. 27–41. Springer Verlag, Berlin, Heidelberg, New York, Tokyo.

Prast, H., Grass, K., and Philippu, A. (1997). The ultradian EEG rhythm coincides temporally with the ultradian rhythm of histamine release in the posterior hypothalamus. *Naunyn Schmiedebergs Arch. Pharmacol.* **356**(4), 526–528.

Preiss, G., and Polosa, C. (1974). Patterns of sympathetic neuron activity associated with Mayer waves. *Am. J. Physiol.* **226**(3), 724–730.

Ranson, S., and Magoun, H. (1939). The hypothalamus. *Ergeb. Physiol.* **41,** 56–163.

Rao, S., and Potdar, A. (1970). Nasal airflow with body in various positions. *J. Appl. Physiol.* **28**(2), 162–165.

Rao, U., Dahl, R. E., Ryan, N. D., Birmaher, B., Williamson, D. E., Giles, D. E., Rao, R., Kaufman, J., and Nelson, B. (1996). The relationship between longitudinal clinical course and sleep and cortisol changes in adolescent depression. *Biol. Psychiatry* **40**(6), 474–484.

Rasmussen, D. D., and Malven, P. V. (1981). Relationship between rhythmic motor activity and plasma luteinizing hormone in ovariectomized sheep. *Neuroendocrinology* **32**(6), 364–369.

Rattenborg, N. C., Amlaner, C. J., and Lima, S. L. (2000). Behavioral, neurophysiological and evolutionary perspectives on unihemispheric sleep. *Neurosci. Biobehav. Rev.* **24**(8), 817–842.

Ray, W. J., and Cole, H. W. (1985a). EEG activity during cognitive processing: Influence of attentional factors. *Int. J. Psychophysiol.* **3**(1), 43–48.

Ray, W. J., and Cole, H. W. (1985b). EEG alpha activity reflects attentional demands, and beta activity reflects emotional and cognitive processes. *Science* **228**(4700), 750–752.

Rebert, C. S., and Low, D. W. (1978). Differential hemispheric activation during complex visuomotor performance. *Electroencephalogr. Clin. Neurophysiol.* **44**(6), 724–734.

Reid, S. A., Duke, L. M., and Allen, J. J. (1998). Resting frontal electroencephalographic asymmetry in depression: Inconsistencies suggest the need to identify mediating factors. *Psychophysiology* **35**(4), 389–404.

Reinberg, A., Motohashi, Y., Bourdeleau, P., Andlauer, P., Lévi, F., and Bicakova-Rocher, A. (1988). Alteration of period and amplitude of circadian rhythms in shift workers. With special reference to temperature, right and left hand grip strength. *Eur. J. Appl. Physiol. Occup. Physiol.* **57**(1), 15–25.

Reivich, M., Gur, R., and Alavi, A. (1983). Positron emission tomographic studies of sensory stimuli, cognitive processes and anxiety. *Hum. Neurobiol.* **2**(1), 25–33.

Renoux, G., Biziere, K., Renoux, M., Guillaumin, J. M., and Degenne, D. (1983). A balanced brain asymmetry modulates T cell-mediated events. *J. Neuroimmunol.* **5**(3), 227–238.

Rice, C., Baio, J., Van Naarden Braun, K., Doernberg, N., Pettygrove, S., Cunniff, C., Meaney, J., Newschaffer, C., *et al.* (2007). Prevalence of autism spectrum disorders—autism and developmental disabilities monitoring network, six sites, United States, 2000. *Morb. Mortal. World Wide* **56**(SS01), 1–11.

Richter, C. P. (1980). Growth hormone 3.6-h pulsatile secretion and feeding times have similar periods in rats. *Am. J. Physiol.* **239**(1), E1–E2.

Riga, I. N. (1957). The neuro-reflex syndrome of unilateral nasal obstruction; preliminary note. *Rev. Otoneuroophtalmol.* **29**(6), 325–335.

Risberg, J., and Prohovnik, I. (1983). Cortical processing of visual and tactile stimuli studied by non-invasive rCBF measurements. *Hum. Neurobiol.* **2**(1), 5–10.

Robin, P. E., and Shortridge, R. T. (1979). Lateralisation of tumours of the nasal cavity and paranasal sinuses and its relationship to aetiology. *Lancet* **1**(8118), 695–696.

Rossi, G., and Rosadini, G. (1967). Experimental analysis of cerebral dominance in man. *In* "Brain Mechanisms Underlying Speech and Language" (I. Darley, Ed.), pp. 167–184. Grune and Stratton, New York.

Roszman, T., Cross, R., Brooks, W., and Markesbery, W. (1985). Neuroimmunomodulation: Effects of neural lesions on cellular immunity. *In* "Neural Modulation of Immunity" (R. Guillemin, M. Cohen, and T. Melnechuk, Eds.), pp. 95–109. Raven Press, New York.

Roszman, T. L., and Brooks, W. H. (1985). Neural modulation of immune function. *J. Neuroimmunol.* **10**(1), 59–69.

Roth, C., Achermann, P., and Borbely, A. A. (1999). Frequency and state specific hemispheric asymmetries in the human sleep EEG. *Neurosci. Lett.* **271**(3), 139–142.

Rush, A. J., Erman, M. K., Giles, D. E., Schlesser, M. A., Carpenter, G., Vasavada, N., and Roffwarg, H. P. (1986). Polysomnographic findings in recently drug-free and clinically remitted depressed patients. *Arch. Gen. Psychiatry* **43**(9), 878–884.

Rush, A. J., George, M. S., Sackeim, H. A., Marangell, L. B., Husain, M. M., Giller, C., Nahas, Z., Haines, S., Simpson, R. K., Jr., and Goodman, R. (2000). Vagus nerve stimulation (VNS) for treatment-resistant depressions: A multicenter study. *Biol. Psychiatry* **47**(4), 276–286.

Rush, A. J., Marangell, L. B., Sackeim, H. A., George, M. S., Brannan, S. K., and Davis, S. M. (2005). Vagus nerve stimulation for treatment-resistant depression: A randomized, controlled acute phase trial. *Biol. Psychiatry* **58**(5), 347–354.

Sackeim, H. A., Rush, A. J., George, M. S., Marangell, L. B., Husain, M. M., Nahas, Z., Johnson, C. R., Seidman, S., Giller, C., Haines, S., Simpson, R. K., Jr., and Goodman, R. R. (2001). Vagus nerve stimulation (VNS) for treatment-resistant depression: Efficacy, side effects, and predictors of outcome. *Neuropsychopharmacology* **25**(5), 713–728.

Sackeim, H. A., Rush, A. J., Marangell, L. B., George, M. S., and Brannan, S. K. (2004). "Long-term antidepressant effects of vagus nerve stimulation (VNS) in treatment-resistant depression." 43rd American College of Neuropsychopharmacology Annual Meeting, San Juan, PR.

Salinsky, M. C., Uthman, B. M., Ristanovic, R. K., Wernicke, J. F., and Tarver, W. B. (1996). Vagus nerve stimulation for the treatment of medically intractable seizures. Results of a 1-year open-extension trial. Vagus Nerve Stimulation Study Group. *Arch. Neurol.* **53**(11), 1176–1180.

Salomon, R. M., Kennedy, J. S., Johnson, B. W., Urbano Blackford, J., Schmidt, D. E., Kwentus, J., Gwirtsman, H. E., Gouda, J. F., and Shiavi, R. G. (2005). Treatment enhances ultradian rhythms of CSF monoamine metabolites in patients with major depressive episodes. *Neuropsychopharmacology* **30**(11), 2082–2091.

Samzelius-Lejdstrom, I. (1939). Researches with the bilateral troncopneumograph on the movements of the respiratory mechanisms during breathing. *Acta. Otolaryngol. suppl.* **35,** 3–104.

Sanders, B., Lattimore, C., Smith, K., and Dierker, L. (1994). Forced single-nostril breathing and cognition. *Percept. Mot. Skills* **79**(3 Pt. 2), 1499–1506.

Sanders, S. W., and Moore, J. G. (1992). Gastrointestinal chronopharmacology: Physiology, pharmacology and therapeutic implications. *Pharmacol. Ther.* **54**(1), 1–15.

Saper, C. B. (1985). Organization of cerebral cortical afferent systems in the rat. II. Hypothalamocortical projections. *J. Comp. Neurol.* **237**(1), 21–46.

Saper, C. B., Loewy, A. D., Swanson, L. W., and Cowan, W. M. (1976). Direct hypothalamo-autonomic connections. *Brain Res.* **117**(2), 305–312.

Sarne, Y., Lavie, P., Oksenberg, A., Gordon, C., and Luboshitzky, R. (1981). Episodic secretion of humoral endorphin in sleep. *Neuroendocrinol. Lett.* **3,** 365–374.

Schiavi, R. C., Davis, D. M., Fogel, M., White, D., Edwards, A., Igel, G., Szechter, R., and Fisher, C. (1977). Luteinizing hormone and testosterone during nocturnal sleep: Relation to penile tumescent cycles. *Arch. Sex. Behav.* **6**(2), 97–104.

Schiff, B. B., and Rump, S. A. (1995). Asymmetrical hemispheric activation and emotion: The effects of unilateral forced nostril breathing. *Brain Cogn.* **29**(3), 217–231.

Schofl, C., Becker, C., Prank, K., von zur Muhlen, A., and Brabant, G. (1997). Twenty-four-hour rhythms of plasma catecholamines and their relation to cardiovascular parameters in healthy young men. *Eur. J. Endocrinol.* **137**(6), 675–683.

Searleman, A., Hornung, D. E., Stein, E., and Brzuszkiewicz, L. (2005). Nostril dominance: Differences in nasal airflow and preferred handedness. *Laterality* **10**(2), 111–120.

Selye, H. (1946). The general adaptation syndrome and the diseases of adaptation. *J. Clin. Endocrinol.* **6,** 117–230.

Selye, H. (1950a). Stress and the general adaptation syndrome. *Br. Med. J.* **1**(4667), 1383–1392.

Selye, H. (1950b). Diseases of adaptation. *Wis. Med. J.* **49**(6), 515–516.

Selye, H. (1950c). Diseases of adaptation and ACTH and cortisone therapy. *An. R. Acad. Nac. Med. (Madr.)* **67**(4), 634–649.

Selye, H., and Fortier, C. (1950). Adaptive reaction to stress. *Psychosom. Med.* **12**(3), 149–157.

Senie, R. T., Rosen, P. P., Lesser, M. L., Snyder, R. E., Schottenfeld, D., and Duthie, K (1980). Epidemiology of breast carcinoma II: Factors related to the predominance of left-sided disease. *Cancer* **46**(7), 1705–1713.

Serafetinides, E., Shurley, J., and Brooks, R. (1972). Electroencephalogram of the pilot whale, Globicephala scammoni, in wakefulness and sleep: Lateralization aspects. *Int. J. Psychophysiol.* **2,** 129–135.

Sercer, A. (1930). Research on the homolateral reflex of the nasal cavity on the lung. *Acta Otolaryngol.* **14,** 82–90.

Servit, Z., Kristof, M., and Strejckova, A. (1981). Activating effect of nasal and oral hyperventilation on epileptic electrographic phenomena: Reflex mechanisms of nasal origin. *Epilepsia* **22**(3), 321–329.

Shannahoff-Khalsa, D. (1991a). Lateralized rhythms of the central and autonomic nervous systems. *Int. J. Psychophysiol.* **11**(3), 225–251.

Shannahoff-Khalsa, D. (1993). The ultradian rhythm of alternating cerebral hemispheric activity. *Int. J. Neurosci.* **70**(3–4), 285–298.

Shannahoff-Khalsa, D. (1997). "Yogic Techniques are Effective in the Treatment of Obsessive Compulsive Disorders." Marcel Dekker Inc., New York.

Shannahoff-Khalsa, D. (2001). Unilateral forced nostril breathing: Basic science, clinical trials, and selected advanced techniques. *Subtle Energies Energy Med. J.* **12**(2), 79–106.

Shannahoff-Khalsa, D. (2003). Kundalini Yoga meditation techniques in the treatment of obsessive compulsive and OC spectrum disorders. *Brief Treat. Crisis Interv.* **3**(3), 369–382.

Shannahoff-Khalsa, D. (2006). "Kundalini Yoga Meditation: Techniques Specific for Psychiatric Disorders, Couples Therapy, and Personal Growth." W. W. Norton & Company, New York, London.

Shannahoff-Khalsa, D., Ray, L., Levine, S., Gallen, C., Schwartz, B. J., and Sidorowich, J. J. (1999). Randomized controlled trial of yogic meditation techniques for patients with obsessive compulsive disorders. *CNS Spectrums: Int. J. Neuropsychiatr. Med.* **4**(12), 34–46.

Shannahoff-Khalsa, D. S. (1991b). Stress technology medicine, a new paradigm for stress and considerations for self-regulation. *In* "Stress: Neurobiology and Neuroendocrinology" (M. Brown, G. Koob, and C. Rivier, Eds.), pp. 647–686. Marcel Dekker Inc., New York.

Shannahoff-Khalsa, D. S. (2004). An introduction to Kundalini yoga meditation techniques that are specific for the treatment of psychiatric disorders. *J. Altern. Complement. Med.* **10**(1), 91–101.

Shannahoff-Khalsa, D. S. (2005). Patient perspectives: Kundalini yoga meditation techniques for psycho-oncology and as potential therapies for cancer. *Integr. Cancer Ther.* **4**(1), 87–100.

Shannahoff-Khalsa, D. S. (2007). Selective unilateral autonomic activation: Implications for psychiatry (a review article), CNS Spectrums. *Int. J. Neuropsychiatr. Med.* **12**(8), pp. 625–634.

Shannahoff-Khalsa, D. S., and Beckett, L. R. (1996). Clinical case report: Efficacy of yogic techniques in the treatment of obsessive compulsive disorders. *Int. J. Neurosci.* **85**(1–2), 1–17.

Shannahoff-Khalsa, D. S., and Kennedy, B. (1993). The effects of unilateral forced nostril breathing on the heart. *Int. J. Neurosci.* **73**(1–2), 47–60.

Shannahoff-Khalsa, D. S., and Yates, F. E. (2000). Ultradian sleep rhythms of lateral EEG, autonomic, and cardiovascular activity are coupled in humans. *Int. J. Neurosci.* **101**(1–4), 21–43.

Shannahoff-Khalsa, D. S., Boyle, M. R., and Buebel, M. E. (1991). The effects of unilateral forced nostril breathing on cognition. *Int. J. Neurosci.* **57**(3–4), 239–249.

Shannahoff-Khalsa, D. S., Gillin, J. C., Yates, F. E., Schlosser, A., and Zawadzki, E. M. (2001). Ultradian rhythms of alternating cerebral hemispheric EEG dominance are coupled to rapid eye movement and non-rapid eye movement stage 4 sleep in humans. *Sleep Med.* **2**(4), 333–346.

Shannahoff-Khalsa, D. S., Kennedy, B., Yates, F. E., and Ziegler, M. G. (1996). Ultradian rhythms of autonomic, cardiovascular, and neuroendocrine systems are related in humans. *Am. J. Physiol.* **270**(4 Pt. 2), R873–R887.

Shannahoff-Khalsa, D. S., Kennedy, B., Yates, F. E., and Ziegler, M. G. (1997). Low-frequency ultradian insulin rhythms are coupled to cardiovascular, autonomic, and neuroendocrine rhythms. *Am. J. Physiol.* **272**(3 Pt. 2), R962–R968.

Shannahoff-Khalsa, D. S., Sramek, B. B., Kennel, M. B., and Jamieson, S. W. (2004). Hemodynamic observations on a yogic breathing technique claimed to help eliminate and prevent heart attacks: A pilot study. *J. Altern. Complement. Med.* **10**(5), 757–766.

Shapiro, C. M., Catterall, J. R., Montgomery, I., Raab, G. M., and Douglas, N. J. (1986). Do asthmatics suffer bronchoconstriction during rapid eye movement sleep? *Br. Med. J. (Clin. Res. Ed.)* **292**(6529), 1161–1164.

Shapiro, E. T., Tillil, H., Polonsky, K. S., Fang, V. S., Rubenstein, A. H., and Van Cauter, E. (1988). Oscillations in insulin secretion during constant glucose infusion in normal man: Relationship to changes in plasma glucose. *J. Clin. Endocrinol. Metab.* **67**(2), 307–314.

Shimada, S. G., and Marsh, D. J. (1979). Oscillations in mean arterial blood pressure in conscious dogs. *Circ. Res.* **44**(5), 692–700.

Shurley, J., Serafetinides, E., Brooks, R., Elsner, R., and Kenney, D. (1969). Sleep in Cetaceans. I. The pilot whale, Globicephala scammoni. *Psychophysiology* **6,** 230.

Simon, C., Brandenberger, G., and Follenius, M. (1987). Ultradian oscillations of plasma glucose, insulin, and C-peptide in man during continuous enteral nutrition. *J. Clin. Endocrinol. Metab.* **64**(4), 669–674.

Snyder, F., Hobson, J. A., and Goldfrank, F. (1963). Blood Pressure Changes During Human Sleep. *Science* **142,** 1313–1314.

Sonnenberg, G. E., Hoffmann, R. G., Johnson, C. P., and Kissebah, A. H. (1992). Low- and high-frequency insulin secretion pulses in normal subjects and pancreas transplant recipients: Role of extrinsic innervation. *J. Clin. Invest.* **90**(2), 545–553.

Sperry, R. W. (1964). The great cerebral commissure. *Sci. Am.* **210,** 42–52.

Springorum, P. W., and Centenera, D. (1938). Die verschiedene Beteiligung beider Nieren an Diureseanderungen und vasomotorishen Reaktionen. *Pflugers Arch* **239,** 440–450.

Stagner, J. I., and Samols, E. (1985). Role of intrapancreatic ganglia in regulation of periodic insular secretions. *Am. J. Physiol.* **248**(5 Pt. 1), E522–E530.

Stancak, A., Honig, J., Wackermann, J., Lepicovska, V., and Dostalek, C. (1991). Effects of unilateral nostril breathing on respiration, heart rhythm, and brain electrical activity. *Neurosciences* **17,** 409–417.

Stein, M. (1985). Bereavement, Depression, Stress, and Immunity. *In* "Neural Modulation of Immunity" (R. Guillemin, M. Cohen, and T. Melnechuk, Eds.), pp. 29–44. Raven Press, New York.

Sterman, M. (1967). Relationship of intrauterine fetal activity to maternal sleep stage. *Exp. Neurol.* **19**(Suppl. 4), 98–106.

Stoksted, P. (1953). Rhinometric measurements for determination of the nasal cycle. *Acta Otolaryngol. Suppl.* **109,** 159–175.

Stoksted, P. (1960). Obstructions in the nose and their influence on the pulmonary functions. *Acta Otorhinolar.* **158**(Suppl.), 110.

Swanson, L. W. (1987). The hypothalamus. *In* "Handbook of Chemical Neuroanatomy, Vol. 5, Integrated Systems of the CNS" (A. Bjorkland, T. Hokfelt, and L. Swanson, Eds.), pp. 1–124. Elsevier Science, Amsterdam.

Takagi, K., and Kobayasi, S. (1955). Skin pressure-vegetative reflex. *Acta Med. Biol.* **4,** 31–57.

Takagi, K., and Sakurai, T. (1950). A sweat reflex due to pressure on the body surface. *Jap. J. Physiol.* **1,** 22–28.

Takahashi, Y., Kipnis, D. M., and Daughaday, W. H. (1968). Growth hormone secretion during sleep. *J. Clin. Invest.* **47**(9), 2079–2090.

Tarouini, B., Lombardi, P., Pernice, L., Andraoli, F., März, W., Cornélissen, G., and Halberg, F. (1986). "Ultradian structure of gastric pH at night." 54th Annual Spring Meeting St. Cloud State University, St. Cloud, Minnesota, Minnesota Academy of Science.

Telles, S., Nagarathna, R., and Nagendra, H. R. (1994). Breathing through a particular nostril can alter metabolism and autonomic activities. *Indian J. Physiol. Pharmacol.* **38**(2), 133–137.

Telles, S., Nagarathna, R., and Nagendra, H. R. (1996). Physiological measures of right nostril breathing. *J. Altern. Complement. Med.* **2**(4), 479–484.

Terzian, H. (1964). Behavioural and EEG effects of intracarotid sodium amytal injection. *Acta Neurochir. (Wien.)* **12,** 230–239.

Totterdell, P. (1995). Effects of depressed affect on diurnal and ultradian variations in mood in a healthy sample. *Chronobiol. Int.* **12**(4), 278–289.

Tsuji, Y., and Kobayashi, T. (1988). Short and long ultradian EEG components in daytime arousal. *Electroencephalogr. Clin. Neurophysiol.* **70**(2), 110–117.

Tucker, D. M. (1981). Lateral brain function, emotion, and conceptualization. *Psychol. Bull.* **89**(1), 19–46.

Van Cauter, E. (1990). Diurnal and ultradian rhythms in human endocrine function: A minireview. *Horm. Res.* **34**(2), 45–53.

Van Cauter, E., and Honinckx, E. (Cauter 1985). Pulsatility of pituitary hormones. *In* "Ultradian Rhythms in Physiology and Behavior" (H. Schultz and P. Lavie, Eds.), pp. 41–60. Springer-Verlag, Berlin.

Veldhuis, J. D., and Johnson, M. L. (1988). Operating characteristics of the hypothalamo-pituitary-gonadal axis in men: Circadian, ultradian, and pulsatile release of prolactin and its temporal coupling with luteinizing hormone. *J. Clin. Endocrinol. Metab.* **67**(1), 116–123.

Veldhuis, J. D., Evans, W. S., Rogol, A. D., Drake, C. R., Thorner, M. O., Merriam, G. R., and Johnson, M. L. (1984). Intensified rates of venous sampling unmask the presence of spontaneous, high-frequency pulsations of luteinizing hormone in man. *J. Clin. Endocrinol. Metab.* **59**(1), 96–102.

Velikonja, D., Weiss, D. S., and Corning, W. C. (1993). The relationship of cortical activation to alternating autonomic activity. *Electroencephalogr. Clin. Neurophysiol.* **87**(1), 38–45.

Vogel, G. W., Vogel, F., McAbee, R. S., and Thurmond, A. J. (1980). Improvement of depression by REM sleep deprivation. New findings and a theory. *Arch. Gen. Psychiatry* **37**(3), 247–253.

Vyazovskiy, V. V., Borbely, A. A., and Tobler, I. (2002). Interhemispheric sleep EEG asymmetry in the rat is enhanced by sleep deprivation. *J. Neurophysiol.* **88**(5), 2280–2286.

Wada, T. (1922). An experimental study of hunger and its relation to activity. *Arch. Psychol. Monogr.* **8,** 1–65.

Watabe, T., Tanaka, K., Kumagae, M., Itoh, S., Hasegawa, M., Horiuchi, T., Miyabe, S., Ohno, H., and Shimizu, N. (1987). Diurnal rhythm of plasma immunoreactive corticotropin-releasing factor in normal subjects. *Life Sci.* **40**(17), 1651–1655.

Watanabe, K., and Hiroshige, T. (1981). Phase relation between episodic fluctuations of spontaneous locomotor activity and plasma corticosterone in rats with suprachiasmatic nuclei lesions. *Neuroendocrinology* **33**(1), 52–59.

Webster, W. (1977). Hemispheric asymmetry in cats. *In* "Lateralization in the Nervous System" (S. Harnad, R. Doty, L. Goldstein, J. Jaynes, and G. Krauthamer, Eds.), pp. 471–480. Academic Press, New York.

Wefelmeyer, T., and Kuhs, H. (1996). Diurnal mood variation in melancholic patients and healthy controls. *Psychopathology* **29**(3), 184–192.

Weigle, D. S. (1987). Pulsatile secretion of fuel-regulatory hormones. *Diabetes* **36**(6), 764–775.

Weitzman, E. D. (1976a). Biologic rhythms and hormone secretion patterns. *Hosp. Pract.* **11**(8), 79–86.

Weitzman, E. D. (1976b). Circadian rhythms and episodic hormone secretion in man. *Annu. Rev. Med.* **27,** 225–243.

Weitzman, E. D., Schaumburg, H., and Fishbein, W. (1966). Plasma 17-hydroxycorticosteroid levels during sleep in man. *J. Clin. Endocrinol. Metab.* **26**(2), 121–127.

Werntz, D. A., Bickford, R. G., Bloom, F. E., and Shannahoff-Khalsa, D. S. (1980). "Cerebral Hemispheric Activity and Autonomic Nervous Function." 10th Annual Meeting Society for Neuroscience, Cincinnati, Ohio, Society for Neuroscience.

Werntz, D. A., Bickford, R. G., Bloom, F. E., and Shannahoff-Khalsa, D. S. (1981). "Selective cortical activation by altering autonomic function." Western EEG Society Meeting, Abstract, Reno, Nevada.

Werntz, D. A., Bickford, R. G., Bloom, F. E., and Shannahoff-Khalsa, D. S. (1983). Alternating cerebral hemispheric activity and the lateralization of autonomic nervous function. *Hum. Neurobiol.* **2**(1), 39–43.

Werntz, D. A., Bickford, R. G., and Shannahoff-Khalsa, D. (1987). Selective hemispheric stimulation by unilateral forced nostril breathing. *Hum. Neurobiol.* **6**(3), 165–171.

Wilson, J. B. (1986). Thirty one years of herpes zoster in a rural practice. *Br. Med. J. (Clin Res Ed)* **293**(6558), 1349–1351.

Wotzilka, G., and Schramek, J. (1930). Tierexperimentelle Untersuchungen uber den Weg des Inspirationsstromes jeder Nasenseite in die Lunge. *Mschr. Ohrenheilk.* **64,** 580–585.

Zabielski, R. (2004). Reefs in experimental gastroenterology—cyclic activities of the gastrointestinal tract. *J. Physiol. Pharmacol.* **55**(Suppl. 2), 19–32.

# INDEX

**T**



**U**



**V**

**Y**

# CONTENTS OF RECENT VOLUMES

## Volume 39



## Volume 40

## Volume 41

## Volume 42



## Volume 43



## Volume 44

## Volume 45

## Volume 46

## Volume 47



## Volume 48

## Volume 49



## Volume 50

## Volume 51

## Volume 52



## Volume 53

## Volume 54



## Volume 55

## Volume 56



## Volume 57



## Volume 58



## Volume 59

## Volume 60



## Volume 61

## Volume 62



## Volume 63



## Volume 64

## Volume 65



## Volume 66

## Volume 70



## Volume 71

## Volume 72



## Volume 73

## Volume 74

## Volume 75



## Volume 76

## Volume 77



## Volume 78

## Volume 79

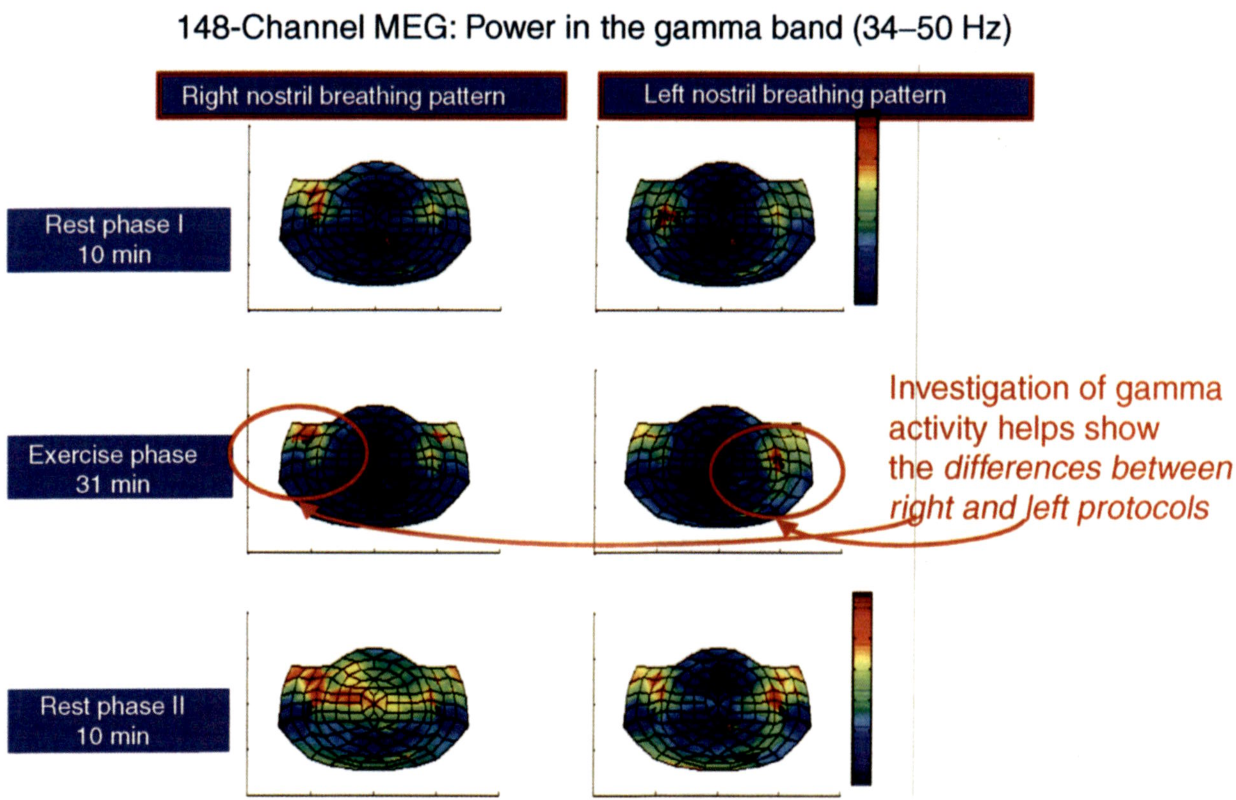


SHANNAHOFF-KHALSA, SECTION V.A., FIG. 37. (See Legend in Text.)

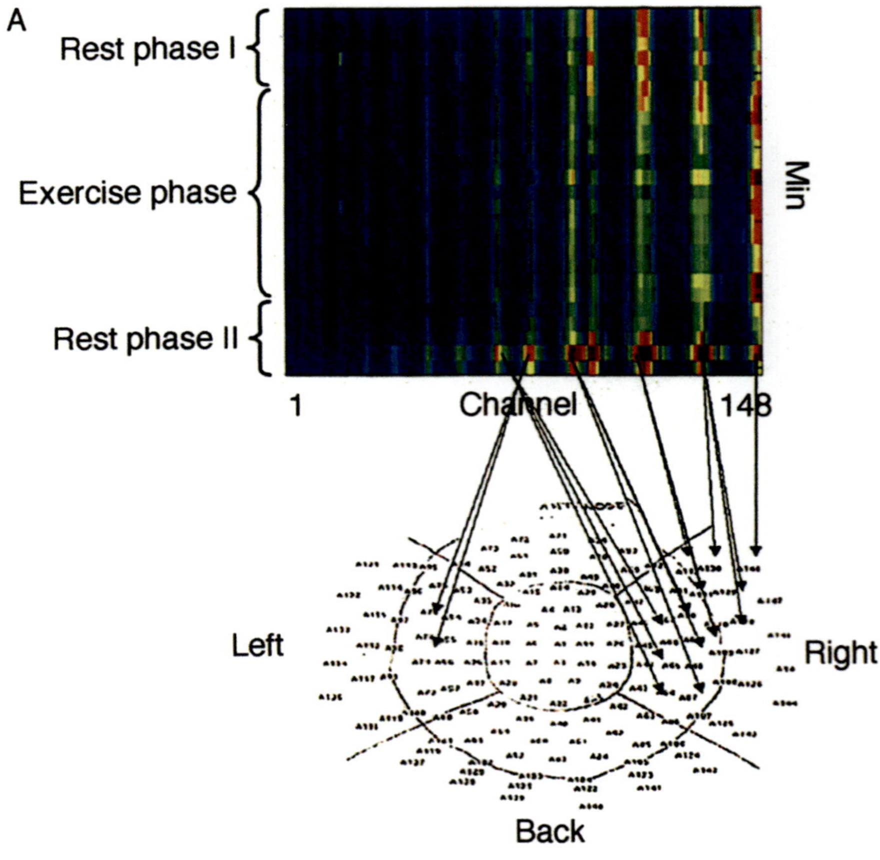


SHANNAHOFF-KHALSA, SECTION V.A., FIG. 38A (LEFT NOSTRIL).

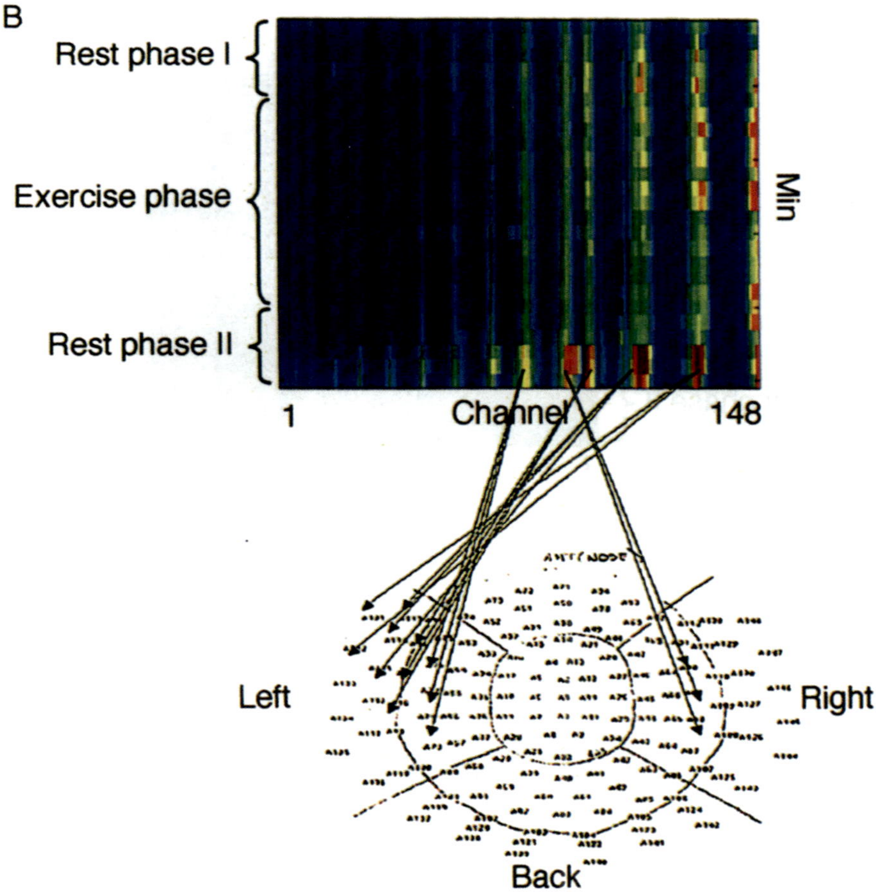


SHANNAHOFF-KHALSA, SECTION V.A., FIG. 38B (RIGHT NOSTRIL). (See Legend in Text.)

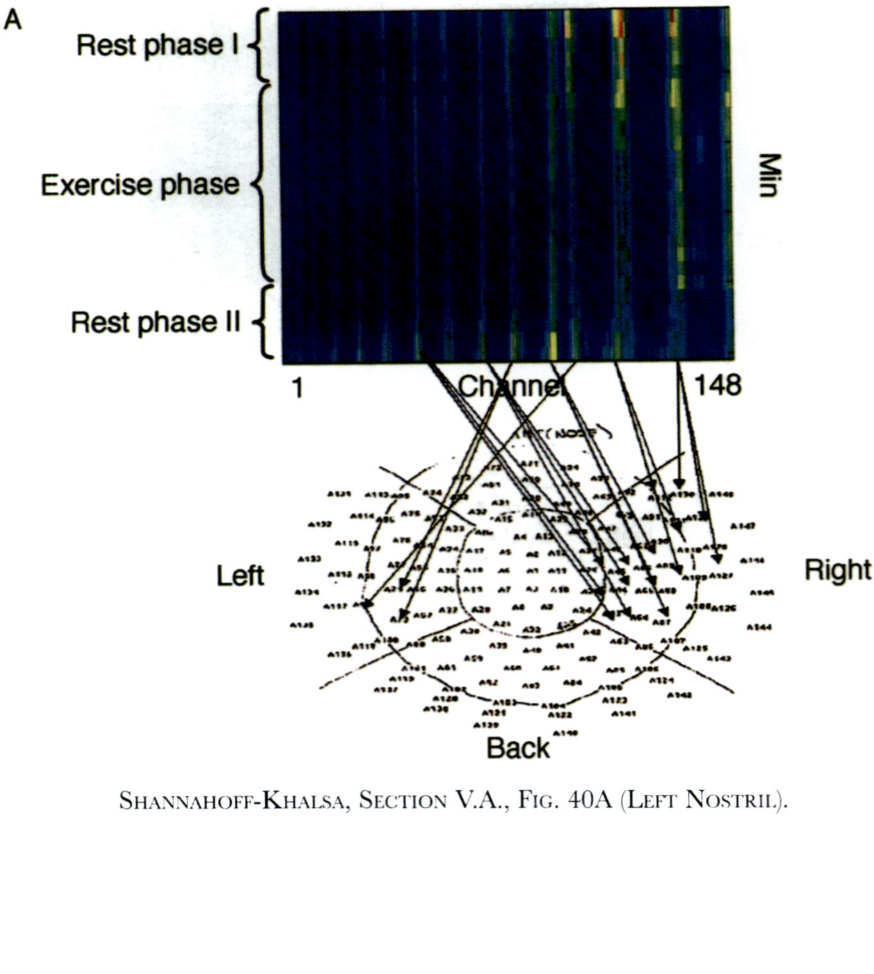


SHANNAHOFF-KHALSA, SECTION V.A., FIG. 40A (LEFT NOSTRIL).

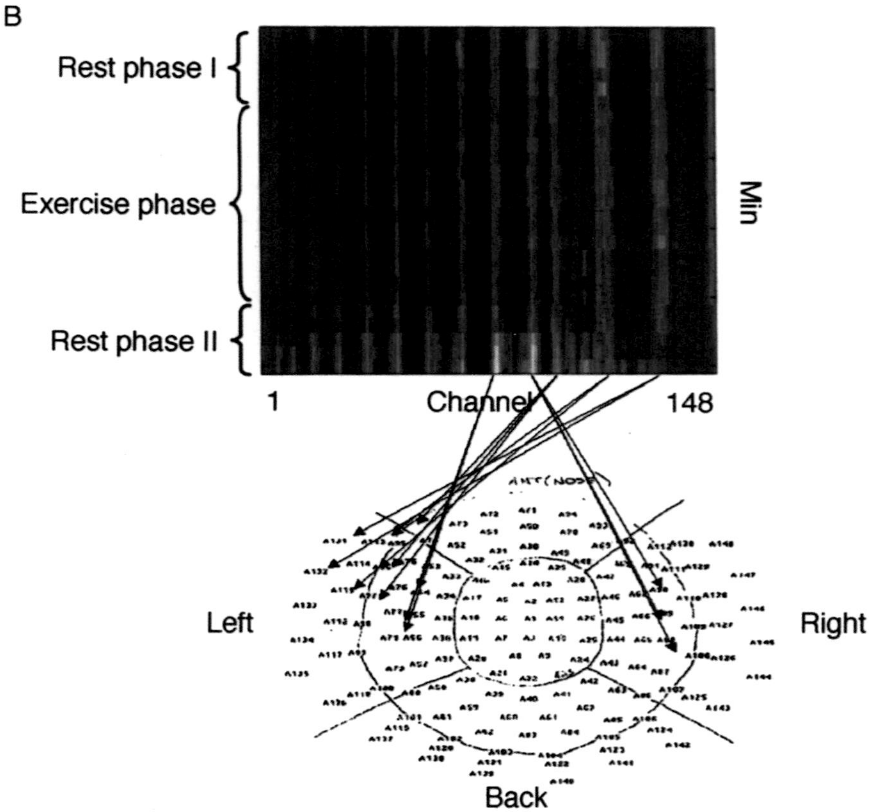


Shannahoff-Khalsa, Section V.A., Fig. 40B (Right Nostril). (See Legend in Text.)

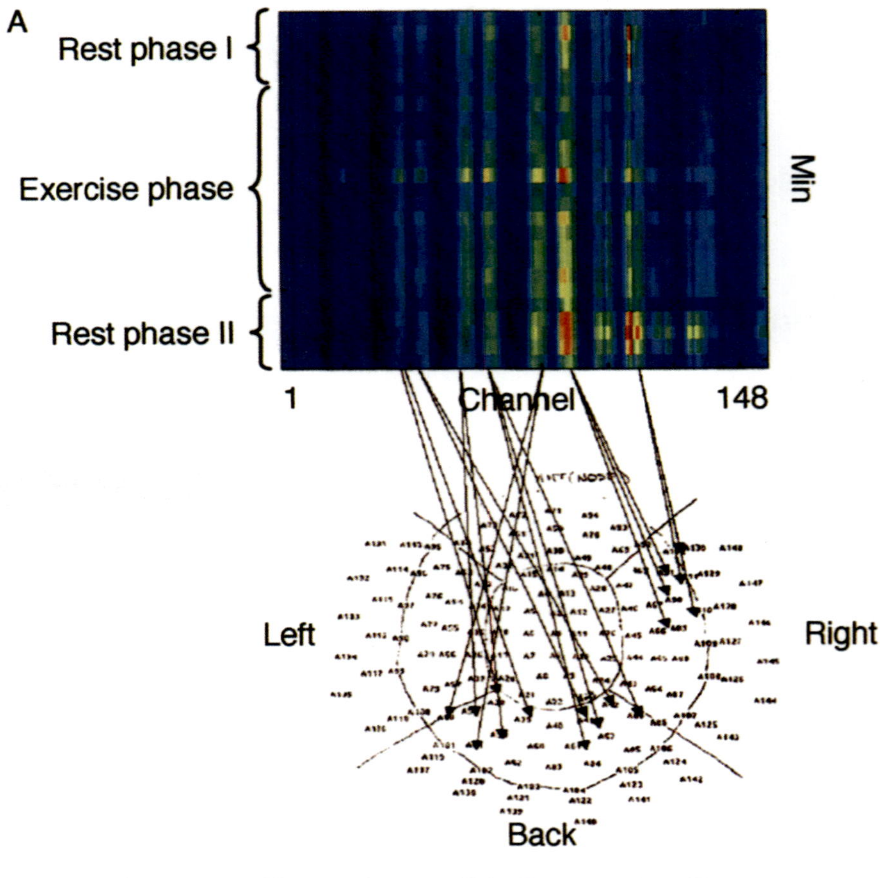


SHANNAHOFF-KHALSA, SECTION V.A., FIG. 41A (LEFT NOSTRIL).

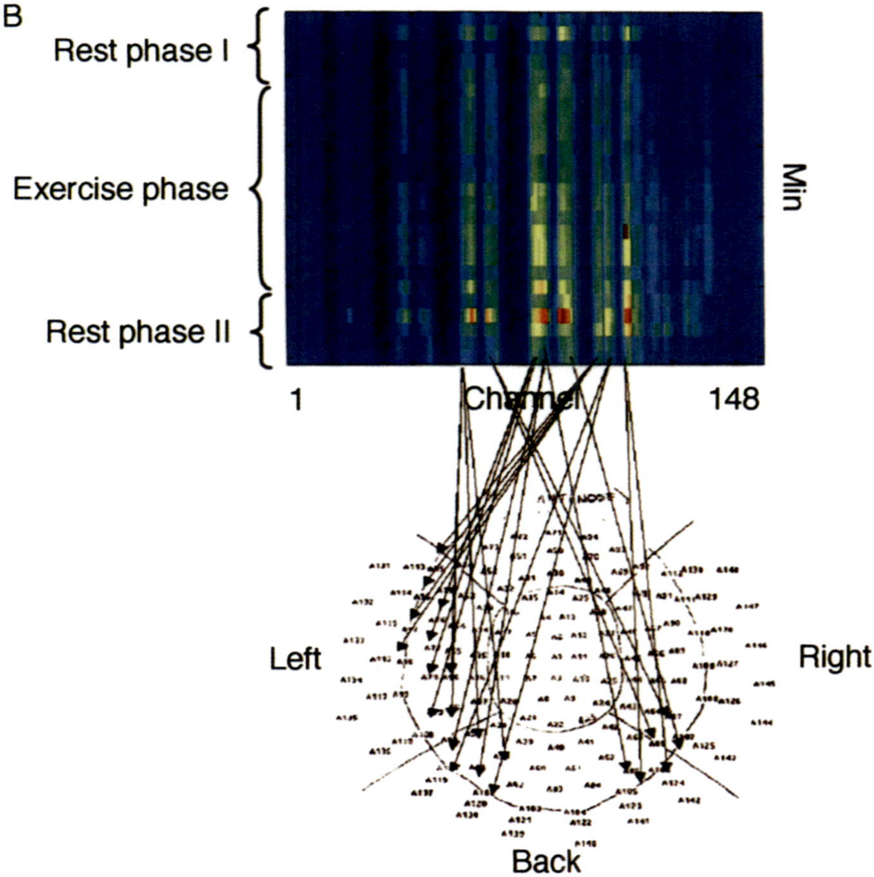


SHANNAHOFF-KHALSA, SECTION V.A., FIG. 41B (RIGHT NOSTRIL). (See Legend in Text.)

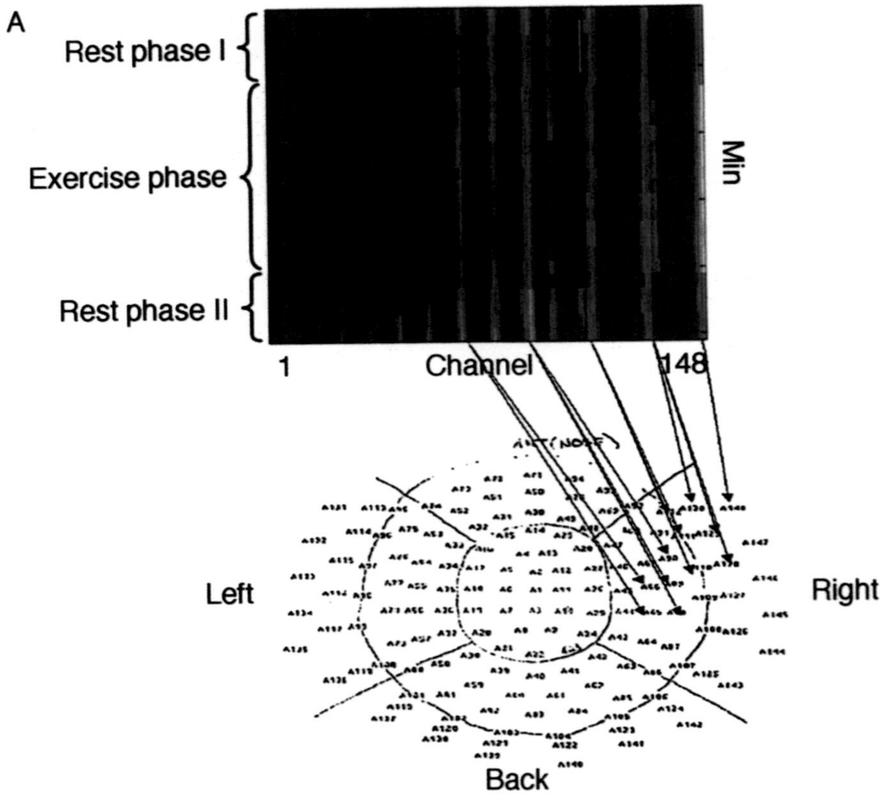


Shannahoff-Khalsa, Section V.A., Fig. 42A (Left Nostril).

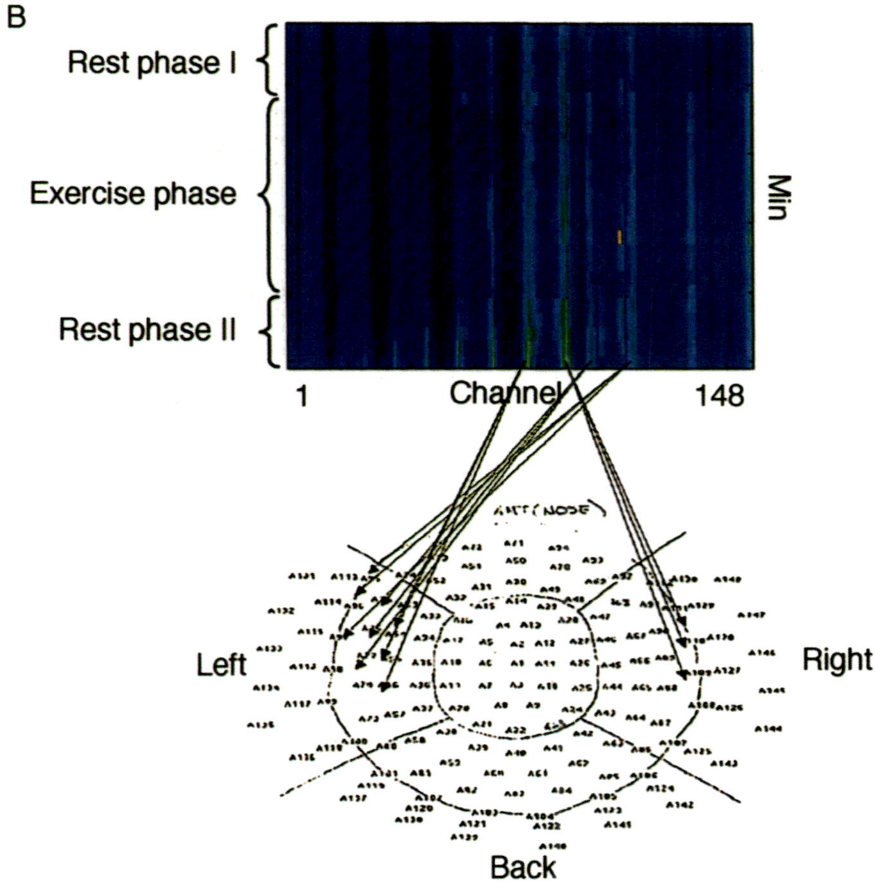


SHANNAHOFF-KHALSA, SECTION V.A., FIG. 42B (RIGHT NOSTRIL). (See Legend in Text.)

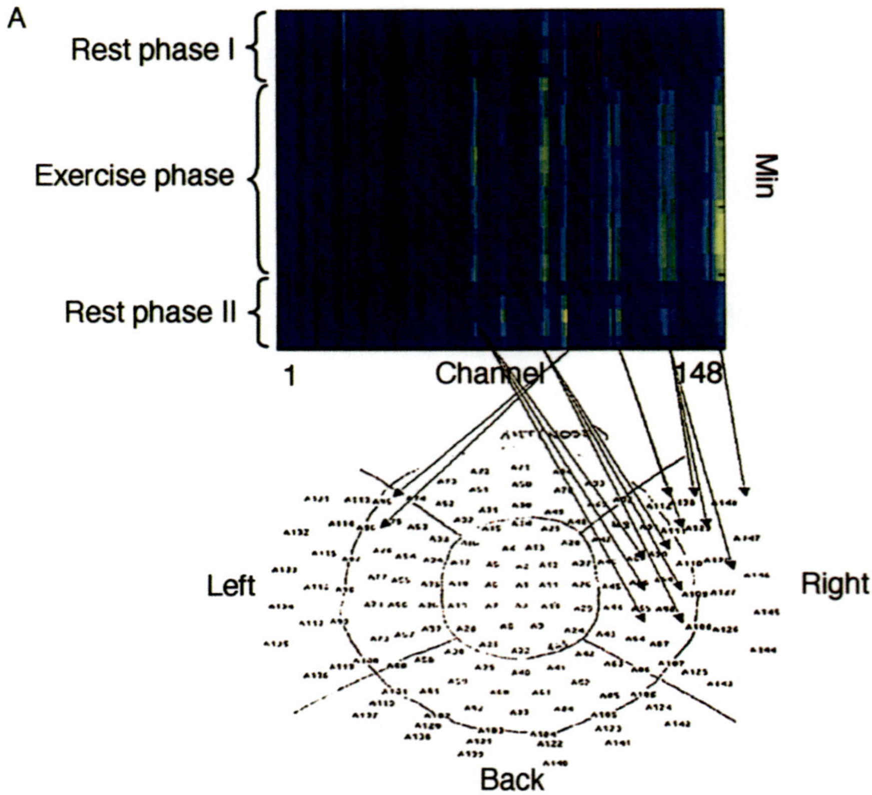


SHANNAHOFF-KHALSA, SECTION V.A., FIG. 43A (LEFT NOSTRIL).

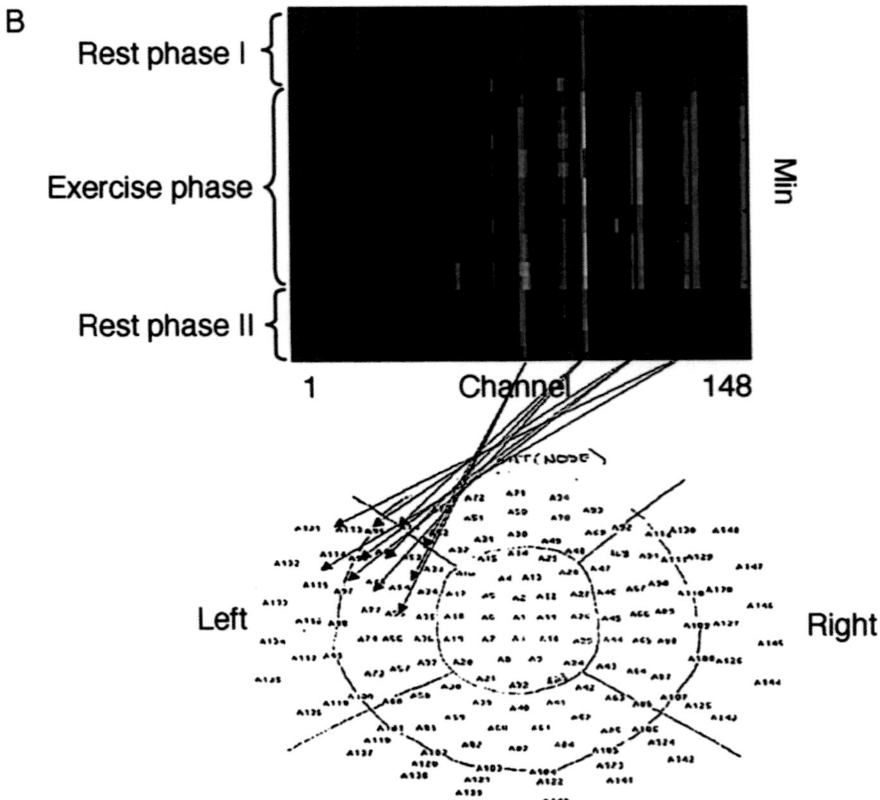


SHANNAHOFF-KHALSA, SECTION V.A., FIG. 43B (RIGHT NOSTRIL). (See Legend in Text.)

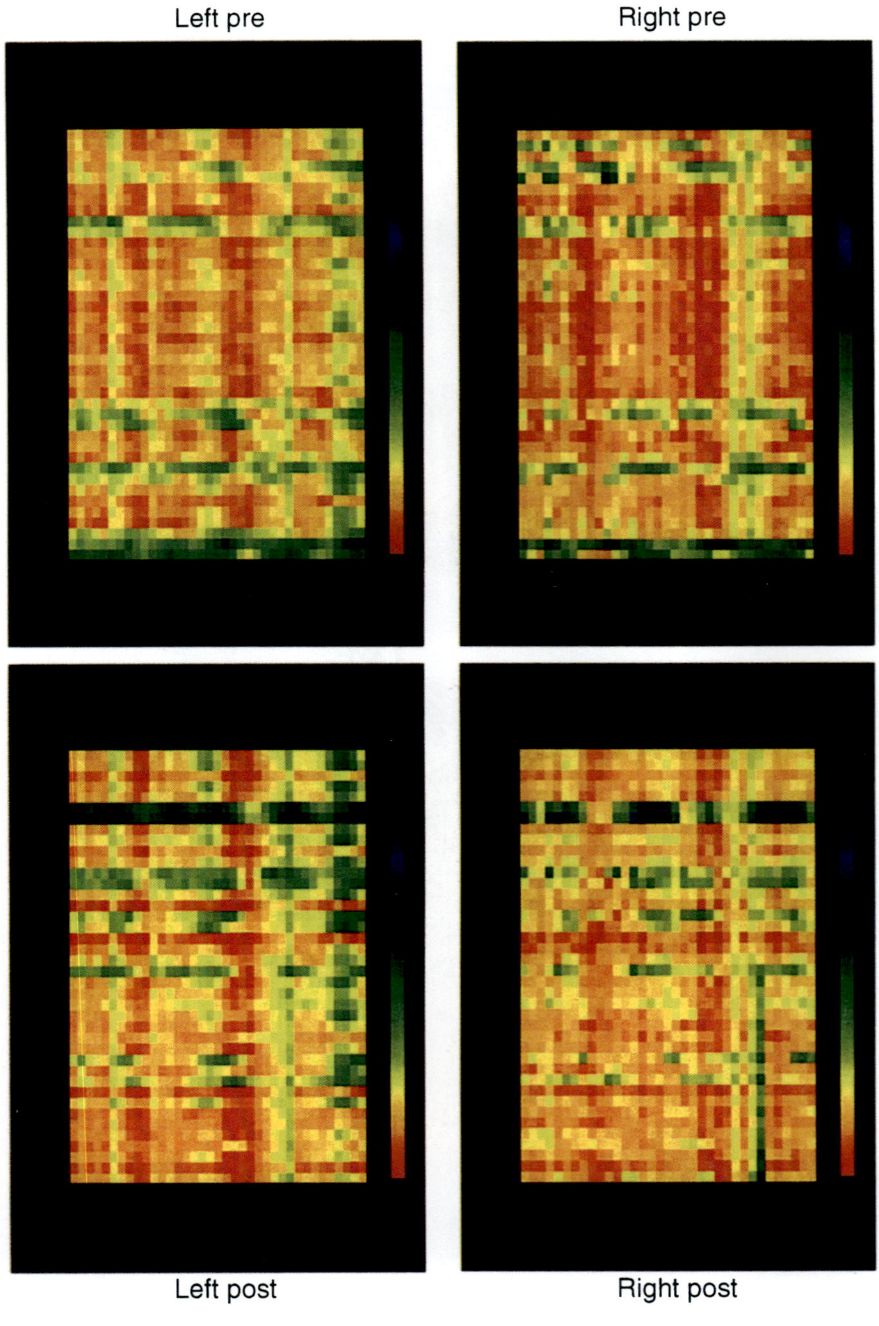


Shannahoff-Khalsa, Section V.A., Fig. 44. (See Legend in Text.)

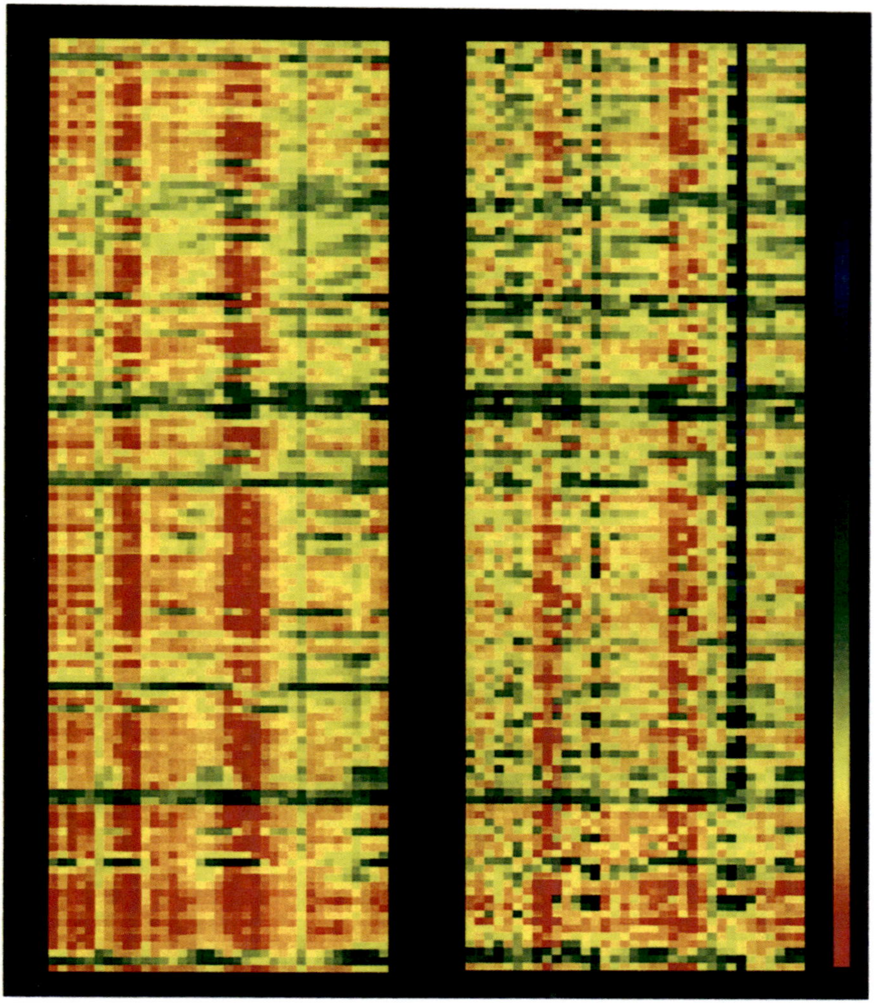

Shannahoff-Khalsa, Section V.A., Fig. 45. (See Legend in Text.)

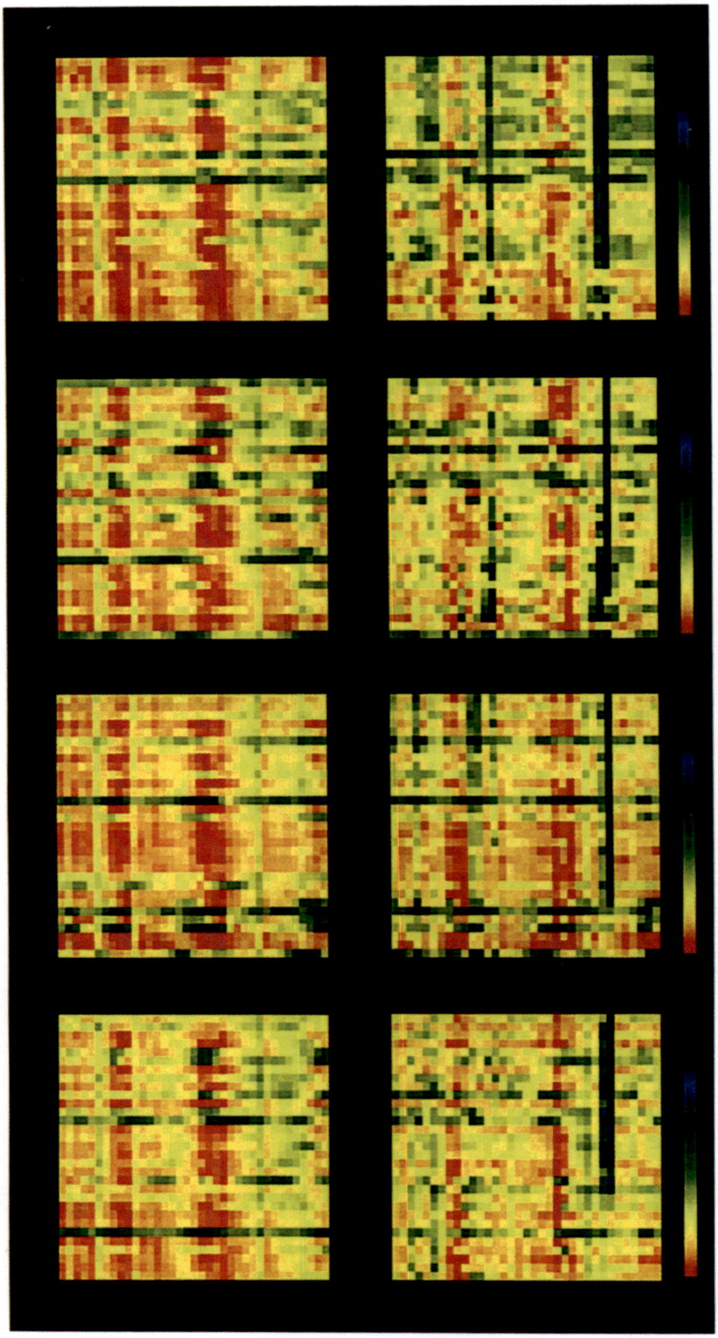

Shannahoff-Khalsa, Section V.A., Fig. 46. (See Legend in Text.)

Kolibri 360 GmbH
Ferdinand-Jühlke-Straße 7
99095 Erfurt, Deutschland
produktsicherheit@kolibri360.de